Y0-CQS-638

Drug Treatment of
Mental Disorders

Edited by

Lance L. Simpson
Columbia University
College of Physicians and Surgeons
New York, New York

Raven Press ▪ New York

DRUG TREATMENT
OF MENTAL DISORDERS

Preface

There is a sad irony that must be borne in mind by anyone who prepares a medical textbook; namely, as the comprehensiveness of the text increases, the likelihood that anyone will read it decreases. This irony stems from the fact that physicians and medical investigators are so pressed for time that they cannot indulge themselves in reading lengthy treatises. That fact has been a major consideration in establishing the scope and content of this volume. Only those drugs that are used often and with notable therapeutic success are considered. Within this context, each drug is described in accordance with our current knowledge of its basic and clinical pharmacology. Emphasis is placed on those aspects of drug action that have therapeutic significance. Whenever appropriate, current thoughts on the biological basis of mental illness are discussed, with the intent of promoting the idea that specific drugs should be used to remedy or offset specific disorders.

In the preparation of this text, I have been immeasurably aided by many persons. I am indebted to the authors, all of whom generously agreed to prepare chapters. I am especially grateful to my assistant, Mrs. Ruby Hough, whose efforts were indispensable. Finally, I appreciate the confidence of Dr. Alan M. Edelson, President of Raven Press, who suggested that the volume be assembled. These persons deserve whatever praise may accrue to the book.

Lance L. Simpson
New York City
(*July 1975*)

Contents

Special Topics

Contributors

Thomas A. Ban
Department of Psychiatry
McGill University
Montreal, Quebec

Frank M. Berger
Department of Psychiatry
University of Louisville
Louisville, Kentucky 40208

Phillip H. Bookman
Department of Medical Research
Hoffmann–La Roche, Inc.
Nutley, New Jersey 07110

Bruce Cabot
Department of Pharmacology
Columbia University
College of Physicians & Surgeons
New York, New York 10032

Magda Campbell
Department of Psychiatry
New York University Medical Center
New York, New York 10016

Jonathan O. Cole
Boston State Hospital
Boston, Massachusetts 02124

John M. Davis
Illinois State Psychiatric Institute
Chicago, Illinois 60612

Carl Eisdorfer
Department of Psychiatry and Behavioral
  Sciences
University of Washington School of Medicine
Seattle, Washington 98195

Ronald R. Fieve
Department of Psychiatry
Columbia University
College of Physicians & Surgeons
New York, New York 10032

Samuel Gershon
Department of Psychiatry
New York University Medical Center
New York, New York 10016

Leo E. Hollister
Veterans Administration Hospital
Palo Alto, California 94304

John S. Kaufmann
Departments of Medicine and Pharmacology
Bowman Gray School of Medicine
Winston Salem, North Carolina 27103

Seymour S. Kety   Department of Psychiatry
                             Harvard Medical School
                             Boston, Massachusetts 02114

Donald F. Klein   Long Island Jewish-Hillside Medical Center
                             Glen Oaks, New York 11004

J. Hillary Lee   Rockland State Hospital
                             Orangeburg, New York 10962

Dennis L. Murphy   Laboratory of Clinical Science
                             National Institute of Mental Health
                             Bethesda, Maryland 20014

John C. Pecknold   Department of Psychiatry
                             McGill University
                             Montreal, Quebec

Lowell O. Randall   Department of Medical Research
                             Hoffmann–La Roche, Inc.
                             Nutley, New Jersey 07110

Murray Raskind   Department of Psychiatry and Behavioral
                                Sciences
                             University of Washington School of Medicine
                             Seattle, Washington 98195

Gerard Selzer   Department of Psychiatry
                             New York University Medical Center
                             New York, New York 10016

Baron Shopsin   Department of Psychiatry
                             New York University Medical Center
                             New York, New York 10016

George M. Simpson   Rockland State Hospital
                             Orangeburg, New York 10962

Lance L. Simpson   Department of Pharmacology
                             Columbia University
                             College of Physicians & Surgeons
                             New York, New York 10032

Arthur M. Small   Department of Psychiatry
                             New York University Medical Center
                             New York, New York 10016

Chapter 1

Recent Genetic and Biochemical Approaches to Schizophrenia

Seymour S. Kety

During the past decade it has become more evident and more widely acknowledged that there are important biological substrates for the major mental illnesses—schizophrenia and the affective disorders. This is probably attributable to independent areas of scientific findings involving genetics and pharmacology. Compelling evidence has been accumulating to support the importance of genetic factors in the etiology of the major psychoses. In addition, a substantial number of drugs have been discovered that have more specific and beneficial effects in these disorders than have ever been available before. The impressive growth of fundamental knowledge regarding the nervous system and its interrelationships with behavior has permitted elucidation of the neural mechanisms by which these drugs may produce their therapeutic effects. This in turn has given rise to parsimonious and credible hypotheses regarding biochemical processes that may be affected in psychiatric disorders. These biochemical alterations may represent the expression of a genetic predisposition to mental illness.

GENETIC FACTORS IN SCHIZOPHRENIA[1]

The significance of genetic factors in the transmission of schizophrenia has not been universally accepted. Family members and monozygotic twins of schizophrenics may share many environmental influences in addition to their genetic endowment, so an increased incidence of schizophrenia among them may reflect the operation of one or both of these factors. Moreover, a diagnosis of schizophrenia that cannot be established objectively and is compatible with a fairly wide range of manifestations is apt to increase the ascertainment of illness in other members of the family and the likelihood of its being diagnosed as schizophrenia.

Studies with adopted individuals offer a means of minimizing these sources of error. Since an adoptee receives his genetic endowment from one family but his life experience as a member of another, it may be possible to dis-

---

[1] This section is based on studies carried out in collaboration with David Rosenthal, Paul Wender, Fini Schulsinger, and Bjørn Jacobsen (Kety, Rosenthal, Wender, and Schulsinger, 1968; Rosenthal, Wender, Kety, Schulsinger, Welner, and Østergaard, 1968; Kety, Rosenthal, Wender, Schulsinger, and Jacobsen, 1975).

entangle genetic and environmental factors by studies based on such individuals and their biological and adoptive families. If a total population of adoptees can be surveyed in whom schizophrenia in the biological relatives occurs after the time of adoption and is not a basis for the transfer, where the mental status of the biological relatives and the adoptees are largely unknown to each other, and where independent diagnoses in each population can be made without that information, it should be possible to reduce to a minimum many types of selective ascertainment and diagnostic bias.

In 1963 my colleagues and I began to collect a total sample of adults legally adopted at an early age by individuals not biologically related to them. We began with all of the legal adoptions granted in the city and county of Copenhagen from the beginning of 1924 to the end of 1947, rejecting those who had been adopted by biological relatives; this yielded a total of 5,483 adoptees. For the purposes of the study we included as "definite schizophrenia" three subtypes defined in the diagnostic manual of the American Psychiatric Association: chronic schizophrenia, latent (ambulatory or borderline) schizophrenia, and acute schizophrenic reaction. Thirty-three schizophrenic "index" adoptees were selected by independent review of the abstracts of the institutional records of the 507 adoptees who had at one time or another been admitted to a mental institution. Unanimous agreement on a diagnosis of chronic, latent, or acute schizophrenia was arrived at among four raters. A control group was selected from the adoptees who had not been admitted to a psychiatric facility; the controls were matched with each index case on the basis of age, sex, socioeconomic class of the rearing family, and time spent with biological relatives, in child-care institutions, or in foster homes before transfer to the adopting family.

Our first report of prevalence and type of mental illness in the relatives was based simply on an examination of institutional records available for the biological and adoptive parents, siblings, and half-siblings of the index and control adoptees. These were identified through the adoption records and the Folkeregister. Abstracts of the hospital records were made, translated into English, and edited to remove any information that would suggest whether a subject was related to an index case or to a control, or was a biological or adoptive relative; then independent diagnoses were made by each of the four raters. A consensus diagnosis was arrived at by conference among the raters.

We previously developed the concept of a "schizophrenia spectrum" of disorders presumably related to schizophrenia and including, besides the three forms of schizophrenia we had accepted in the selection of index cases, a category of "uncertain schizophrenia." This was the best diagnosis that could be made, although from the information we had we could not be certain. In addition, we developed the category of "schizoid or inadequate personality," which appeared to have certain characteristics related to schizophrenia but which were of a milder extent.

A statistically significant concentration of "schizophrenia spectrum" disorders was found among the biological relatives of index cases as compared to the biological relatives of controls. In contrast, the adoptive relatives for both the index and the control group showed a low incidence of schizophrenia spectrum disorders, with no significant difference between them (Kety et al., 1968). In fact, the number of illnesses we found in the relatives was too small to permit a further breakdown of the schizophrenia spectrum.

At this juncture we had secured little information about the environment of the probands other than the presence or absence of mental illness in their adopted relatives. In an earlier study (Rosenthal et al., 1968) we suggested that there might be many more schizophrenics and individuals within the schizophrenia spectrum than merely those who had been hospitalized at one time or another. Therefore we felt that it would be important to carry out complete psychiatric interviews of all relatives. This might permit a more exhaustive survey of the population with regard to schizophrenia and other psychiatric diagnoses, and it might provide more information about life experience in the genesis of these disorders. We secured the collaboration of Dr. Bjørn Jacobsen, a Danish psychiatrist, who agreed to carry out the interviews and spent the greater part of the next 2 yr doing so.

A total of 512 relatives were identified through the population records; of these, 119 had died and 29 had emigrated or disappeared. There was an interesting and highly significant difference in the death rates between the biological relatives (35) of index cases and the biological relatives (13) of controls ($p = 0.0004$). That difference is probably accounted for by suicide and accidental and other traumatic deaths. Of the remaining 360 relatives, more than 90% participated in an exhaustive psychiatric interview conducted by Jacobsen, who had not known the relationship of any subject to a proband. Practically all of the biological relatives themselves did not know of the relationship and so did not inform the examiner. Extensive summaries of these interviews were then prepared and edited to remove any clues that would permit guessing the relationship of the subject to a proband; they were then read independently by three raters, each of whom independently recorded his best psychiatric diagnosis for each subject from a list of possible diagnoses covering the entire range listed in the *Diagnostic and Statistical Manual* (*DSM-II*) of the American Psychiatric Association, ranging from "no mental disorder" to "chronic schizophrenia." After that, a consensus was arrived at among the raters, the code was broken, and the subjects were allocated to their respective four groups: biological or adoptive relatives of schizophrenic index adoptees, and biological or adoptive relatives of control adoptees.

Of these four populations, one is different from the rest in being genetically related to a person with schizophrenia with whom they have not lived, i.e., the biological relatives of the index cases. With regard to mental illness other than schizophrenia these relatives do not differ from the rest (Table 1), but with regard to schizophrenia they show a higher incidence of illness (Table 2). For chronic schizophrenia the prevalence in the biological relatives of index

TABLE 1. *Consensus diagnoses outside the schizophrenia spectrum in biological and adoptive relatives*

	Interviewed relatives (%)[a]			
	Index group		Control group	
Diagnosis	Biological (N = 81)	Adoptive (N = 31)	Biological (N = 121)	Adoptive (N = 41)
Psychiatrically normal	37	36	41	27
Organic illness	9	16	5	15
Neurotic illness	5	10	5	5
Affective illness	2	3	9	7
Personality disorder	33	26	32	37
All nonschizophrenic diagnoses	49	55	51	63

[a] The Ns represent interviewed relatives whose consensus diagnoses were outside the schizophrenia spectrum.

cases is 2.9% (five of 173 relatives) compared with 0.6% in the other three categories combined (two of 339 relatives); for latent schizophrenia it is 3.5% (six of 173 relatives) compared with 1.2% (four of 339 relatives); and for uncertain schizophrenia it is 7.5% (13 of 173 relatives) compared with 2% (seven of 339 relatives). For any of these diagnoses of schizophrenic illness, the prevalence in those genetically related to the schizophrenic index cases is 13.9% (24 of 173 relatives) compared to 2.7% (two of 74 relatives) in their adoptive relatives, or 3.8% (13 of 339 relatives) in all subjects not genetically related to an index case (Table 2). The difference between the group genetically related to the schizophrenic index cases and those not so

TABLE 2. *Prevalence of schizophrenia spectrum disorders in the biological and adoptive relatives of schizophrenic index and control subjects*

		Diagnosis of schizophrenia in relatives							
	Relatives identified (No.)	Chronic		Latent		Uncertain		Total	
Type of relative		No.	%	No.	%	No.	%	No.	%
Biological relatives of schizophrenic adoptees	173	5[a]	2.9	6	3.5	13[b]	7.5	24[c]	13.9
Biological relatives of control adoptees	174	0	—	3	1.7	3	1.7	6	3.4
Adoptive relatives of schizophrenic adoptees	74	1	1.4	0	—	1	1.4	2	2.7
Adoptive relatives of control adoptees	91	1	1.1	1	1.1	3	3.3	5	5.5

[a] p < 0.05. Significances apply to differences between biological relatives of schizophrenic adoptees and biological relatives of controls; other differences were not significant.
[b] p < 0.01.
[c] p < 0.001.

related is highly significant statistically and speaks for the operation of genetic factors in the transmission of schizophrenia. The diagnosis of schizoid or inadequate personality was made rather frequently among biological relatives of both index and control adoptees (7.5%).

The evidence thus far presented is compatible with genetic transmission of schizophrenia but is not entirely conclusive, since there are possible environmental factors such as *in utero* influences, birth trauma, and early mothering experiences which have not been ruled out. However, there were 127 biological paternal half-siblings of index cases and controls, and these could help to settle the question since the biological paternal half-siblings did not share the same mother, neonatal mothering experience, or postnatal environment with their adopted half-siblings. The only thing they shared was the same

TABLE 3. *Schizophrenic illness in the biological paternal half-siblings of index and control groups*

| | Biological paternal half-siblings | | | |
| | Index group (N = 63) | | Control group (N = 64) | |
Diagnosis	No.	%	No.	%
Definite schizophrenia	8	13[a]	1	1.6
Definite or uncertain schizophrenia	14	22[b]	2	3.0

[a] p = 0.015. Significances apply to differences between index and control groups, by Fisher's exact probability test.
[b] p = 0.001.

father and a certain amount of genetic overlap. The number of paternal half-siblings is almost identical for index cases and controls, but the number of those who were diagnosed as having definite or uncertain schizophrenia is markedly different, with 14 among the half-siblings of the index cases and only two among the half-siblings of controls ($p = 0.001$). There is a similar incidence if we restrict the diagnosis to definite schizophrenia (Table 3). We regard this as compelling evidence that genetic factors operate significantly in the transmission of schizophrenia.

These data do not permit the conclusion that schizophrenia is a unitary disorder, since they are equally compatible with a syndrome of multiple etiologies and different modes of genetic transmission. Although the 24 diagnoses of definite or uncertain schizophrenia were distributed among the biological relatives of 17 of the index probands, there were 16 who had no diagnoses of schizophrenic illness in their biological relatives. The possibility that there are at least two forms of schizophrenia—one in which there is a strong genetic basis and one in which there is little or no genetic basis—is compatible with our data.

These data do not imply that genetic factors and the biological processes involved in their expression are the only important influences in the etiology and pathogenesis of schizophrenia. We are currently engaged in analyzing the interviews with respect to experiential factors and their possible interaction with biological vulnerability. This may help us to decide which factors make possible or prevent the development of schizophrenia.

CURRENT NEUROCHEMICAL HYPOTHESES OF SCHIZOPHRENIA

The idea of a biochemical basis for psychosis is not new. The Hippocratic physicians postulated that mental illness resided in the brain and was the result of chemical disturbances there. During the last century Thudichum restated that hypothesis, suggesting that many forms of insanity were probably the result of "toxic substances fermented within the brain." Interestingly, and fortunately for those who followed him, he did not spend his time looking for those postulated toxic substances. Instead, he recognized that their discovery, if they existed, would require a great deal of information about the normal biochemistry of the brain. His important contributions were in that area.

Until fairly recently, however, the field of biological psychiatry was characterized by a large number of rather premature and simplistic attacks on the major psychoses, elaborated before there was enough substantive knowledge from which to proceed. The optimistic results reported were often the result of dietary, drug, or other nondisease variables that were inadequately controlled (Kety, 1959). Meanwhile there has been a remarkable increase in fundamental knowledge of the biochemistry of the brain, the physiology and pharmacology of the synapse, and the relationships between these and behavior—with the result that a few more cautious hypotheses have begun to emerge. These have represented not great leaps from insufficient basic information but rather short and logical steps contributed by many individuals. Two hypotheses relating to the biological substrates of schizophrenia are the foci of considerable current research activity.

Transmethylation

In 1952 Harley-Mason (Osmond and Smythies, 1952) speculated that the newly delineated process of biological transmethylation might somehow be involved in schizophrenia. He was impressed that many hallucinogens were methylated substances, and that one of these, mescaline, would result from the O-methylation of dopamine at the 3, 4, and 5 positions. Although O-methylation of catecholamines had not yet been described, he postulated that such might occur in the body and that in schizophrenia there might be an accumulation of hallucinogenic methylated metabolites. He singled out one substance, 3,4-dimethoxyphenylethylamine, as being of special interest, since this compound had been reported to produce catatonic behavior in animals.

This hypothesis received its first test in the administration of niacinamide in large doses to schizophrenics. The rationale was that this substance would be methylated and would thereby competitively divert the biological trans-methylation process away from the production of hallucinogenic substances. Unfortunately the striking therapeutic results initially reported have not been confirmed in a substantial number of controlled trials. Since it has been shown that the administration of niacinamide to animals does not significantly de-press brain levels of S-adenosylmethionine, the major methyl donor in the brain, niacinamide is not an effective methyl acceptor and its administration does not constitute a test of the transmethylation hypothesis.

In 1961 the hypothesis was tested in another manner (Pollin, Cardon, and Kety, 1961), this time by administering methionine in conjunction with a monoamine oxidase (MAO) inhibitor to schizophrenic patients. In approxi-mately one-third of the patients there was a brief exacerbation of psychosis, a phenomenon that has been reported in several subsequent studies. In one of these (Antun, Burnett, Cooper, Daly, Smythies, and Zealley, 1971), it was found that methionine alone, without MAO inhibition, can produce the same manifestation in schizophrenics. Although it is difficult to exclude the possi-bility that the methionine has produced a toxic psychosis superimposed on schizophrenia, it should be noted that normal subjects who receive the same dose of methionine do not experience a psychotic reaction. The results in schizophrenic patients are compatible with the transmethylation hypothesis, although alternative possibilities have not been ruled out. The ability of large doses of methionine to elevate S-adenosylmethionine levels in the brain, and reports that methionine administration in schizophrenics caused an increase in the excretion of dimethyltryptamine, a well-known hallucinogen, were compatible with the hypothesis, although the latter finding has not been firmly established by unassailable analytical techniques.

In 1962 a substance which produced a pink spot on paper chromatography and was identified as 3,4-dimethoxyphenylethylamine was reported in the urine of schizophrenic patients (Friedhoff and Van Winkle, 1962). This re-port was followed by a large number of attempted replications, most of which were successful in demonstrating the pink spot in the urine of schizophrenics and to a considerably lesser extent in the urine of nonschizophrenics. How-ever, the fact that phenothiazines produced metabolites which also gave a pink spot in a similar position confused the issue. More recently 3,4-dimeth-oxyphenylethylamine has been demonstrated by mass fragmentography in the urine of normals and schizophrenics, and evidence indicated that it is ex-ogenous in origin. The issue has not yet been resolved.

There is evidence that the enzyme indoleamine-N-methyltransferase is present in the brain (Saavedra, Coyle, and Axelrod, 1973). This enzyme is capable of methylating tryptamine to dimethyltryptamine, although it does not methylate serotonin. Several studies have reported finding methylated indoleamines in the blood or urine of schizophrenics, and some have suggested a correlation with the intensity of psychosis occurring either spontaneously or in association with the ingestion of methyl donors. There have been few studies with unassailable analytical techniques such as mass fragmentography.

Dopamine Hypothesis

Pharmacology offers two approaches to the pathogenesis of a disorder. One is to investigate the mechanism of action of drugs which ameliorate the disorder, and the other is to examine the actions of drugs which produce or mimic the disorder. In the case of schizophrenia, both of these approaches have been actively pursued.

Since the discovery in 1951 that chlorpromazine was beneficial in the treatment of schizophrenic patients, a number of phenothiazine derivatives have been prepared, many of which have antipsychotic properties. Somewhat later haloperidol, a butyrophenone not chemically related to the phenothiazines, was also found to be effective in the treatment of schizophrenics. As both groups of drugs became widely used, it soon became evident that an important side effect of both was the development of symptoms like those of Parkinson's disease. With the elucidation of the dopamine-containing nigrostriatal pathway and the discovery that dopamine was deficient in the caudate nucleus of patients suffering from Parkinson's disease, an action on that amine became a possibility for explaining the extrapyramidal effects of the antipsychotic drugs. In 1963 Carlsson and Lindqvist first suggested that these drugs acted by blocking dopamine receptors (Carlsson and Lindqvist, 1973). They found that chlorpromazine and haloperidol increased the levels of dopamine metabolites in the brain, whereas promethazine, a phenothiazine drug not effective in schizophrenia, did not. With remarkable insight Carlsson and Lindqvist speculated that dopamine release was increased in the case of the active antipsychotic drugs and that it was brought about by some feedback mechanism in response to a blockade of dopamine receptors. Since that observation it has been established that the postulated blockade of dopamine receptors does in fact occur. Several pharmacological studies have confirmed the increased synthesis and turnover of dopamine in the brain in response to psychoactive congeners, and a blockade of dopamine receptors has been demonstrated physiologically by microelectrode recording and biochemically on dopamine-sensitive adenylate cyclase of brain.

Matthysse (1973) pointed out that the phenothiazines have a notoriously wide spectrum of effects, and that a criterion for the mechanism involved in antipsychotic activity would be the ability of that criterion to discriminate between effective and ineffective phenothiazines and butyrophenones. That criterion has been met to a considerable extent in the case of dopamine receptor blockade.

Although the phenothiazines were at first thought to be useful merely as "tranquilizers" of disturbed behavior, it eventually became apparent that they had rather specific effects on the cardinal features of schizophrenia. Whereas sedative agents (e.g., the barbiturates) or antianxiety drugs (e.g., diazepam) were no more effective than placebo in the treatment of schizophrenia, chlorpromazine in large-scale controlled studies produced significant improvement in thought disorder, blunted affect, withdrawal, and autistic behavior—all cardinal features of schizophrenia as described by Bleuler. The ability of these agents to activate withdrawn patients and bring the characteristic flat affect toward normal is hardly a sedative or tranquilizing effect. More likely, these drugs are highly specific and act at some central nervous system site involved in the manifestation of psychotic behavior.

In addition to drugs which act to relieve psychosis, there are also drugs that evoke psychosis. For example, lysergic acid diethylamide (LSD) has long been known to produce a toxic psychosis thought to resemble schizophrenia. The psychosis induced by overdosage of amphetamine, however, is much closer to schizophrenia. In fact, even experienced clinicians have confused amphetamine-induced psychosis with endogenous psychosis. Chronic amphetamine toxicity is characterized by a paranoid psychosis with auditory hallucinations and stereotyped behavior but with little delirium or confusion. Schizophrenic patients have been reported readily able to recognize an LSD psychosis as different from their usual symptoms, but were unable to differentiate an amphetamine psychosis. Furthermore, amphetamine, methylphenidate, and L-DOPA can precipitate active schizophrenia in schizophrenic patients enjoying remission.

There is evidence to suggest that the psychosis due to amphetamine is mediated through release and potentiation of dopamine at its receptors in the brain. The stereotyped behavior induced in animals by amphetamine can be prevented by lesions of dopamine pathways. Dopamine itself or apomorphine, which is known to stimulate dopamine receptors, produces stereotypy when injected in the brain. Furthermore, dopamine receptor blockers, (e.g., the antipsychotic drugs) abort amphetamine-induced stereotypy.

There is thus a remarkable convergence on the part of several agents on dopamine synapses in the brain. The drug that produces a psychosis most closely resembling schizophrenia appears to act by potentiating dopamine at its synapses in the brain, whereas a large number of drugs in two distinct chemical classes which have in common their ability to block dopamine receptors also have quite specific effects on the cardinal features of schizophrenia. This has led to the hypothesis that an overactivity of dopamine synapses may play a crucial role in the pathogenesis of schizophrenia.

Dopamine: Norepinephrine Imbalance?

Although hyperactivity of dopamine could explain certain features of schizophrenia (e.g., stereotyped behavior, paranoid delusions, and auditory hallucinations), it would hardly in itself account for some of the others, e.g., anhedonia, withdrawal and autism, or flatness of affect. These manifestations appear to involve behavioral components which in animals have been related to the activity of norepinephrine. For example, there is considerable indirect evidence that norepinephrine pathways are involved in appetitive or reward behavior, exploratory activity, and elevated mood. It is possible then that the corresponding manifestations of anhedonia, withdrawal, and flatness of affect represent an insufficiency of norepinephrine at its synapses in schizophrenia. A parsimonious mechanism exists that could produce both the increase in dopamine activity and the decrease in norepinephrine activity which the more complete explanation of schizophrenic symptoms would require. That mechanism may be the enzyme dopamine-β-hydroxylase, which converts dopamine to norepinephrine at the noradrenergic nerve endings in the brain. A throttling of that enzyme could conceivably result in the release of dopamine at the expense of norepinephrine (see Wise and Stein, 1973; but see also Wyatt, Schwartz, Erdely, and Barchas, 1975).

There are other findings related to schizophrenia which involve serotonin, histamine, or acetylcholine, although these findings are few and their significance remains to be determined. A reciprocal relationship between cholinergic and catecholaminergic pathways is suggested by the ability of physostigmine, an acetylcholinesterase inhibitor, to prevent the acute exacerbation of psychosis that can be precipitated in schizophrenics by methylphenidate. An insensitivity of schizophrenics to histamine, as evidenced by diminution in the wheal produced by that amine, has not yet been explained.

One of the most striking findings to emerge from biological research in schizophrenia is that by Wyatt and collaborators (Wyatt, Murphy, Belmaker, Cohen, Donnelly, and Pollin, 1973), who reported a significantly diminished level of MAO in the platelets of schizophrenic patients. This finding has assumed greater significance in conjunction with their observation that the diminution in that enzyme holds true even for the nonschizophrenic monozygotic twin in pairs discordant for schizophrenia. This finding—which should be free of the influence of drugs, institutionalization, and other nondisease variables which often confuse the interpretation—suggests that the reduced level of the enzyme in schizophrenia is a genetic characteristic. If this characteristic were also to involve MAO in the brain, its relevance to behavioral and mental alterations would be quite clear. Unfortunately the results obtained in five studies which included assays of MAO in the brain of schizophrenics are not consistent.

CONCLUDING REMARKS

There has been an opportunity here for only a cursory review of some of the highlights of current biochemical approaches to schizophrenia. For a more comprehensive picture of the contributions of a large number of investigators to the catecholamines of the brain and their relationship to be-havior, psychopharmacology, and quite possibly to schizophrenia, the reader is referred to the proceedings of a recent conference (Matthysse and Kety, 1975).

Although biochemistry is not a complete explanation of behavior, mood, cognition, or their disturbances in the major psychoses, it is apparent that considerable progress has been made in recent years. The relevance of certain areas of fundamental research, notably the synaptic functions of the biogenic amines and their relationships to behavior, have become more clearly estab-lished, and a modicum of cautious optimism seems warranted.

REFERENCES

Antun, F. T., Burnett, G. B., Cooper, A. J., Daly, R. J., Smythies, J. R., and Zealley, A. K. (1971): The effects of l-methionine (without MAOI) in schizophrenia. *J. Psychiatr. Res.,* 8:63–71.

Carlsson, A., and Lindqvist, M. (1963): Effect of chlorpromazine or haloperidol on formation of 3-methoxytryptamine and normetanephrine in mouse brain. *Acta Pharmacol. Toxicol.,* 20:140.

Friedhoff, A. J., and Van Winkle, E. (1962): Characteristics of an amine found in urine of schizophrenic patients. *J. Nerv. Ment. Dis.,* 135:550–555.

Kety, S. S. (1959): Biochemical theories of schizophrenia: A two-part critical review of current theories and of the evidence used to support them. *Science,* 129:1528–1532, 1590–1596.

Kety, S. S., Rosenthal, D., Wender, P. H., and Schulsinger, F. (1968): The types and prevalence of mental illness in the biological and adoptive families of adopted schizophrenics. In: *The Transmission of Schizophrenia,* edited by D. Rosenthal and S. S. Kety, pp. 345–362. Pergamon Press, Oxford.

Kety, S. S., Rosenthal, D., Wender, P. H., Schulsinger, F., and Jacobsen, B. (1975): Mental illness in the biological and adoptive families of adopted individuals who have become schizophrenic: a preliminary report based upon psychiatric interviews. In: *Genetics and Psychopathology,* edited by R. Fieve, H. Brill, and D. Rosenthal. Johns Hopkins Press, Baltimore (*in press*).

Matthysse, S. (1973): Antipsychotic drug actions: A clue to the neuropathology of schizophrenia? *Fed. Proc.,* 32:200–205.

Matthysse, S., and Kety, S. S, editors (1975): *Symposium on Catecholamines and their Enzymes in the Neuropathology of Schizophrenia.* Pergamon Press, Oxford.

Osmond, H., and Smythies, J. (1952): Schizophrenia: A new approach. *J. Ment. Sci.,* 98:309–315.

Pollin, W., Cardon, P. V., and Kety, S. S. (1961): Effects of amino acid feedings in schizophrenic patients treated with iproniazid. *Science,* 133:104–105.

Rosenthal, D., Wender, P. H., Kety, S. S., Schulsinger, F., Welner, J., and Østergaard, L. (1968): Schizophrenic offspring reared in adoptive homes. In: *The Transmission of Schizophrenia,* edited by D. Rosenthal and S. Kety, pp. 377–391. Pergamon Press, Oxford.

Saavedra, J. M., Coyle, J. T., and Axelrod, J. (1973): The distribution and properties of the non-specific N-methyltransferase in brain. *J. Neurochem.,* 20:743–752.

Wise, C. D., and Stein, L. (1973): Dopamine beta-oxidase deficits in the brains of schizophrenic patients. *Science,* 181:344.

Wyatt, R. J., Murphy, D. L., Belmaker, R., Cohen, S., Donnelly, C. H., and Pollin, W. (1973): Reduced monoamine oxidase activity in platelets: A possible genetic marker for vulnerability to schizophrenia. *Science,* 179:916.

Wyatt, R. J., Schwartz, M. A., Erdely, E., and Barchas, J. D. (1975): Dopamine beta-hydroxylase activity in brains of chronic schizophrenic patients. *Science,* 187:368–369.

Chapter 2

Phenothiazines

Jonathan O. Cole

This is a most appropriate time to write a chapter on the clinical psychopharmacology of the antipsychotic phenothiazine drugs. Chlorpromazine has now come of age in several respects. To begin with, chlorpromazine was first used in psychiatric patients more than 20 years ago. In the second place, an excellent history of its discovery and early use has been prepared by Dr. Judith Swazey (1974). Lastly, the Smith Kline & French Laboratories' patent on this drug in the United States has now expired, and several generic chlorpromazines are currently being prepared for market.

Since chlorpromazine in particular and the many subsequent antipsychotic drugs in general have had profound effects on American and indeed on international psychiatry, reducing the lengths of hospitalization for schizophrenic patients and permitting many patients to be handled in the community in ways not heretofore even anticipated, it is remarkable that no Nobel Prize in medicine has been awarded to the discoverers of chlorpromazine. After reading Swazey's book and thinking about the matter, one may speculate concerning the reasons for the lack of an award for such a significant medical, psychiatric, and social development. First, the original discovery of the chemical was made by a drug industry chemist rather than by a university-affiliated basic scientist. Secondly, the drug was not synthesized for the purpose for which it is now used. It was one of a series of antihistamine-like drugs that turned out to have a wide range of autonomic blocking effects, principally α-adrenergic. It was introduced into human medicine as an adjunct to anesthesia by Henri Laborit, a French anesthetist working in a naval hospital. His status in academic French medicine may resemble that of a present-day United States Naval anesthesiologist working in Portsmouth, Virginia. To make matters worse, the theories of traumatic surgical shock on which Laborit based his use of chlorpromazine are far from being generally accepted as correct. He may therefore have discovered a very useful drug for the wrong reasons!

Laborit's observation that patients who received chlorpromazine were more tranquil after surgery than other comparable surgical patients was followed up by a psychiatric colleague working in a nearby hospital. This psychiatrist never pursued his own early report on a limited number of cases. The work of Delay and Deniker at St. Anne's Hospital in Paris which followed shortly thereafter and which really made the clinical effects of chlorpromazine known to world psychiatry therefore did not constitute a major discovery; their clinical observations were not based on any theory but were purely empirical, checking out an interesting result found by a colleague.

Be that as it may, the discovery of chlorpromazine was a great and important event in psychiatry. It has led to the testing and synthesis of a wide variety of other related and unrelated chemical compounds with similar pharmacological properties. Interestingly enough, imipramine, the first tricyclic antidepressant, was synthesized as a potential antipsychotic chlorpromazine-like drug. There are at least 13 useful antipsychotic phenothiazine derivatives currently available for routine prescription use in the United States.

BASIC PHARMACOLOGY

Although there are many phenothiazine drugs, they all have the same basic structure (Fig. 1). The structure has been modified in many ways in order to

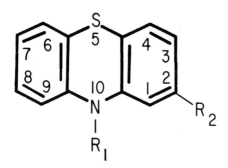

FIG. 1. Basic structure of the phenothiazine molecule. Different phenothiazines of clinical interest have substituents added at the 10 position (R_1) and the 2 position (R_2).

generate newer or better antipsychotic drugs. The hope of developing newer compounds has frequently been realized; that of developing better compounds has not. We currently have many phenothiazines of equivalent antipsychotic potency.

The available phenothiazines can be grouped into three chemical categories, each differing in terms of the substituents attached to the phenothiazine nucleus. Accordingly they are identified as aminoalkyl (or aliphatic), piperidyl, and piperazinyl phenothiazines. Examples of each of these compounds are illustrated in Fig. 2.

The phenothiazines are among the most ubiquitously acting drugs in all of pharmacology. To a greater or lesser extent, they exert actions on every organ system in the body. Indeed, there is an entire spectrum of actions which these drugs exert on the nervous system alone. Of these, the only one that appears to correlate well with antipsychotic activity is blockade of dopamine-mediated synaptic transmission (Matthysse, 1973). Blocking dopamine transmission may also be the mechanism by which these drugs evoke certain neurological disorders, e.g., pseudoparkinsonism. Although there is intense interest in the effects of phenothiazines on synaptic transmission, a precise role for dopamine in the etiology of schizophrenia has not been established.

There has been a substantial effort to correlate blood levels of various phenothiazines with the therapeutic response these drugs produce (Forrest, Carr, and Usdin, 1974). Unfortunately the work has met with only limited success. Major difficulties encountered are: (1) there is an extraordinary

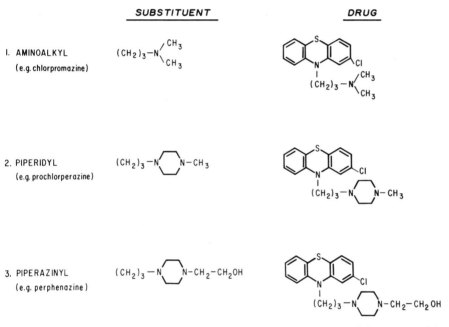

FIG. 2. The three major classes of phenothiazine antipsychotic drugs. The classes differ in terms of the substituent group added at the 10 position of the phenothiazine nucleus (Fig. 1).

array of phenothiazine metabolites; (2) therapeutic response does not bear any simple relationship to blood levels of phenothiazines or their metabolites; and (3) patients may continue to show beneficial effects from the drugs long after dosing has been discontinued. Perhaps the only conclusion to be drawn is that there is still much to be learned about the pharmacology of phenothiazines.

PHENOTHIAZINE USE IN PSYCHOTIC PATIENTS

The major use of phenothiazines in psychiatry is for treatment of schizophrenia. Although these drugs may have limited utility in other psychiatric disorders, this chapter focuses on the treatment of psychosis.

Efficacy

Although some previously marketed phenothiazines (e.g., mepazine and promazine) are significantly less effective than the other active antipsychotic phenothiazines, all the drugs currently available are probably equally effective in the treatment of acute and chronic schizophrenia (Cole and Davis, 1975). Studies attempting to compare these medications in clinical trials in acute or chronic schizophrenic patients usually conclude that the drugs have an essentially identical effect. The minor variations found from study to study are very likely manifestations of the laws of probability rather than reflections of real differences between drugs.

A good deal of effort has been expended in looking for "the right phenothiazine for the right patient." When this is viewed as a problem of identifying unique predictors of drug response within groups of schizophrenic patients, the outcome has often been intellectually stimulating but neither reproducible nor clinically useful. Predictors in large-scale Veterans Administration (VA) and National Institute of Mental Health (NIMH) collaborative studies have generally been unreplicatable (Goldberg, Frosch, Drossman, Schooler, and Johnson, 1972).

The more conventional clinical stereotypic ideas about the drugs—e.g., chlorpromazine has a sedative effect whereas trifluoperazine is activating— may have a very limited basis in fact. Furthermore, the phenomena behind such general impressions usually do not support differential use in treatment. Chlorpromazine is in fact one of the more sedative of the phenothiazines when first given. Thioridazine is also relatively sedative; but the sedative effect of either drug is probably of relatively short duration after any given dose, lasting perhaps 4 to 6 hr, whereas the antipsychotic effect lasts for days and possibly weeks. Less-sedative phenothiazines (e.g., trifluoperazine or fluphenazine) still cause sedation in some patients on acute administration or even on chronic administration; but when the sedation does occur, it is short-lived. The more potent piperazine phenothiazines (e.g., trifluoperazine or fluphenazine) do "stimulate" some patients. However, in my experience this stimulation generally takes the form of restlessness caused by akathisia rather than useful psychomotor activation. Chlorpromazine itself, however sedative it may be acutely, is significantly better than placebo in treating retarded, withdrawn, underactive, acute schizophrenics. Trifluoperazine is fine for treating overactive, disturbed schizophrenics. I have found no convincing evidence that there is a significant difference between any of these drugs when used over a several-day or several-week period.

Studies are just beginning to look at differences between the phenothiazines in less stereotypic situations. For example, a study that compared mesoridazine with chlorpromazine (both given intramuscularly for 24 hr) to acutely disturbed, newly admitted patients showed mesoridazine to be significantly superior to chlorpromazine in degree of symptom reduction in several areas of schizophrenic psychopathology (Hamid and Wertz, 1973). This difference in efficacy may well be due to differences in side effects. Chlorpromazine probably causes much more marked sedation and hypotension than does mesoridazine when given intramuscularly in doses sufficient to control psychotic excitement. Therefore patients may not tolerate doses of chlorpromazine sufficient to benefit their psychosis maximally within the first 24 hr, whereas they may tolerate mesoridazine. If my interpretation of this study is correct, then drugs which have relatively little autonomic blocking activity should be superior in the short-term control of psychotic behavior. Studies on the antipsychotic butyrophenones have tended to support this prediction (Slotnick, 1971; Anderson and Kuehnle, 1974).

In general, one can say about the efficacy of the phenothiazines as a group that they produce relatively more symptom reduction during the first week of treatment than in subsequent weeks, with the majority of the improvement occurring in the average patient by 6 weeks. Some further slight improvement may occur by 13 weeks, but there is very little thereafter. Core symptoms of schizophrenia (e.g., apathy, withdrawal, retardation, hebephrenic giggling and grimacing) show the greatest drug-placebo difference in acute studies. These symptoms show almost no change on placebo and modest change on drug. Secondary symptoms (e.g., delusions, hallucinations, hostility) show rather more change on placebo but substantially more on drugs. However, the drug-placebo difference with the primary symptoms is greater than that seen with the secondary symptoms. Nevertheless, the degree of overall improvement in drug-treated patients is greater for the secondary symptoms (Goldberg, Klerman, and Cole, 1965).

Treatment Resistant Patients

Some apparently schizophrenic patients remain disturbed and psychotic even after very large doses of phenothiazines have been administered for prolonged periods of time. What can one do in such cases? As noted by Klein and Davis (1969) the first thing to do in such cases is to be sure that the patient is actually taking his medication. If the patient has been receiving pills or tablets, one should shift to liquid or injectable medication. If this produces no change, a higher dose of the same medication may be tried. High-dosage regimens will probably be of limited value in chronic patients. An NIMH collaborative study showed that increased improvement with dosages of 2,000 mg chlorpromazine occurred only in patients under 40 who had been hospitalized less than 10 years; older, chronically hospitalized patients did not improve (Prien and Cole, 1968). Even with the younger patients the degree of benefit was relatively modest.

Monroe (1970) reported benefits in severely disturbed, schizophrenic patients when diazepam or diphenylhydantoin was added to their treatment regimen. This procedure is based on the premise that abnormal neurological foci may have been activated by the phenothiazines, which generally lower convulsive thresholds and might activate brain abnormalities. Another study (Van Putten, Mutalipassi, and Malkin, 1974) suggests that a trial of intramuscular benztropine be given to determine whether some of the disturbed behavior is actually akathisia rather than psychosis. A toxic delirium secondary to antiparkinsonian drugs should also be considered. On occasion chronically psychotic patients appear to do better on no drug than on phenothiazines, and rare patients do better on diazepam or even on antidepressants than on antipsychotic drugs. Electroconvulsive therapy (ECT) is an established clinical treatment for disturbed schizophrenic behavior, and there is even a modicum of evidence that ECT plus phenothiazines might produce a slightly better long-term outcome in schizophrenic patients than phenothiazines alone (Smith, Surphlis, Gynther, and Shimkunas, 1967).

Some patients are simply chronically and quietly psychotic, but inadequately responsive to treatment. A recent study in ambulatory patients at Boston State Hospital suggests that changing such patients to new phenothiazines may not always be beneficial. In a small study in which patients living in sheltered environments in the community were randomly assigned to chlorpromazine, thiothixene, or "doctor's choice" (the medication they were on at the time the study was initiated), the patients on doctor's choice medication did better overall in terms of absence of relapse than did either of the other two groups (Gardos, 1974). Selected patients in the other two groups did relatively well, but on the average the two groups transferred to chlorpromazine or thiothixene showed a higher incidence of psychotic relapse than did the doctor's choice group. Changing drugs in chronic patients is not without modest risk.

As a final note, the treatment-resistant schizophrenic patient is seen often enough to make one worry about the adequacy of our antipsychotic drugs. These agents are a great improvement over treatments available before 1952, but they are by no means either infallible or ideal. They are probably best thought of as psychotostatic rather than truly curative. This coupled with the fact that many patients are rather seriously impaired psychosocially before developing an acute schizophrenic episode helps us to understand why drug treatment is not a full solution for the troubles of psychiatry in general or schizophrenia in particular.

LONG-ACTING INJECTABLE PHENOTHIAZINES

There are currently on the market in the United States two preparations—fluphenazine enanthate and fluphenazine decanoate—which are given by injection and have a duration of antipsychotic action that is probably 2 to 4 weeks. Since schizophrenic patients do not usually relapse abruptly when a drug is discontinued, it is very difficult to obtain clear and accurate assessments of the duration of action of long-acting injectable antipsychotic drugs.

In general, both drugs are effective and useful (Groves and Mandel, 1975). An early presumption that the decanoate was likely to cause fewer side effects and to have a longer duration of antipsychotic action still remains to be firmly demonstrated.

Both drugs have a unique technological advantage. In chronic ambulatory or even chronic hospitalized patients known to be resistant to regular antipsychotic drug ingestion, the injection of a long-acting drug every 2 to 4 weeks is clearly much more effective than oral medication in keeping the patient free of increased psychosis. Furthermore, the drug may be administered to ambulatory patients in the home by visiting nurses rather than requiring them to return compulsively to the clinic for their injections.

These drugs are clearly better than placebo in home treatment of acutely psychotic individuals (Goldberg, DiMascio, and Chaudhary, 1970). They may also be used as an initial treatment for newly hospitalized psychotic patients. In one study they were somewhat more effective than chlorpromazine (Chien and Cole, 1973), although the mean chlorpromazine dosage used was 325 mg/day, which is rather low.

The incidence of serious adverse effects from the use of these long-acting injectable drugs has been remarkably low. Early fears that patients would become actively allergic to a depot drug that could not be removed from the body have proved baseless. Nevertheless, these drugs cause more extrapyramidal side effects than do conventional oral phenothiazines. It appears that in many patients the drug level in the blood drops sufficiently during the 2 to 4 weeks between injections to leave the patient liable to a recurrence of dystonia or parkinsonism after reinjection. With oral medication the drug remains at a relatively high and stable level in the blood, and the patient tends not to develop neurological side effects once the initial introductory period of drug administration has passed.

For patients who do not tolerate depot phenothiazines well, the best approach to ensuring reliable drug ingestion is administration of the entire daily dose at bedtime in liquid form, with supervision by responsible relatives. Education through group therapy or other approaches aimed at shaping better drug-taking behavior in chronic schizophrenic patients has not been adequately tested but might well be effective.

PHENOTHIAZINE USE IN NONPSYCHOTIC PATIENTS

There is modest evidence that phenothiazines are better than placebo in the treatment of geriatric psychiatric patients with such psychotic behavior as agitation, restlessness, delusions or hallucinations, or thought disorder (Cole and Stotsky, 1974). The drugs do not help the memory deficit. Geriatric patients take far lower doses than young adult schizophrenics. Thioridazine dosages of 25 to 100 mg/day are more usual than higher dosages. In elderly patients it is wise to begin with a small minimal dose of phenothiazine and raise it gradually as needed. Such patients develop hypotension and ataxia very easily; such side effects can lead to falls and fractures in the elderly. Nevertheless, agitated or hyperaroused elderly patients clearly can benefit from the use of phenothiazine drugs and should not be deprived of adequate dosages when necessary. Dosages must be raised carefully and with close observation.

The drugs have also been used in anxious outpatients. The evidence here is mixed, but on the average phenothiazines are probably somewhat better than placebo in the treatment of anxiety. They are likely not as effective as chlordiazepoxide, diazepam, or similar antianxiety drugs. They may well differ from the benzodiazepines in that they lack any disinhibiting effect; they may in fact be more likely to reduce anxiety while decreasing activity and adventurousness, whereas drugs like diazepam may decrease the anxiety while increasing motor activity and adventurousness. In some patients an increase in activity and a decrease in inhibition is clinically desirable; in others such a shift might well be a disaster. For this reason there may be occasional out-patients in whom nonsedative antianxiety drugs are needed. Given such pa-tients, it may well be that tricyclic antidepressants (e.g., doxepin) or non-phenothiazine antianxiety agents (e.g., hydroxyzine) may be preferable to the phenothiazines. There have been a few cases of tardive dyskinesia in neurotic patients receiving relatively low doses of phenothiazines, which makes one hesitate to use these drugs in such patients, except when they clearly have *not* responded adequately to other available antianxiety agents and *do* re-spond well to phenothiazines.

The drugs are also used in the treatment of patients with personality dis-orders or other characterological nonpsychotic problems. There is some evi-dence (Klein and Davis, 1969) that drugs such as thioridazine are effective in emotionally unstable character disorders that alternate rapidly from giddy euphoria to suicidal depression. However, such persons, even though they gain mood stability on phenothiazines, generally do not like the drug's effects and often do not take it after leaving the hospital.

The use of phenothiazine drugs (e.g., chlorpromazine intramuscularly) as a form of behavior control for institutionalized juvenile delinquents is even more dubious. The drug is probably not particularly effective except as a sedative in such conditions. It is certainly unpleasant and aversive. It may well be necessary in some highly unstable delinquents with marked behavioral ab-normalities to try a formal clinical trial on one of the oral phenothiazines. However, such a trial should be carried out with proper observation and as part of an integrated treatment program rather than as a series of treatment-unrelated acute dosings of malefactors.

There is good evidence that chlorpromazine and thioridazine may be ef-fective in some kinds of depression. Chlorpromazine seems to be particularly effective in agitated depressions (Klein and Davis, 1969) and thioridazine in anxious depressions (Hollister, 1973). It may well be that other phenothiazines in lower dosages are useful in some depressions. The effect of chlor-promazine in agitated depression is worthy of more detailed scrutiny. The drug improves severely agitated depressions but is inclined to worsen the psychopathology of depressed patients who do not show initial agitation.

Most of these drugs of course are excellent antiemetics. One drug in this general class, levomepromazine, even appears to be an analgesic. Thiorida-zine could conceivably be used in the treatment of premature ejaculation, since an early effect of this drug is to postpone or eventually prevent ejacula-tion without interfering initially with erectile potency. This would be turning the sexual side effect of thioridazine (impotence) from a liability into an asset, but I know of no evidence that the drug has been effectively used in this manner.

SIDE EFFECTS

From Acute Administration

Since the various phenothiazines apparently are almost always identically effective clinically, the major differences between them lie in the area of side effects (Hollister, 1973; Cole and Davis, 1975). A gross and very approxi-mate continuum can be constructed, with thioridazine to the left and fluphena-zine to the right, listing the drugs in crude order of increasing potency from thioridazine to chlorpromazine to perphenazine to fluphenazine. On this same crude diagram, sedation would be greatest at the thioridazine end and least at the fluphenazine end, while neurological side effects would order them-selves in the opposite direction. Thioridazine and chlorpromazine also have more autonomic and perhaps more endocrine side effects than do the high-potency piperazine phenothiazines. The implications of this are fairly clear. A person who shows a blood pressure drop on one of the more autonomically active phenothiazines (e.g., thioridazine or chlorpromazine) may show little or no hypotension when shifted to one of the piperazines. Similarly a patient distressed by extrapyramidal side effects with fluphenazine may not show such side effects if shifted to thioridazine.

Within this framework is a separate issue on which there are essentially no data. When given single doses of chlorpromazine, normal subjects find the experience very uncomfortable; they seem to be less distressed by equivalent antipsychotic dosages of the higher-potency phenothiazines. Schizophrenics seem to learn to tolerate either type of phenothiazine relatively well. How-ever, schizophrenic patients in the community often stop taking their medica-tion. Do they do this in the same manner that most other kinds of medical patients stop taking their long-term medications? Do they do it because of increasing psychosis? Do they do it because they intensely dislike the sub-jective states induced by the drug? To my knowledge, no one except Van Putten (1974) has ever considered the consumer acceptability aspect of the phenothiazines. A comparable but more extensive study in ambulatory patients should be done.

Although drowsiness, lethargy, and malaise are sometimes induced by the more autonomic phenothiazines, these side effects may not be the only reason for patient rejection of phenothiazine medications. A recent study showed that many chronic patients suffered severely from dysphoria, restlessness, and agitation while on phenothiazines, all of which were very nicely relieved by antiparkinsonian drugs (Van Putten et al., 1974). Therefore some of the unpleasantness patients feel while on phenothiazines may in fact be more subtle forms of the neurological side effects that are more common with the high-potency piperazine drugs. A description of the main neurological side effects caused by these drugs is probably worth repeating, even at this late date.

Dystonia is an acute, rigid or slowly fluctuating spasm, usually of the muscles of the neck, face, and tongue, causing this area to be held in a tight and unusual position. This side effect tends to appear during the first few days of treatment and is seen most commonly with the piperazine drugs. It is rapidly relieved by antiparkinsonian drugs given intramuscularly, by intravenous caffeine sodium benzoate or diphenhydramine, and probably by a variety of other drugs.

Pseudoparkinsonism usually appears a little later in treatment and is characterized by stiffness, shuffling gait, mask-like facies, drooling, and cogwheel rigidity in the extremities. Tremor, the usual sign of naturally occurring parkinsonism, is less clearly a trademark of this side effect syndrome because tremor is so commonly present in psychiatric patients with or without pseudoparkinsonism. These symptoms also respond reasonably well to antiparkinsonian agents.

Akathisia is sometimes known as the "restless leg syndrome." It is manifested by a feeling of acute discomfort in the muscles of the extremities and sometimes of the whole body, and it can be relieved only by movement. Patients therefore get up and down frequently, move their legs and feet up and down, pace to and fro, and appear generally restless and agitated. The movements may well have a driven quality that is not common in agitation due to inner psychic distress. When asked, the patients describe the motions as being due to discomfort in the muscles and usually do not relate it to inner psychic conflicts or preoccupations. The proof of the diagnosis is its relief by antiparkinsonian agents.

Sometimes patients are given increasing doses of the offending phenothiazine drug to relieve their "agitation." Paradoxically, this treatment sometimes works because as the dose of antipsychotic agent is raised higher and higher a threshold at which neurological side effects of this sort disappear is often passed. If the treating clinician is in doubt, the issue of akathisia can often be resolved by a therapeutic test with a single dose of an injectable antiparkinsonian agent. This should reduce akathisia but not affect psychically-induced agitation.

Many clinicians, including renowned experts in clinical psychopharmacology, endorse the prophylactic use of antiparkinsonian drugs along with phenothiazines to prevent or minimize the development of neurological side effects. I disagree with this position, and agree with Hollister's (1973) view on the matter. Giving two drugs when one will do is always unwise and can lead to more side effects. The antiparkinsonian agents themselves can induce a variety of side effects, including dry mouth, blurred vision, urinary retention, exacerbation of narrow-angle glaucoma, bowel stasis, confusion, and toxic delirium of the atropine type. In addition, I know of no clear evidence that antiparkinsonian agents are in fact effectively prophylactic in preventing neurological side effects. In a study carried out at Boston State Hospital in patients receiving repeated doses of fluphenazine enanthate at biweekly intervals, we found that prophylactic administration of an antiparkinsonian drug did not significantly affect the incidence of neurological side effects (Chien, DiMascio, and Cole, 1974). There was a slight trend for the neurological reactions to be less severe when they did occur. On the other hand, antiparkinsonian drugs *do* work when given acutely to relieve emerging neurological side effects.

At the other end of this issue, there is ample evidence from controlled studies that patients maintained on antiparkinsonian drugs for more than 3 months are very unlikely to have neurological side effects recur when the antiparkinsonian agents are discontinued. Only about 10% of such patients have any further trouble (Orlov, Kasparian, DiMascio, and Cole, 1971; Klett and Caffey, 1972). Therefore, I would discontinue antiparkinsonian agents a few days after the neurological side effects have come under control and give them again only if side effects recur. Two recent studies encourage me in this position. One by Lasagna's group at Rochester showed that chlorpromazine blood levels were significantly reduced when patients also received trihexyphenidyl (Rivera-Camlimlim, Castaneda, and Lasagna, 1973). Another study by Singh and Smith (1973) showed that acute schizophrenic patients stabilized on haloperidol and beginning to improve substantially became markedly worse when benztropine was administered. The antiparkinsonian drugs therefore may interfere with the therapeutic efficacy of antipsychotic drugs; the evidence for this is suggestive but not conclusive and certainly requires further study.

There are a few special side effects or related issues that pertain to the use of some individual phenothiazines. For example, it is well documented that thioridazine can cause retinitis pigmentosa with possible irreversible blindness at doses over 800 to 1,000 mg/day (Shader, Appleton, and DiMascio, 1970). Higher doses of this drug are therefore to be avoided, although using a higher dose of the drug for a short time could conceivably be justified in an acutely psychotic patient who was known not to tolerate other antipsychotic drugs. Thioridazine is also more likely to cause characteristic changes in the electrocardiogram (ECG) than are other phenothiazines. The significance of these changes is unclear (Ayd, 1970). Until we have data on the real incidence of adverse cardiovascular events in patients receiving thioridazine and compare them with the incidence of comparable events in patients on other phenothiazines, we will not know whether to be worried by the ECG changes induced by thioridazine. Since thioridazine is widely believed to be the best phenothiazine for use in geriatric psychiatric patients—although the efficacy of haloperidol and acetophenazine is somewhat better documented in such conditions (Cole and Stotsky, 1974)—it seems likely that thioridazine does not routinely induce any dramatic cardiovascular ill effects; were it otherwise, geriatric patients would have frequent adverse cardiovascular reactions.

Chlorpromazine is unique among the phenothiazines for causing marked photosensitivity. Patients receiving chlorpromazine in the summer are likely to develop severe sunburns after relatively short exposure to the sun. Although this can be prevented by using special salves that block the ultraviolet rays of the sun, it seems simpler to use some other phenothiazine in these patients. Jaundice is probably more commonly observed with chlorpromazine than with the other drugs; this was certainly true during the 1950s. More recently the incidence of jaundice in chlorpromazine-treated patients is estimated by Hollister (1973) as being approximately one in a thousand patients treated.

From Long-Term Administration

For the first 10 to 15 yr that phenothiazine derivatives were used in psychiatry, almost no long-term side effects were even suspected. Pregnancy with these drugs appeared then and now to be an uncomplicated event, except for the rare infant born with an acute dystonic reaction, which rapidly passes as his blood phenothiazine level drops. This condition can be treated in the same way as acute dystonic reactions in adult psychiatric patients. More recently there have been suspicions that sudden death occurs more frequently in patients on chronic maintenance phenothiazine treatment than was the case in the days before phenothiazine treatment was instituted. Unfortunately the data are obscure and controversial (Moore and Book, 1970). Some studies have shown no change in the incidence of such deaths in psychiatric hospitals since phenothiazines were introduced, and others have demonstrated an increase. The differences are not great, and certainly sudden deaths of unknown cause have been occurring in schizophrenics for years.

Approximately 10 years ago chronic patients began to show pigmentation in the eye and the skin (Greiner and Berry, 1964). The skin pigmentation was of a grayish, brownish, sometimes purplish hue and occurred in those areas of the skin exposed to light and sun. It appears to be associated either only or chiefly with chlorpromazine administration and fades when the administration of high-dosage phenothiazines is stopped. It appears to have no special consequence for the patient other than its modestly unattractive appearance.

Eye changes have also been described in patients exposed to high-dosage chlorpromazine treatment for either short or long periods (Prien, DeLong, Cole, and Levine, 1970). The acute effects of high-dosage chlorpromazine treatment appear to be pigmentary deposits in the anterior layers of the cornea, with some cloudy swelling. The chronic version of this problem is the appearance of granular deposits in the posterior surface of the cornea and anterior surface of the lens. These deposits are almost always detected only on slitlamp examination by an ophthalmologist. More rarely they are detected by the cloudiness of the cornea and lens when a light is flashed into the patient's eye. I know of only one apocryphal case of actual visual impairment resulting from these deposits. I have never heard of a case in which visual impairment was first reported by a patient who then was shown to have clear granular deposits in the eye on slitlamp examination. It is my opinion therefore that patients receiving maintenance phenothiazine treatment do *not* need routine slitlamp examinations or even routine ophthalmological examination. Annual physical examinations in such patients that include checking for cloudiness of the lens or cornea could serve as a preliminary screen. If cloudiness is observed, then an ophthalmological examination is obviously necessary. Even if cloudiness is found, no special clinical action needs to be taken other than probably decreasing the phenothiazine dosage, assuming that antipsychotic drug treatment is still clearly indicated. In patients studied to date, the chlorpromazine dosage appeared to be the major determinant of the presence of such ophthalmological pigmentation.

The major and most troublesome chronic side effect from prolonged use of the phenothiazines is tardive dyskinesia (Marsden, Tarsy, and Baldessarini, 1975). The term means "late-appearing abnormal movements" and as such is reasonably descriptive. The movements, which are most commonly seen in chronic psychiatric patients who are often old and often with some element of organic brain disease with or without concurrent schizophrenia, manifest themselves most frequently by abnormal movements of the tongue, mouth, jaw, and lips. Vermicular movements of the tongue, chronic irregular chewing movements of the jaws, tongue protrusion, or smacking or puckering of the lips are relatively frequent manifestations. This may extend to grimaces involving the whole face, with irregular protrusion of the tongue. Irregular, somewhat explosive speech may be associated with it, as may irregularities in breathing and swallowing, although the latter are uncommon. Neck twisting, body rocking, or rhythmic pelvic movements may accompany the syndrome or be its principal manifestation. Similarly, choreoathetotic movements of the hands and arms and akathisia-like movements of the hands and arms and akathisia-like stamping, jiggling, or twisting movements of the legs and ankles may occur.

Unfortunately the condition was overlooked for many years, probably because abnormal movements have been common in chronic psychiatric patients for centuries. A senile chorea manifested by chewing movements was observed in the elderly long before phenothiazines were ever used; and the line between some of the abnormal movements seen in patients with presumed tardive dyskinesia and the rocking movements seen in chronically institutionalized mental retardates or chronically psychotic patients in the predrug era is hard to define. Nevertheless, movements of this sort are now relatively common on chronic wards in mental hospitals. Perhaps a third of the most regressed or senile patients in the wards at Boston State Hospital show some abnormal movements that may well be considered tardive dyskinesia, and a smaller number of patients are quite clearly and visibly affected by the syndrome. Ambulatory psychotic patients in the community not infrequently show similar movements; and the syndrome has been seen, though very rarely, in neurotic patients receiving phenothiazines or other antipsychotic drugs for relatively short periods of time. A similar syndrome has been informally described in acute patients who may have received antipsychotic drugs for only a few months; the abnormal movements in these patients last a few days, weeks, or months and subsequently disappear entirely. In old, chronic patients the movements sometimes disappear, whereas in other patients they seem to persist for years rather than months and may well be permanent. Luckily the syndrome generally is not progressive and is remarkably unbothersome to the patients involved, who frequently claim total ignorance of movements quite visible to others or report no distress or bother concerning the movements. This general unconcern has been observed in chronically hospitalized patients and may not be as characteristic of patients in the community.

Unfortunately, although claims have been made that tardive dyskinesia is more common in patients given high doses of antipsychotic drugs or those who showed neurological side effects quite prominently early in their treatment with such drugs, these claims have not been adequately substantiated to date; the condition has been described in patients receiving the whole spectrum of available antipsychotic drugs, including reserpine and thioridazine as well as the more potent piperazine phenothiazines. Therefore there is no rational basis for preferring one phenothiazine to another in terms of its low likelihood of causing tardive dyskinesia. Neither is it clear that intermittent drug treatment is less likely than continuous drug treatment to lead to tardive dyskinesia. It is not known whether giving large doses of phenothiazines early to attempt a rapid cure of schizophrenia is good or bad in the long run. Obviously, however, the message is that phenothiazines and other related antipsychotic drugs should be used judiciously and only when necessary.

Physicians should be alert to the early signs of tardive dyskinesia, which may include athetoid movements of the hands, vermicular movements of the tongue, or tics of the lips or jaw. When such movements are observed phenothiazine administration should be stopped and the patient observed. Not infrequently if the patient is developing a dyskinesia, the movements become worse when the antipsychotic drug is stopped. The movements seem to be caused by dopaminergic overactivity in the basal ganglia. The phenothiazine drugs block dopamine receptors and decrease dopaminergic activity and therefore suppress the abnormal movements of tardive dyskinesia (Kazamatsuri, Chien, and Cole, 1972). When the drug is stopped, the movements may blossom forth. In patients with severe abnormal movements, the physician may have no choice at the moment other than reinstitution of antipsychotic drug treatment; in fact, he may be driven to choose a drug particularly high in neurological side effects to achieve maximal parkinsonian freezing. It should be noted that the antiparkinsonian drugs make these dyskinesias worse.

In a single limited study haloperidol was administered for 20 weeks to patients with pre-existing tardive dyskinesia; the movements were suppressed by haloperidol, although the dose had to be raised part way through the 20-week period; when haloperidol was stopped at the end of the study, the movements were no worse than they had been at the beginning (Kazamatsuri et al., 1972). It may be that the abnormal condition comes on suddenly in an all-or-none fashion rather than being quietly progressive with continuing phenothiazine dosage. Certainly its appearance seems to have a strong element of individual vulnerability rather than being a common or unavoidable occurrence in all patients. Sadly enough, there is currently no well-documented and effective treatment of the abnormal movements other than the use of antipsychotic drugs, which presumably cause the condition in the first place.

Some patients with clearly abnormal movements may continue to be very psychotic, thus placing the physician in the highly uncomfortable position of having to choose between controlling the psychosis and risking the development of further neurological abnormalities. As in many other areas of medicine, one must weigh the relative degree of evil involved in the two alternatives; I believe many psychiatrists opt for controlling the psychosis and hope to avoid further potential, but not certain, neurological impairment.

SUMMARY

The available antipsychotic phenothiazines all appear to be essentially equal in potency for many purposes, and particularly for the treatment of schizophrenia. They differ fairly widely in side effects, and there may be particular reasons for using one or another of them in a particular context. The side effects of these drugs are generally not serious in the short run. Antiparkinsonian agents are useful in the treatment of neurological side effects but are probably less useful in preventing them. The long-term prophylactic use of antiparkinsonian agents in combination with phenothiazines should be discouraged. Although the drugs are clearly much more effective than placebo in the treatment of schizophrenia, they are not generally curative and often only stabilize the patient in a state of limited psychosis in which other ambulatory and psychosocial treatment procedures may be applied.

More recently long-term neurological side effects have been associated with phenothiazine use. Currently the implications of such side effects for the treatment of schizophrenic patients are obscure. There appears to be no specific way to use antipsychotic drugs that avoids the occurrence of tardive dyskinesia, and in most cases the severity of the psychosis makes the use of phenothiazines or equivalent antipsychotic drugs mandatory.

TREATMENT SUMMARY

Generic name	Trade name	Daily dosage range (mg)[a]	Dosage equivalent to 300 mg chlorpromazine[b]
Aminoalkyl			
Chlorpromazine	Thorazine	100–1,000	300
Triflupromazine	Vesprin	20–150	100
Piperidyl			
Thioridazine	Mellaril	30–800[c]	300
Mesoridazine	Serentil	50–400	150
Piperacetazine	Quide	20–160	30
Piperazinyl			
Trifluoperazine	Stelazine	2–30	25
Perphenazine	Trilafon	2–64	28
Carphenazine	Proketazine	25–400	75
Acetophenazine	Tindal	40–80	50
Butaperazine	Repoise	30–50	30
Prochlorperazine	Compazine	15–125	60
Thiopropazate	Dartal	6–30	30
Fluphenazine	Prolixin	0.5–20	6

[a] Dosage range for the treatment of psychosis.

[b] Dosage equivalents prepared by Dr. George Gardos, Boston State Hospital, on the basis of clinical experience and other available estimates.

[c] Mandatory upper limit because of retinitis pigmentosa.

REFERENCES

Anderson, W. H., and Kuehnle, J. C. (1974): Strategies for the treatment of acute psychosis. *J.A.M.A.*, 229:1884–1889.

Ayd, F. A. (1970): Cardiovascular effects of phenothiazines. *Int. Drug Ther. Newslett.*, 5:1–8.

Chien, C. P., and Cole, J. O. (1973): Depot phenothiazine treatment in acute psychosis: A sequential comparative clinical study. *Am. J. Psychiatry*, 130:13–19.

Chien, C. P., DiMascio, A., and Cole, J. O. (1974): Antiparkinson agents and depot phenothiazine. *Am. J. Psychiatry*, 131:86–90.

Cole, J. O., and Davis, J. M. (1975): Antipsychotic agents. In: *Comprehensive Textbook of Psychiatry,* edited by A. M. Freedman, H. I. Kaplan, and B. J. Sadock. Williams and Wilkins, Baltimore.

Cole, J. O., and Stotsky, B. A. (1974): Improving psychiatric drug therapy: A matter of dosage and choice. *Geriatrics,* 83:74–78.

Forrest, I. S., Carr, C. J., and Usdin, E. (1974): *Phenothiazines and Structurally Related Drugs.* Raven Press, New York.

Gardos, G. (1974): Are antipsychotic drugs interchangeable? *J. Nerv. Ment. Dis.,* 159:343–348.

Goldberg, H., DiMascio, A., and Chaudhary, B. (1970): A clinical evaluation of fluphenazine enanthate. *Dis. Nerv. Syst.,* 31 (Suppl.):46–47.

Goldberg, S. C., Frosch, W. A., Drossman, A. K., Schooler, N. R., and Johnson, G. F. S. (1972): Prediction of response to phenothiazines in schizophrenia: A cross validation study. *Arch. Gen. Psychiatry,* 26:367–373.

Goldberg, S. C., Klerman, G. L., and Cole, J. O. (1965): Changes in schizophrenic psychopathology and ward behavior as a function of phenothiazine treatment. *Br. J. Psychiatry,* 3:120–133.

Greiner, A. C., and Berry, K. (1964): Skin pigmentation and corneal and lens opacities with prolonged chlorpromazine therapy. *Can. Med. Assoc. J.,* 90:663–665.

Groves, J. E., and Mandel, M. R. (1975): The long acting phenothiazines. *Arch Gen. Psychiatry (in press).*

Hamid, T., and Wertz, W. (1973): Mesoridazine versus chlorpromazine in acute schizophrenia. *Am. J. Psychiatry,* 130:689–692.

Hollister, L. (1973): *Clinical Use of Psychotherapeutic Drugs.* Charles C Thomas, Springfield, Ill.

Kazamatsuri, H., Chien, C. P., and Cole, J. O. (1972): Treatment of tardive dyskinesia. II. Short term efficacy of dopamine-blocking agents, haloperidol and thiopropazate. *Arch. Gen. Psychiatry,* 27:100–103.

Klein, D. F., and Davis, J. (1969): *Diagnosis and Drug Treatment of Psychiatric Disorders,* pp. 139–173. Williams & Wilkins, Baltimore.

Klett, C. J., and Caffey, E. M., Jr. (1972): Evaluating the long-term need for antiparkinson drugs by chronic schizophrenics. *Arch. Gen. Psychiatry,* 26:374–379.

Marsden, C. D., Tarsy, D., and Baldessarini, R. J. (1975): Spontaneous and drug-induced movement disorders in psychotic patients. In: *Psychiatric Complications of Neurological Diseases,* edited by D. F. Benson and D. Blumer. Grune & Stratton, New York *(in press).*

Matthysse, S. (1973): Antipsychotic drug actions: A clue to the neuropathology of schizophrenia? *Fed. Proc.,* 32:200–205.

Monroe, R. (1970): *Episodic Behavioral Disorders.* Harvard University Press, Cambridge.

Moore, M. T., and Book, M. H. (1970): Sudden death in phenothiazine therapy. *Psychiatr. Q.,* 44:389–395.

Orlov, P., Kasparian, G., DiMascio, A., and Cole, J. O. (1971): Withdrawal of antiparkinson drugs. *Arch. Gen. Psychiatry,* 25:410–412.

Prien, R. F., and Cole, J. O. (1968): High dose chlorpromazine therapy in chronic schizophrenia. *Arch. Gen. Psychiatry,* 18:402–495.

Prien, R. F., DeLong, S. L., Cole, J. O., and Levine, J. (1970): Ocular changes occurring with prolonged high dose chlorpromazine therapy. *Arch. Gen. Psychiatry,* 23:464–467.

Rivera-Camlimlim, L., Castaneda, L., and Lasagna, L. (1973): Effects of mode of management on plasma chlorpromazine in psychiatric patients. *Clin. Pharmacol. Ther.,* 14:978–986.

Shader, R. I., Appleton, W. S., and DiMascio, A. (1970): Ophthalmological (pigmentary) changes. In: *Psychotropic Drug Side Effects,* edited by R. I. Shader and A. DiMascio, pp. 107–116. Williams & Wilkins, Baltimore.

Singh, M. M., and Smith, J. M. (1973): Reversal of some therapeutic effects of an antipsychotic agent by an antiparkinsonism agent. *J. Nerv. Ment. Dis.,* 157:50–58.

Slotnick, V. B. (1971): Management of the acutely agitated psychiatric patient with parenteral neuroleptics: A comparative symptom effectiveness profile of haloperidol and chlorpromazine. Presented at the Fifth World Congress of Psychiatry, Mexico.

Smith, K., Surphlis, W., Gynther, M., and Shimkunas, A. (1967): ECT-chlorpromazine and chlorpromazine compared in the treatment of schizophrenia. *J. Nerv. Ment. Dis.,* 144:284–290.

Swazey, J. (1974): *Chlorpromazine: The History of the Psychiatric Discovery.* MIT Press, Cambridge, Mass.

Van Putten, T. (1974): Why do schizophrenic patients refuse to take their drugs? *Arch. Gen. Psychiatry,* 31:67–72.

Van Putten, T., Mutalipassi, L., and Malkin, M. (1974): Phenothiazine induced decompensation. *Arch. Gen. Psychiatry,* 30:102–105.

Chapter 3

Thioxanthenes

George M. Simpson and J. Hillary Lee

The first thioxanthene derivatives were synthesized in the laboratories of H. Lundbeck and Company during the late 1950s. The first report on the synthesis and pharmacology appeared in 1958 (Peterson, Lassen, Holm, Kopf, and Møller Nielsen, 1958) and was followed by a report on the pharmacological characteristics of 66 new thioxanthenes (Møller Nielsen, Hougs, Lassen, Holm, and Petersen, 1962). To date, many different thioxanthenes have been synthesized, although only four have been marketed; chlorprothixene (Taractan) and thiothixene (Navane) are the only ones available in the United States. Clopenthixol and flupenthixol, the latter in both an oral and depot form, are available in several other countries.

CHEMISTRY

The thioxanthenes, like the phenothiazines, consist of a triple-ring, heterocyclic nucleus; the thioxanthenes differ from the phenothiazines in that the nitrogen (N) atom in the phenothiazine nucleus (position 10) is replaced by a carbon (C) atom (Fig. 1). Those thioxanthenes with central nervous system (CNS) activity are characterized by a double bond between the C10 and the side chain as well as specific substitutions in position 2. The ac-

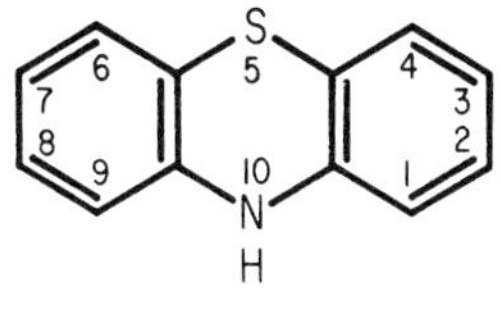

PHENOTHIAZINE NUCLEUS

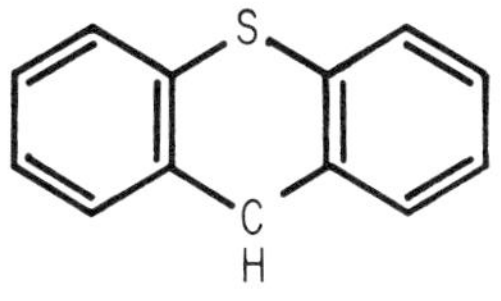

FIG. 1. Basic structure of the phenothiazine and thioxanthene molecules. Note that the thioxanthenes are structural derivatives of the phenothiazines.

THIOXANTHENE NUCLEUS

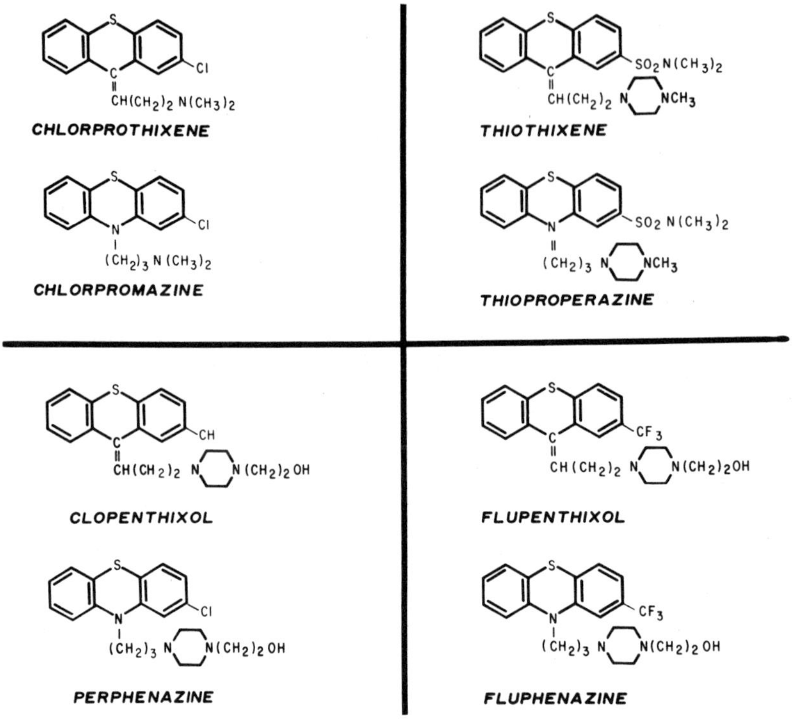

FIG. 2. Structure of the four major thioxanthenes and their phenothiazine analogues.

tive derivatives have a three-carbon side chain terminating in an amine grouping. Because of a double bond at the C10 in substituted thioxanthenes, two isomers of each thioxanthene (*cis* and *trans*) can be formed. Following isolation of the two isomers, it was found that the *cis* form is many times more biologically active than the *trans* form. (Initially the active isomer was thought to be the *trans* form, but subsequent X-ray crystallography demonstrated that the *cis* has the active isomer configuration.) The chemical structures of the four thioxanthenes demonstrated to have therapeutic activity are shown in Fig. 2 with their phenothiazine analogues.

PHARMACOLOGY

Compounds with documented antipsychotic activity have specific effects on a variety of parameters that can be assessed in animals. The screening profile used for potential neuroleptics (antipsychotic drugs) includes decreased motility, selective inhibition of conditioned avoidance responses, antagonism of amphetamine-induced stereotypies and of apomorphine-induced emesis, production of catalepsy, potentiation of analgesics and hypnotics, and a taming effect. Although the known neuroleptics have these effects in varying degrees, it is not known how directly related or essential each "animal" characteristic is for the therapeutic effect observed in patients.

The profile of the thioxanthenes is similar to those of other neuroleptics in terms of the above pharmacological parameters; like the phenothiazines, the different thioxanthenes exert their various pharmacological activities to differing degrees. Thiothixene produces selective inhibition of the conditioned avoidance response (i.e., it leaves the escape response intact), whereas the same dosages of chlorprothixene and clopenthixol interfere with both avoidance and escape. A similar profile appears with their phenothiazine analogues; i.e., thioproperazine, the thiothixene analogue, affects only the avoidance response, whereas chlorpromazine, the chlorprothixene analogue, is less selective (Weissman, 1974). Thiothixene is also similar to thioproperazine in that it is an extremely potent antiemetic and an active blocker of amphetamine stereotypies in comparison to chlorpromazine (Weissman, 1974).

Møller Nielsen, Pedersen, Nymark, Franck, Boech, Fjalland, and Christensen (1973) compared the effects of chlorprothixene, clopenthixol, and flupenthixol with those of fluphenazine, perphenazine, chlorpromazine, and haloperidol on motility, catalepsy, apomorphine vomiting, and amphetamine stereotypies. They found that chlorprothixene is quite similar to chlorpromazine in that it has a weak cataleptogenic effect, weak apomorphine vomiting antagonism, and weak amphetamine stereotypy antagonism. It differed from chlorpromazine in that it had a strong inhibiting effect on motility.

Clopenthixol is more potent than chlorprothixene in its cataleptogenic effect, antiemetic effect, and amphetamine stereotypy antagonism. Its analogue perphenazine is a somewhat more potent cataleptogenic agent, although the two drugs are similar on other variables. Flupenthixol is similar to clopenthixol and closer to haloperidol than chlorpromazine in most of its pharmacological effects. For a more extensive review of the chemistry and pharmacology of the thioxanthenes, the reader is referred to the article by Petersen and Møller Nielsen (1964).

CLINICAL STUDIES

It is well known that the course of research, particularly clinical trials, is never totally orderly; and although it would be useful to report comparisons between each thioxanthene and its phenothiazine analogue, such data do not exist for all the forms. In the following, a summary of the clinical effects (efficacy, toxicity, unwanted effects) is presented for each compound. An effort has been made to focus primarily on controlled trials, although in many instances there is a paucity of such studies.

Chlorprothixene

Chlorprothixene, the chlorpromazine analogue, was the first thioxanthene derivative demonstrated to be an active antipsychotic agent. The early trials were open, and so in addition to its antipsychotic activity the investigators commented on its sedative properties (Madsen and Ravn, 1959). Most of the subsequent studies with chlorprothixene were also uncontrolled, perhaps because clinical trial methodology was relatively rudimentary at the time this drug was first receiving attention. However, several controlled studies have shown that it is more effective than placebo in the treatment of schizophrenia (Karn, Mead, and Fishman, 1961; Scanlan and May, 1963).

In a double-blind collaborative study (Lasky, Klett, Caffey, Bennett, Rosenblum and Hollister, 1962), six drugs were compared (chlorprothixene, fluphenazine, thioridazine, chlorpromazine, triflupromazine, and reserpine) in 512 newly admitted schizophrenic patients. The statistical analyses of behavior rating scale data revealed a variety of differences among drugs, particularly in syndromes associated with excitement-retardation. A multivariate analysis revealed that reserpine was less effective than the three most effective drugs (chlorpromazine, thioridazine, and fluphenazine). Chlorprothixene had an intermediate effect. The problem of relative efficacy, however, is difficult to assess, even with the best controlled studies, for it is clear that in this study the dosages of drugs were in no way comparable. The average daily dosages were: chlorprothixene 224 mg, chlorpromazine 746 mg, thioridazine 845 mg, fluphenazine 10 mg, triflupromazine 208 mg, and reserpine 6 mg. Also, since most of the work with chlorprothixene was done during the late 1950s and early 1960s, the literature is replete with inconclusive studies. One can conclude only that chlorprothixene is an active antipsychotic agent.

The dosage range for the treatment of schizophrenia is 50 to 1,000 mg/day (mean 400 mg). The side effect profile is similar to that of chlorpromazine, with sedative, autonomic, and cardiovascular effects being most prominent. Early studies (Ravn, 1970) found no evidence of extrapyramidal effects or liver toxicity, but the dosages used in these studies were very low. A definitive evaluation of unwanted effects is still needed.

Thiothixene

Investigations with thiothixene, the thioxanthene analogue of thioproperazine, began during the mid-1960s; since the study designs were somewhat more sophisticated, there is more information available on this compound. Early clinical trials quickly affirmed its antipsychotic activity (Simpson and Iqbal, 1965; Sugerman, Stolberg, and Herrmann, 1965; Gallant, Bishop, and Shelton, 1966), its long-term efficacy in chronic schizophrenia (Angus, Iqbal, Iqbal, and Simpson, 1967), and its value in acute schizophrenia (Overall, Hollister, Shelton, Kimbell, and Pennington, 1967).

A variety of double-blind controlled trials have been carried out and have generated some comparative information, particularly in terms of side effects. In a comparison with thioridazine, Gallant, Bishop, Timmons, and Gould (1966) found thiothixene at dosages of 20 to 30 mg/day to be equivalent in efficacy in chronic schizophrenia to thioridazine at 800 mg/day. Side effects were mild for both drugs: some orthostatic hypotension and extrapyramidal effects were seen with both, and drowsiness occurred only with thioridazine. More recently the same investigators (Dillenkoffer, George, Bishop, and Gallant, 1974) compared the electrocardiographic (ECG) effects of thiothixene and thioridazine in chronic schizophrenic patients. The dosage range for thiothixene was 10 to 40 mg/day, and for thioridazine 200 to 800 mg/day. Both agents were administered according to a fixed-dosage schedule. Only two of the 13 patients on thiothixene had ECG changes. One change was transient, occurring at 10 mg/day and disappearing at higher dosages; the second patient had mild, nonspecific T-wave changes throughout the study. Among the thioridazine group all 13 patients had changes at 400 mg/day. The changes comprised a lengthening of the Q-T intervals and moderate to marked lowering and flattening of T-waves. Routine clinical and side effect assessments were also carried out, and the results were similar to those previously reported.

Denber and Turns (1972) compared thiothixene and trifluoperazine in acute schizophrenic patients and reported that thiothixene is somewhat superior to trifluoperazine, although no statistical procedures were used to evaluate differences. Both drugs were effective in reducing psychotic symptomatology. The most frequent unwanted effect for both drugs was rigidity; the incidence of other unwanted effects was similar for the two compounds, with autonomic and extrapyramidal signs occurring most frequently.

Whereas most drug trials focus on changes in symptomatology, Gardos, Finnerty, and Cole (1970) compared the effects of thiothixene and trifluoperazine on movement in a step system, a behavioral measure. A step system comprises different levels of adjustment ranging, for example, from no work assignment, to increasing hours of work per week, to work outside the hospital. As the level of work adjustment increases (from step to step), the privileges and pay also increase, thus providing an incentive for patients to move on to the next step. Reaching the highest step would mean their work adjustment approaches "normal" levels, and at least on this parameter the patients could be considered ready for discharge. The authors reported that thiothixene produced slightly higher mean step scores than did trifluoperazine, and they related this to its hypothesized "activating" properties. However, the differences between drugs never reached the accepted level of significance, making such conclusions tenuous.

The therapeutic dosage range for the treatment of schizophrenia is 10 to 60 mg/day. Unwanted effects are similar to the higher-potency phenothiazines, with extrapyramidal effects more preponderant than the sedative effects.

Clopenthixol

Clopenthixol is not on the market in the United States, and therefore only a brief summary of its clinical characteristics is presented. The early evaluations of clopenthixol carried out in the United States and abroad indicated that it is an active antipsychotic agent (Ban, Ferguson, and Lehmann, 1963; Simpson, Angus, and Iqbal, 1966; Sugerman, Lichtigfeld, and Herrmann, 1966; Wolpert, Sheppard, and Merlis, 1967). In a controlled comparison with perphenazine, Dehnel, Vestre, and Schiele (1968) found essentially no difference clinically between the two compounds (the mean clopenthixol dosage was 132 mg, and perphenazine 51 mg). In terms of side effects, there was no difference between the two drugs on the most frequent side effects, i.e., insomnia, drowsiness, and restlessness.

Clopenthixol appears to be a moderately potent antipsychotic agent on a molar basis (dosage range up to 150 mg). Its unwanted effects consist primarily of extrapyramidal symptoms. Although it was clinically effective on both a short- and a long-term basis (Simpson, Arengo, Angus, Beckles, and Rochlin, 1972; Saletu, Itil, Arat, and Akpinar, 1973) it produced a somewhat higher than expected incidence of laboratory abnormalities, and so marketing was not pursued in the United States.

Flupenthixol

Flupenthixol, which is not marketed in the United States, appears to be an active antipsychotic agent. It is available in both oral and long-acting forms; most work has been done with the latter. Unfortunately no well-controlled trials (using a placebo or a comparative drug) with either form have been reported. The clinical studies, however, suggest that the average dosage for the depot form is 40 mg every 2 weeks, although some investigators have used up to 120 mg. Side effects appear to be primarily extrapyramidal in nature. The possibility that it has antidepressant properties has been raised, as it has with other thioxanthenes (*vide infra*).

SPECIAL STUDIES

Electroencephalography

Saletu and co-workers (1973) studied changes in electroencephalographic (EEG) variables during a 1-year trial of clopenthixol. They found an increase in slow and a decrease in fast activity; a decrease in average frequency, frequency deviation, and β-bursts; and an increase in rhythmical activity. They reported that these changes were similar to the EEG characteristics of other neuroleptics in chronic schizophrenia.

In another study Itil, Patterson, Keskiner, and Holden (1974) compared the effects of haloperidol, fluphenazine, and thiothixene on EEG records. The study employed a double-blind multiple-crossover design with 2-month placebo periods between each 3-month drug trial. The effects of the three prototypic compounds on EEG were similar. There was a decrease of delta, an increase of theta and alpha, and a decrease in very fast beta in comparison with the placebo period. Sleep recordings were also done, and again there was no difference in the effects of the three neuroleptics on the EEG variables.

Antidepressant Effects

In early work with the thioxanthenes, investigators frequently noted an "activation" effect, particularly at lower dosages. This led to a substantial literature (and controversy) over their role as antidepressants. Here the studies evaluating the activating and/or antidepressant activities of chlorprothixene, thiothixene, and flupenthixol are presented with an emphasis on controlled studies.

Chlorprothixene

In some early, uncontrolled studies (Madsen and Ravn, 1959), chlorprothixene was reported to have possible antidepressant activity, and several controlled studies have been carried out to evaluate this possibility in depressed patients. Hutchinson and Smedberg (1963) compared electroconvulsive therapy (ECT) and six different drugs (imipramine, tranylcypromine, amitriptyline, pheniprazine, phenelzine, and chlorprothixene) in depression. The investigator was blind as to which treatment each patient was receiving. ECT was significantly better than the drug treatments, but among the drugs only one comparison was significant (imipramine and tranylcypromine were better than amitriptyline, pheniprazine, phenelzine, and chlorprothixene). In fact, chlorprothixene produced the least amount of improvement. In another study, Lodge Patch, Pitt, and Yeo (1967) compared imipramine and chlorprothixene in moderately severe depressions using a crossover design. They found a time effect in that more improvement occurred before the crossover than after, regardless of which drug was used first. Although drug comparisons were not significant, the authors reported that the results tended to favor imipramine; it was clearly more effective in the older patients. The authors noted the limitations of the crossover design because of the order effect. In addition, a crossover procedure is not the design of choice for a time-limited illness such as depression. These two studies suggest that chlorprothixene has some beneficial effect in depression, although this effect only approaches and certainly does not surpass the results with orthodox antidepressants.

Thiothixene

The activating and antidepressant properties of thiothixene have received more attention than similar properties in any other thioxanthene. The early clinical trials (Angus et al., 1967; Hekimian, Gershon, and Floyd, 1967) suggested that this compound has a bimodal action, with activation at low dosages and an antipsychotic effect at high dosages. Several trials have been carried out in an attempt to verify this effect.

DiMascio and Demirgian (1972) compared the workshop performance of a group of schizophrenics who were placed on thiothixene with that of another group who continued their prior medication (mainly chlorpromazine and thioridazine). They found an increase in output with thiothixene in contrast with a decrease in the group whose medication was unchanged. This was interpreted as supporting an activation effect for thiothixene. The study was not blind, and although the authors emphasized the objective nature of the dependent variable there may have been more interest in the thiothixene group, even in terms of the need for dosage regulation, which may have contributed to the difference. Another variable that may have influenced the results and which was not assessed was adverse side effects. It is possible that the sedative effects so characteristic of chlorpromazine and thioridazine may have been interfering with workshop performance, while the relative absence of such effects with thiothixene enabled the patients to work unhindered.

Gardos and Cole (1973) reviewed the clinical efficacy literature with thiothixene in schizophrenia, thus determining the optimal dosage, evidence of activation, and the presence of side effects indicative of central nervous system stimulation for each study. They found that the slope of the regression line relating optimal dosage with the latter two measures was negative, suggesting more activation was associated with low dosages and less activation with high dosages. This relationship was discussed as evidence for a bimodal action of thiothixene, and the procedure was suggested as a model to evaluate the presence of similar activity in other compounds. However, an earlier study (Simpson, Angus, Edwards, Go, and Lee, 1972) which examined the possibility of a bimodal effect of thiothixene in schizophrenia produced essentially negative results.

There have been two controlled studies in which the antidepressant properties of thiothixene were compared directly with a standard antidepressant in depressed patients. Kiev (1972) compared thiothixene and protriptyline in outpatient psychotic depressions. The thiothixene group received a mean daily dosage of 13.5 mg, and the protriptyline group 22.9 mg. Both drugs produced improvement; thiothixene patients achieved significantly better scores than the protriptyline group on one of the four Hamilton factors (agitated depression) and a greater "continuing" effect on the anxiety factor. Despite the double-blind design, the unwanted effects may well have "broken the code." Approximately half of the 25 patients on thiothixene complained of tremor and restlessness; a similar proportion of the 25 protriptyline patients reported dry mouth.

In the second controlled study (Simpson et al., 1972), thiothixene and amitriptyline were compared in newly admitted patients with endogenous depressions. The mean thiothixene dosage was 9 mg/day, and the mean amitriptyline dosage 215 mg/day. Significant improvement was noted on 13 of the 22 Hamilton items with amitriptyline, and on three items with thiothixene. Four of the 40 drug comparisons were significant, all in favor of amitriptyline. The data from these two studies suggest that thiothixene does produce improvement in depression, but the results in terms of its relative efficacy in comparison with standard antidepressants are somewhat contradictory.

Flupenthixol

Flupenthixol first received attention as an antidepressant in 1969 (Reiter, 1969). In this anecdotal report (without systematic evaluations, statistical analyses, or even a comparison agent), flupenthixol was reported to be as effective as other antidepressants (none was included in the trial), to be without side effects, and to produce a rapid remission (within 1 day to 1 week). Mersky (1971) in a follow-up letter also commented on its rapid onset of therapeutic effect, although only 24 of his 53 depressed patients (albeit chronic) responded. Another letter (Hall and Coleman, 1973) reported favorably on the antidepressant effects of the compound. While each of the three reports indicated either the value of or need for a controlled study, none of the investigators expressed any reservations concerning their conclusions. Despite these enthusiastic claims, a reasoned evaluation of flupenthixol's value in depression will be possible only when well-designed, controlled studies are carried out.

In conclusion, the evidence from controlled studies suggests that chlorprothixene and thiothixene can effect improvement in depression. However, in view of the possible tardive dyskinesia-producing potential of neuroleptics, before they can be touted as a treatment of choice they must be shown not only to be equal to conventional treatments but to exceed them in efficacy. This is a particularly important consideration in the older depressed patient who, because of the recurring nature of his illness, usually requires maintenance therapy. In these patients both age and the continued exposure to neuroleptics increase the likelihood of dyskinetic symptoms.

INDICATIONS AND USAGE

It should be emphasized that the treatment recommendations here cover all patients, whether they be in or out of hospital. Maintenance dosages in particular may be equally high in either situation. In acute treatment obviously one would be more careful about rapid dosage increases. In a poorly controlled situation such as an outpatient clinic, side effects that are not readily or rapidly dealt with may lead to a discontented patient refusing to take medication.

Chlorprothixene

Chlorprothixene is primarily indicated for the treatment of schizophrenia or other psychotic states. It may be effective in depression but is not recommended for this condition. Chlorprothixene can be helpful in the treatment of schizophrenia in dosages of 25 mg t.i.d. or q.i.d., up to several hundred milligrams two or three times a day. The dosage of all antipsychotic agents varies tremendously among individuals, and therefore fixed dosage regimens are not recommended. Patients should be treated according to their symptomatology but ordinarily are first given a low dosage if symptoms are minor or not adversely interfering with the patient or with other patients on the ward. Thus a starting dose of 25 mg t.i.d. or q.i.d. could be used for a quiet, withdrawn, hallucinating, newly admitted patient or a patient in a day hospital. The dosage might be increased rapidly to levels as high as 1,000 mg, depending on the side effects and the onset of behavioral improvement. No precise maximum dosage can be recommended because occasional patients require dosages even above what might seem to be the top limit. As soon as improvement is obtained, the dosage can be slowly reduced to a maintenance level, which is often approximately half of the initial therapeutic level; this dosage should be adjusted gradually and can be given on a once-a-day regimen at bedtime. Dosages over 2 g daily are not recommended since the anticholinergic effect of this drug produces extreme dry mouth, constipation, and pupillary dilation. In addition, if a patient has not responded at levels as high as this, then a change to a more potent drug is wise.

Small dosages should be used for elderly patients; the cardiovascular effects (i.e., the ability of the drug to produce hypotension and tachycardia) have an important bearing on the dosage used. Indeed, a more potent antipsychotic agent is recommended in such patients in order to avoid adverse cardiovascular effects, e.g., hypotension. Despite this, chlorprothixene is frequently used in the elderly because of a reportedly lower incidence of extrapyramidal effects.

In the acute patient who is very excited, parenteral chlorprothixene may be used in dosages of 25 to 50 mg, which can be repeated as required until the patient is manageable. One can capitalize on its powerful sedative effect, as well as the ultimate antipsychotic effect. The injection is relatively painless and can be repeated several times a day if required prior to the institution of oral therapy.

Thiothixene

Thiothixene has been recommended for a wide variety of psychotic states including organic psychoses, schizophrenia, and psychotic depressions. We do not recommend its use in the latter condition. As already mentioned, antipsychotic drugs may have a beneficial effect on depressions, but the frequency of depression in the elderly and their proneness to tardive dyskinesia should make the clinician wary of using a neuroleptic. We have seen approximately 20 patients suffering from neither schizophrenia nor organic psychoses who had severe, disturbing, and in some cases crippling tardive dyskinesias. Many of these patients had involutional melancholia and could have been adequately treated with tricyclic antidepressants or even ECT.

Small dosages of thiothixene have been found beneficial in the organic psychoses; thus 2 mg t.i.d. for a starting dose with an upper limit of 12 mg/day have been found helpful in diseases of the senium. Higher dosages could be used, but the likelihood of extrapyramidal effects developing must be taken into consideration. This is particularly important because the combination of an antipsychotic agent and an antiparkinsonian agent should be avoided if possible in the elderly. These patients are more prone to toxic confusional states due to antiparkinsonian agents as well as other side effects due to anticholinergic drugs. A maintenance dose of 6 to 8 mg/day is usually adequate for elderly patients.

As with all thioxanthenes, the major indication for thiothixene is the treatment of schizophrenia. Dosages of up to 60 mg/day are recommended, although even higher dosages may be required in some patients. Again, the dosage is variable and depends on the sensitivity of each patient to side effects and to the onset of behavioral improvement. There is also considerable evidence that parenteral thiothixene has both a sedating and an antipsychotic effect, so it can be used in the initial treatment of very overactive, excited patients whether they are schizophrenic or manic. Dosages of 2, 4, and even as high as 6 or 8 mg may be used at one time and then repeated two or three times a day. This should produce a calming effect rapidly. Thereafter an oral dose can be introduced that initially might be approximately twice the parenteral dosage; later it is increased or decreased according to the patient's needs. For instance, in very overactive, excited patients, a dosage regimen of 5 mg t.i.d. rapidly increased to 20 mg t.i.d. on the second or third day may be utilized. In quieter patients a slower incremental regimen can be instituted. In the former regimen the likelihood of extrapyramidal reactions, particularly dystonic reactions, is increased; however, if one is aware of this possibility and recognizes that the condition rapidly responds to antiparkinsonian medication, it is not a contraindication. Again, after a patient is stabilized and the symptoms have remitted, the dosage can be slowly reduced to approximately half the initial dosage, the reduced level then serving as maintenance therapy. The actual length of maintenance therapy depends on the severity of the illness and the frequency of the episodes. In all cases the lowest possible dosage should be used. This can be given once a day, at bedtime, which is more economical. Furthermore, a simple regimen may mean that the drug is taken more reliably.

TREATMENT SUMMARY

Generic name	Trade name	Daily dosage range (mg)[a]
Chlorprothixene	Taractan	100–1,000
Thiothixene	Navane	20–60

[a] Dosage range for the treatment of psychosis.

REFERENCES

Angus, J. W. S., Iqbal, F., Iqbal, J., and Simpson, G. M. (1967): A year's trial of thiothixene in chronic schizophrenia. *Int. J. Neuropsychiatry,* 3:408–412.

Ban, T. A., Ferguson, K., and Lehmann, H. E. (1963): The effect of clopenthixol on chronic psychiatric patients. *Am. J. Psychiatry,* 119:984–985.

Dehnel, L. L., Vestre, N. D., and Schiele, B. C. (1968): A controlled comparison of clopenthixol and perphenazine in chronic schizophrenic population. *Curr. Ther. Res.,* 10:169–176.

Denber, H. C. B., and Turns, D. (1972): Double-blind comparison of thiothixene and trifluoperazine in acute schizophrenia. *Psychosomatics,* 13:100–104.

Dillenkoffer, R. L., George, R. B., Bishop, M. P., and Gallant, D. M. (1974): Electro-cardiographic evaluation of thiothixene: A double-blind comparison with thioridazine. In: *Thiothixene and the Thioxanthenes,* edited by I. S. Forrest, C. J. Carr, and E. Usdin. Raven Press, New York.

DiMascio, A., and Demirgian, E. (1972): Study of the activating properties of thiothixene. *Psychosomatics,* 13:105–108.

Gallant, D. M., Bishop, M. P., and Shelton, W. (1966): A preliminary evaluation of P-4657B: A thioxanthene derivative. *Am. J. Psychiatry,* 123:345–346.

Gallant, D. M., Bishop, M. P., Timmons, E., and Gould, A. R. (1966): Thiothixene (P-4657B): A controlled evaluation in chronic schizophrenic patients. *Curr. Ther. Res.,* 8:153–158.

Gardos, G., and Cole, J. O. (1973): The dual action of thiothixene. *Arch. Gen. Psychiatry,* 29:222–225.

Gardos, G., Finnerty, R. J., and Cole, J. O. (1970): Thiothixene and trifluoperazine in a step system. *Psychosomatics,* 11:36–40.

Hall, P., and Coleman, J. (1973): Flupenthixol in the treatment of depressive states. *Br. J. Psychiatry,* 122:120–121.

Hekimian, L. J., Gershon, S., and Floyd, A. (1967): Some clinical and physiologic effects of a thioxanthene derivative, thiothixene (P-4657B) in 20 newly hospitalized male schizophrenics. *J. Clin. Pharmacol.,* 7:52–57.

Hutchinson, J. T., and Smedberg, D. (1963): Treatment of depression: A comparative study of E.C.T. and six drugs. *Br. J. Psychiatry,* 109:536–538.

Itil, T. M., Patterson, C. D., Keskiner, A., and Holden, J. M. (1974): Comparison of phenothiazine and nonphenothiazine neuroleptics according to psychopathology, side effects and computerized EEG. In: *Thiothixene and the Thioxanthenes,* edited by I. S. Forrest, C. J. Carr, and E. Usdin, pp. 35–45. Raven Press, New York.

Karn, W. N., Mead, B. T., and Fishman, J. J. (1961): Double-blind study of chlor-prothixene (Taractan), a panpsychotropic agent. *J. New Drugs,* 1:72–79.

Kiev, A. (1972): Double-blind comparison of thiothixene (Navane) and protriptyline (Vivactil) in psychotic depression. *Dis. Nerv. Syst.,* 11:811–816.

Lasky, J. J., Klett, C. J., Caffey, E. M., Jr., Bennett, J. L., Rosenblum, M. P., and Hollister, L. E. (1962): Drug treatment of schizophrenic patients: A comparative evaluation of chlorpromazine, chlorprothixene, fluphenazine, reserpine, thioridazine and triflupromazine. *Dis. Nerv. Syst.,* 23:698–706.

Lodge Patch, I. C., Pitt, B. M., and Yeo, Y. M. (1967): The direct comparison of antidepressants: Imipramine and chlorprothixene. *J. Psychiatr. Res.,* 5:273–280.

Madsen, E., and Ravn, J. (1959): Preliminary therapeutic experiments with a new psychotropic drug, Truxal. *Nord. Psykiatr. Medlemski,* 13:82.

Mersky, H. (1971): Flupenthixol "Fluanxol." *Br. J. Psychiatry,* 119:230.

Møller Nielsen, I., Hougs, W., Lassen, N., Holm, T., and Petersen, P. V. (1962): Central depressant activity of some thioxanthene derivatives. *Acta Pharmacol. Toxicol. (Kbh.),* 19:87–100.

Møller Nielsen, I., Pedersen, V., Nymark, M., Franck, K. F., Boeck, V., Fjalland, B., and Christensen, A. V. (1973): The comparative pharmacology of flupenthixol and some reference neuroleptics. *Acta Pharmacol. Toxicol. (Kbh.),* 33:353–362.

Overall, J. E., Hollister, L. E., Shelton, J., Kimbell, I., Jr., and Pennington, V. (1967): Broad-spectrum screening of psychotherapeutic drugs: Thiothixene as an antipsychotic and antidepressant. *Clin. Pharmacol. Ther.,* 8:249–255.

Petersen, P. V., Lassen, N., Holm, T., Kopf, R., and Møller Nielsen, I. (1958): Chemical structure and pharmacologic effects of thioxanthene analogues of chlorpromazine, promazine and mephazine. *Arzneim. Forsch.,* 8:395.

Petersen, P. V., and Møller Nielsen, I. (1964): Thioxanthene derivatives. In: *Psychopharmacological Agents,* Vol. 1, edited by M. Gordon. Academic Press, New York.

Ravn, J. (1970): The history of the thioxanthenes. In: *Discoveries in Biological Psychiatry,* edited by F. J. Ayd, Jr. and B. Blackwell. Lippincott, Philadelphia.

Reiter, P. J. (1969): On flupenthixol, an antidepressant of a new chemical group. *Br. J. Psychiatry,* 115:1399–1402.

Saletu, B., Itil, T. M., Arat, M., and Akpinar, S. (1973): Long-term clinical and quantitative EEG effects of clopenthixol in schizophrenics: Clinical-neurophysiological correlations. *Int. Pharmacopsychiatry,* 8:193–207.

Scanlan, E. P., and May, A. E. (1963): A controlled trial of Taractan in chronic schizophrenia. *Br. J. Psychiatry,* 109:418–421.

Simpson, G. M., Angus, J. W. S., Edwards, J. G., Go, S. H., and Lee, J. H. (1972): Role of antidepressants and neuroleptics in the treatment of depression. *Arch. Gen. Psychiatry,* 27:337–345.

Simpson, G. M., Angus, J. W. S., and Iqbal, J. (1966): The effect of clopenthixol on chronic schizophrenia, *Curr. Ther. Res.,* 8:3, 85–91.

Simpson, G. M., Arengo, A. D., Angus, J. W. S., Beckles, E. D., and Rochlin, D. (1972): A one-year trial of clopenthixol in chronic schizophenia. *Can. Psychiatr. Assoc. J.,* 17:321–323.

Simpson, G. M., and Iqbal, J. (1965): A preliminary study of thiothixene in chronic schizophrenics. *Curr. Ther. Res.,* 7:697–700.

Sugerman, A. A., Lichtigfeld, F. J., and Herrmann, J. (1966): A pilot study of clopenthixol in chronic schizophrenics. *Curr. Ther. Res.,* 8:220–224.

Sugerman, A. A., Stolberg, H., and Herrmann, J. (1965): A pilot study of thiothixene in childhood schizophrenia. *Curr. Ther. Res.,* 8:617.

Weissman, A. (1974): Chemical pharmacological, and metabolic considerations on thiothixene. In: *Thioxthixene and the Thioxanthenes,* edited by I. S. Forest, C. J. Carr, and E. Usdin, pp. 1–10. Raven Press, New York.

Wolpert, A., Sheppard, C., and Merlis, S. (1967): An early clinical evaluation of clopenthixol in treatment-resistant female schizophrenic patients. *Am. J. Psychiatry,* 124:156–159.

Chapter 4

Haloperidol and the Butyrophenones

Thomas A. Ban and John C. Pecknold

BUTYROPHENONES AND DIPHENYLBUTYLPIPERIDINES

In the course of systematic efforts to synthesize more potent narcotic analgesics than pethidine (meperidine), the Mannich reaction[1] with normeperidine and acetophenone yielded the propiophenone derivative R951 (Janssen, van de Westeringh, Jageneau, Demoen, Hermans, van Daela, Schellekens, van der Eycken, and Niemegeers, 1959). Lengthening the two-carbon ethylene chain of this propiophenone by one methyl group resulted in the butyrophenone R1187; and replacement of the ester moiety of R1187 by a tertiary alcohol produced the aminoalcohol R1472. Finally, by substituting the ketonic phenyl ring of R1472 with a fluorine atom, and the phenyl ring attached to the piperidine nucleus with a chlorine atom, haloperidol was obtained. Since haloperidol induced cataleptic immobility, inhibited "exploratory," "operant," and (intracranial) "self-stimulating" behavior, and interfered with apomorphine-induced vomiting, amphetamine-induced stereotyped chewing, and norepinephrine-induced mortality, Janssen (1970) suggested that the newly synthesized compound should have neuroleptic (antipsychotic) properties.

Seventeen years have passed since the discovery of the antipsychotic properties of haloperidol, the first neuroleptic butyrophenone preparation, during which time well over 5,000 organic bases related to haloperidol have been prepared by Janssen Pharmaceutica in Beerse (Belgium); more than 100 patents describing various butyrophenones have been obtained; and more than 25 of these compounds have been investigated by psychiatrists, neurologists, anesthesiologists, and clinical pharmacologists. In spite of the large number of psychoactive butyrophenone preparations, only two have been marketed in North America to date (Fig. 1): haloperidol (Haldol) and droperidol (Inapsine).

While haloperidol has been extensively employed with various therapeutic indications, droperidol, because of its rapid onset and relatively short duration of action, is used only as an adjunct to general anesthesia. More recently,

---

[1] Replacement of active hydrogen atoms in organic compounds by aminomethyl or substituted aminomethyl groups via a reaction with formaldehyde and ammonia or a primary or secondary amine.

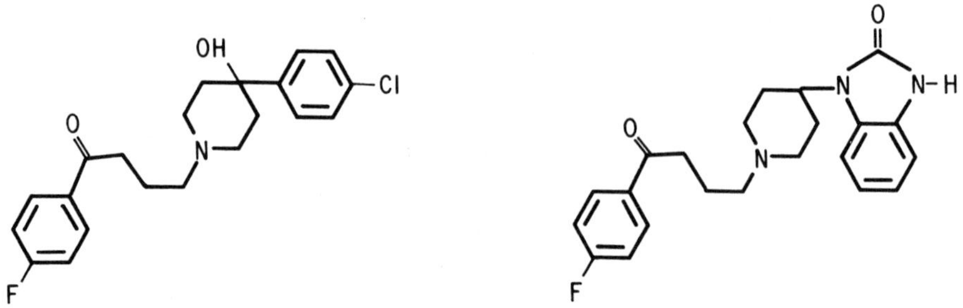

FIG. 1. Structure of the two major butyrophenones.

however, the possibility of employing it in psychiatric emergencies and in the treatment of amphetamine, alcohol, and/or heroin addiction has been raised (Janssen, 1972). Furthermore, in at least one well-designed study consisting of an uncontrolled clinical trial with 67 patients and a comparative study with 45 patients, the effectiveness of droperidol was found to be equal to that of haloperidol in the treatment of schizophrenia (Cocito, Ambrosini, Arate, Berilacqua, and Tortora, 1970).

Replacement of the carbonyl in the propylene chain of the butyrophenone structure by a fluorophenyl resulted in a chemically new group of drugs, usually referred to as diphenylbutylpiperidines. Common characteristics of this new class of neuroleptics are their long duration of action and great specificity for dopamine receptors. Accordingly, pimozide, the best known of the diphenylbutylpiperidine series (Fig. 2), is a long-acting oral neuroleptic

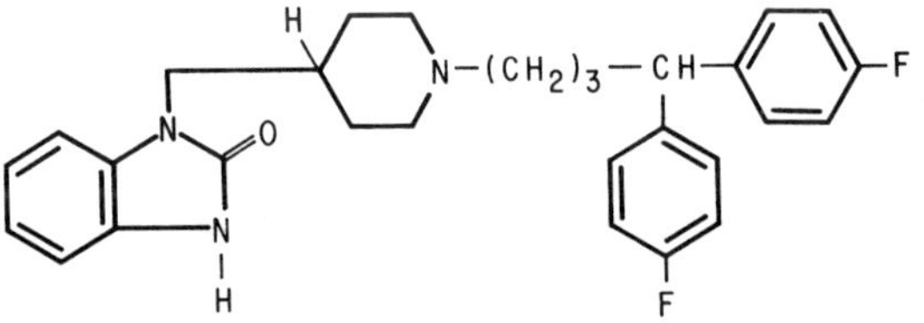

PIMOZIDE

FIG. 2. Structure of pimozide, a diphenylbutylpiperidine derivative.

with a duration of action of 1 day; other diphenylbutylpiperidines have even longer durations of action (Janssen, Niemegeers, and Schellekens, 1965; Villeneuve, Dogan, Lachance, and Proulx, 1970).

METABOLISM OF HALOPERIDOL

Radioisotope studies in rats have shown that haloperidol is rapidly and almost completely absorbed, to the extent that peak serum levels are reached within 2 hr after oral administration. Although relatively high plasma levels are maintained for only about 72 hr, significant concentrations of radio-activity remain in the circulation for 1 week, and traces for at least 1 month, even after the administration of a single dose (Johnson, Charalampous, and Braun, 1967). However, Zingales (1971) found the therapeutic response to haloperidol treatment unrelated to the plasma level of the free, unmetabolized drug.

In radioisotope studies, of all the organs the liver contains the greatest quantity of absorbed radioactivity, reaching a maximum of 15% 3 hr after drug administration; considerably less radioactivity is concentrated in the lungs, kidneys, brain, spleen, and heart (Braun, Kade, and Roscoe, 1967). Janssen and Allewijn (1968) found a linear relationship between dosage and the speed of distribution, metabolism, and excretion of haloperidol. This may explain the relatively low incidence of toxic effects caused by haloperidol in studies in which high initial and/or rapidly increasing dosage schedules are employed (DiMascio, 1972).

Excretion of haloperidol proceeds slowly; thus even when urinary and fecal excretions are combined, less than 50% of the ingested drug is recovered by the end of the first week, and small amounts of radioactivity are excreted for at least 28 days after a single oral dose. Garriotti and Stolman (1971) suggest that haloperidol is extensively metabolized, by various catabolic routes, and very little if any of the free drug is excreted into the urine when administered in the therapeutic dosage range.

PSYCHIATRIC INDICATIONS

Child Psychiatry

Among the various butyrophenone preparations, haloperidol has been extensively employed in child psychiatric practice. While there are indications that the therapeutic activity of haloperidol in overactive, aggressive, assaultive, impulsive, hostile, and/or destructive children of mixed psychiatric diagnosis is superior to chlorpromazine (LeVann, 1969, 1971), fluphenazine (Serrano and Forbis, 1973), thioridazine (Ucer and Kreger, 1969), and other commercially available phenothiazines (Grabowski, 1973), thioridazine was found to be equal to haloperidol in improving "home behavior" (Claghorn, 1972). Neither haloperidol nor chlorpromazine was more effective than an inactive placebo in groups of children and adolescents "usually treated with major tranquilizers" (Lewis and James, 1973). It should be noted, however, that almost half of the children in the latter study were diagnosed as having a neurosis or a reactive situational disorder.

Fluphenzine was compared with haloperidol in two studies concerning the therapy of schizophrenic children. Both drugs in both clinical trials were found to be highly efficacious; in one of the studies (Faretra, Droher, and

Dowling, 1970), however, haloperidol had a faster onset of action with a greater therapeutic effectiveness in "provocativeness" and "autism," and in the other study (Engelhardt, Polizoes, Waizer, and Hoffman, 1973) it produced less extrapyramidal side effects.

Adult Psychiatry

Behavioral Disorders

It has become increasingly evident in recent years that some of the butyrophenones (e.g., haloperidol and droperidol) can interfere with psychological dependence in patients addicted to amphetamine-like stimulants or morphine-like narcotics. On the basis of animal pharmacological findings that morphine withdrawal aggression (in rats) can be aggravated (Karkalas and Lal, 1971; Puri and Lal, 1974) and that self-administration of morphine can be interfered with by dopamine antagonists such as haloperidol and droperidol (Hanson and Cimini, 1973; Smith and Davis, 1973), the possibility of employing haloperidol in the prevention and/or treatment of heroin withdrawal symptoms was raised. In favor of this hypothesis are the findings that administration of haloperidol in the dosage of 1 to 2 mg t.i.d. alleviated the withdrawal symptoms of heroin addiction (Karkalas and Lal, 1971; Friedman and Le-Compt, 1972, 1973). Not only was haloperidol (1 to 2 mg t.i.d.) equal to methadone (10 mg q.i.d.) in alleviating withdrawal symptoms to heroin, but it was also effective in alleviating withdrawal symptoms to methadone (Landsberg, 1973; Patlak, 1973). As far as amphetamine-induced psychosis is concerned, Angrist, Lee, and Gershon (1974) showed that haloperidol produced improvement within an hour of its administration.

Neuroses

In spite of the common contention that the therapeutic indications of neuroleptics in psychiatry are exclusively in the functional psychoses, Gilbert (1969) in a placebo-controlled study revealed that the range of therapeutic activity of haloperidol includes anxiety-tension states. In a 4-week double-blind study with 113 anxious neurotic outpatients, haloperidol was found to be equal or superior to diazepam (Lord and Kidd, 1973) and chlordiazepoxide (Donald, 1967), i.e., standard antianxiety sedative drugs. Furthermore, in double-blind comparisons, haloperidol was found to be equally effective to trifluoperazine (Rossman, Moskowitz, Fleishman, Sheppard, and Merlis, 1970) and pimozide (Kenway, 1973) in the treatment of recurrent anxiety states, and equal or superior to fluphenazine (Ayd, 1972) and thioridazine (Lingi, 1973) in therapy-resistant neurotics. Finally, Rogerson and Butler (1971) found haloperidol better than an inactive placebo, and

Greenberg (1970) found it better than chlordiazepoxide in the treatment of depressive neurotics.

Functional Psychoses

Manic-depressive psychosis

Bobon, Pinchard, Collard, and Bobon (1972)—in their new classification of neuroleptics with special reference to the antimanic, antiautistic, and ataraxic properties of drugs—list droperidol and haloperidol as the compounds with the highest "antimanic potency." The same authors (Bobon and Collard, 1972; Bobon et al., 1972) suggested that droperidol is the model neuroleptic for chemical restraint and the most powerful initial treatment for manic states. They recommend parenteral use of droperidol initially, followed by oral treatment with haloperidol concomitantly with an ataraxic or sedative neuroleptic. On the other hand, Sangiovanni's group found that intramuscular haloperidol was the most rapid way to control aggressive, overactive assaultive manic patients (Sangiovanni, Taylor, Abrams, and Gaztanagna, 1973).

Whereas Angyal (1967) suggested that haloperidol is superior to any other pharmacological and/or physical treatments of mania, Schou (1968) and Prien, Caffey, and Klett (1971) maintain that protracted manic states respond better to lithium than to haloperidol. On the other hand, there is sufficient evidence to believe that acute manic attacks are controlled more rapidly with haloperidol than with lithium. When administered parenterally at 30-min intervals, both haloperidol (5 mg) and chlorpromazine (50 mg) brought about rapid amelioration of mania within an average time of less than 2.5 hr; but of the two, haloperidol appeared to be the safer drug (Man and Chen, 1973). In spite of the fact that both chlorpromazine and haloperidol are effective in controlling mania, Prien et al. (1971) suggest that better control is attained with a combination of lithium and chlorpromazine or haloperidol than any one of the three drugs alone. However, Cohen and Cohen (1974) report irreversible brain damage caused by the combined administration of haloperidol and lithium.

In spite of the favorable therapeutic findings by Inose, Hirata, Kajiwara, Iwata, Tano, Takahashi, Seo, and Sakai (1969), it is usually agreed that haloperidol has no place in the treatment of depressed psychiatric patients. Moreover, it may induce severe depression (Volmat and Allers, 1970; Morgan, 1972; Abuzzahab, 1973).

Schizophrenia

Divry, Bobon, and Collard (1960) found haloperidol therapeutically effective in the schizophrenias in general, and Delay, Pichot, Lemperiere, and Elissalde (1960) found that the therapeutic efficacy of haloperidol is considerably greater in acute and paranoid schizophrenia than in hebephrenic schizophrenia. These findings were further substantiated by the results of

Crane (1967) and Goldstein, Clyde, and Caldwell (1968), which showed
higher mean improvement rates (70% to 75%, respectively) in studies reporting on treatment of acute schizophrenic patients than in those reporting
on treatment of chronic schizophrenic patients (40% to 57%, respectively).
Overactivity, agitation, and paranoid ideation have improved in all clinical
trials in which it has been studied (Crane, 1967).

Parenteral and/or oral haloperidol treatment has been successful in the
rapid control of excitement and severe, disruptive symptoms of schizophrenia
(Oldham and Bott, 1971; Man and Chen, 1973). In a double-blind, placebo-
controlled study, Reschke (1974) found that haloperidol in dosages of 2 or
5 mg is significantly more effective than 1 mg haloperidol, 25 mg chlorpromazine, and placebo. He noted that adequate control was achieved with an
average of 2.5 injections in patients receiving the 5-mg dose, and with an
average of 3.7 injections in patients receiving the 2-mg dose. More recently
a so-called "digitalization method" was described that employed orally administered haloperidol for achieving rapid control (Donlon and Tupin, 1974).

During the 1960s, one of us (T.A.B.), in collaboration with H. E. Lehmann, was engaged in systematic clinical studies with haloperidol. Several
clinical trials were conducted in acute and chronic schizophrenic patients, in
the course of which haloperidol was administered alone or in combination
with other drugs (Ban, 1969). In one of these studies it was found that
therapeutic changes occurred significantly faster with haloperidol than with
chlorpromazine or chlorprothixene in a group of newly admitted schizophrenic
patients (Lehmann, Ban, Matthews, and Garcia-Rill, 1964). This corre-
sponds with Rubin's finding (1971) that the onset of activity of haloperidol
is somewhat faster than that of trifluoperazine. In another study O'Brien,
DiGiacomo, and Webb (1974) found that in a population of hostile, suspicious, acute schizophrenic patients, haloperidol produced significantly more
improvement than trifluoperazine.

In the same series of studies but with chronic schizophrenic patients, the
onset of action of haloperidol was significantly shorter than that of butaperazine (Warnes, Lehmann, Ban, and Lee, 1966); and haloperidol produced
overall improvement in a slightly higher percentage of patients than tri-
fluperazine (Ban and Lehmann, 1967). Similarly, Hollister's group (Hollister, Overall, Caffey, Bennett, Meyer, Kimball, and Honingfeld, 1962)
found haloperidol significantly superior to thiopropazate, and Weston's group
(Weston, Bentley, Unwin, Morris, and Harper, 1973) found it superior to
thioridazine in chronic schizophrenics. On the other hand, in a similar population there was no significant difference between the therapeutic effects of
haloperidol and fluphenazine (Ban and Stonehill, 1964; Hall, Vestre, Schiele,
and Zimmerman, 1968).

There is little evidence that any combination of antipsychotic drugs is
superior to appropriate use of single drugs (Hollister, 1972). On the other

hand there are indications that the addition of α-methyl-*p*-tyrosine (a specific tyrosine hydroxylase inhibitor) and α-methyldopa (a DOPA decarboxylase inhibitor)—substances which interfere with dopamine synthesis—produce marked potentiation of the therapeutic effects of haloperidol and pimozide (Ahlenius and Engel, 1971, 1973; Chouinard, Pinard, Prenoveau, and Tetreault, 1973*a,b*). These findings indicate that interference with dopamine synthesis enhances the therapeutic activity of haloperidol.

Although haloperidol and the other butyrophenone neuroleptics may correct some of the biochemical changes associated with schizophrenia, there is sufficient evidence to believe that discontinuation of haloperidol administration leads to relapse in 73% to 96% of schizophrenic patients. In view of this, it is rather important to know that haloperidol can be administered once a day instead of in divided doses (Ayd, 1973).

Gilles de la Tourette's Disease

A particular indication for haloperidol is Gilles de la Tourette's disease, a relatively rare condition characterized by multiple motor tics and an irresistible compulsion to swear. This uncommon affliction, which usually begins with facial tics (progressing to involve the arms and legs), barking sounds, and coprolalia, has not only attracted much attention but has produced divided opinions as to whether it has a psychodynamic or an organic etiology (Friel, 1973).

Successful treatment with haloperidol was first reported by Seignot (1961), confirmed by Challas and Brauer (1963), and further substantiated by the end of 1972 in at least 18 other reports (Ban, 1973). Since then, six other papers with favorable therapeutic findings have been published (Friel, 1973; Shapiro, Shapiro, and Wayne, 1973; Still and Han, 1973; Ford and Beyer, 1974; Goforth, 1974; Leiman and Nussbaum, 1974). In view of the fact that haloperidol is a potent dopamine receptor blocker, and considering the finding that it is therapeutically effective in the treatment of Gilles de la Tourette's disease, Snyder, Taylor, Coyle, and Meyerhoff (1970) suggest that hyperactivity of the dopaminergic system in the corpus striatum (as predicted by Mahler and Rangell in 1943) has a role in the pathology of this condition. Whether this hyperactivity of the dopaminergic system is produced by enhanced release of dopamine, impaired inactivation of dopamine, or hypersensitivity of the dopamine receptors, however, remains to be determined. In favor of Snyder's hypothesis are the findings that the only neuropathological change described in Gilles de la Tourette's disease is in the corpus striatum (i.e., an increased ratio of small to large neurocytes) and that prolonged haloperiodol treatment results in a decrease in dopamine excretion, corresponding to the decrease in tics per minute (Messiha, Knoop, Vanecko, O'Brien, and Corson, 1971).

Organic Brain Syndromes

Beneficial therapeutic effects with butyrophenones have been reported in both acute and chronic organic brain syndrome patients. Accordingly, the usefulness of haloperidol in the treatment of alcohol withdrawal and delirium tremens was first suggested by Oles (1960), confirmed by Giacobini and Lassenius (1961), and further substantiated in several other reports (Ban, 1973). More recently in a double-blind, comparative study, Ritter and Davidson (1971) found haloperidol and perphenazine equally effective in the treatment of acute alcoholic psychosis, while Palestine (1973) found haloperidol significantly superior to mesoridazine and hydroxyzine in delirium tremens and in treating the alcohol withdrawal syndrome.

Finally, it should be noted that the usefulness of haloperidol in the treatment of Huntington's chorea was first suggested by Olsson (1961), later confirmed by Lecoeur (1965) and Escalar and Majeron (1969), and further substantiated in several other reports (Klawans and Ringel, 1972; Candelise, 1973; Faglioni, Spinnler, and Vignolo, 1973).

Geriatric Psychiatry

In 1961 Gerle, Petersson, and Widmark reported on the use of haloperidol in geriatric patients. In an open study with 10 therapy-refractory geropsychiatric patients, they found that haloperidol (in doses from 0.2 to 0.3 mg b.i.d.) produced marked or moderate improvement in all subjects. These findings were further substantiated by Sugerman, Williams, and Adlerstein (1964) in a two-phase (i.e., open and placebo-controlled, double-blind) study in which haloperidol was successfully administered to 24 elderly patients with chronic brain syndrome in the dosage range of 1 to 4.5 mg/day over a 6-week period. Similar favorable results were obtained by Tobin, Brousseau, and Lorenz (1970) in an open study with 18 hospitalized geriatric patients. Nevertheless, while Tsuang, Lu, Stotsky, and Cole (1971) and Stotsky (1972) found haloperidol equal to thioridazine, and Whanger (1973) found it equal to trifluoperazine, Tewfik's group reported negative therapeutic findings with haloperidol in senile psychosis (Tewfik, Jain, Harcup, and Magowan, 1970).

NONPSYCHIATRIC INDICATIONS

Besides their psychiatric indications, butyrophenones are frequently employed as antiemetic drugs and in the treatment of various neurological disorders. Similarly to chlorpromazine, haloperidol pretreatment protects dogs from apomorphine-induced vomiting (Janssen et al., 1965). Comparing the efficacy of the two drugs, Janssen et al. found that haloperidol was approximately 40 times as potent as chlorpromazine and its duration of action about four times longer. The antiemetic effects of haloperidol have been substantiated in human volunteers "challenged with apomorphine" (Shields, Ballinger, and Hathaway, 1971) and in a double-blind study (Tornetta, 1972) in which haloperidol (0.5, 1, 2, or 4 mg i.m.) prevented postoperative nausea and vomiting. Haloperidol was also effective in cancer patients with nausea and vomiting due to the administration of cytotoxic drugs (Plotkin, Plotkin, and Okun, 1973). Within 2 hr of oral administration of 1.0 or 2.0 mg haloperidol, both the severity of nausea and the frequency of vomiting had been reduced by about 60%, an effect that lasted approximately 6 hr. Finally, Korczyn (1971) reported prompt and sustained abolition of persistent hiccups after administering haloperidol (5 mg t.i.d. orally or parenterally) to patients with lower brainstem disorders, uremia, or extensive burns.

Haloperidol has been successfully employed in a variety of neurological conditions, including hemiballism (Suarez, 1969), spasmodic torticollis (Kivalo and Weckman, 1970; Gilbert, 1971, 1972), and torsion dystonia (Fedi, 1967). Most important, however, are the findings that haloperidol alleviates L-DOPA-induced dyskinesias (Mones, 1972) and choreiform activity (Siegel and Mones, 1971), regardless of whether it is due to Huntington's or Sydenham's chorea (Axley, 1972; Shenker, Grossman, and Klawans, 1973), and regardless of whether it is due to juvenile familial (Lanski, 1972), chronic liver disease (O'Neil, Klawans, and Holmes, 1971), or systemic lupus erythematosus-induced chorea (Heilman, Kohler, and LeMaster, 1971).

An entirely different area in which haloperidol is therapeutically indicated is in the treatment of stutterers and ticquers. Tapia's (1969) favorable therapeutic findings with haloperidol in the treatment of stuttering were further substantiated by Quinn and Peachey (1973) and Wells and Malcolm (1971) in a placebo-controlled 8-week clinical study. Furthermore, in a 3-yr follow-up of this last report, Cookson and Wells (1973) noted that fluency remained improved while on haloperidol. Early clinical findings of Connell, Corbett, Horne, and Matthews (1967) that haloperidol reduces the frequency of tics has also been confirmed (Tapia, 1969).

ADVERSE EFFECTS

Man's (1973) 2-yr study with 64 patients indicated a positive relationship between the occurrence of extrapyramidal signs (76.5%) and improvement rate (78%), but there was no clear-cut relationship between improvement and adverse reactions—including extrapyramidal signs—in Crane's (1967) comprehensive review on haloperidol. In fact, the lowest number of side effects (median 0.4 per patient) occurred in studies with the highest improvement rate (74%); and patients exhibiting an average of more than two side effects were from studies in which less than 53% of the sample was rated as improved. On the other hand, there was a relationship between dosage range and side effects. For doses up to 4 mg/day the median number of side effects was 0.30 per patient; for doses between 4 and 32 mg/day it was 0.60; and there was a sharp increase to 1.41 per patient for doses exceeding 32 mg/day. Increasing the dose of haloperidol to over 16 mg/day did not enhance therapeutic efficacy, but exceeding a dose of 32 mg/day produced a sharp increase in toxicity.

On the basis of a careful analysis of 55 studies, Crane (1967) suggested that the most frequent side effects of haloperidol are parkinsonism (reported in 1,282 patients) and dystonia (225 patients), closely followed by restlessness, including akathisia (221 patients). Similarly the most common side effects were extrapyramidal reactions (40%) in the comprehensive review of Goldstein et al. (1968). Since only two of seven studies reported parkinsonism when haloperidol was administered at a dosage below 4 mg/day, and since 15 of the 25 studies which reported dystonia used doses higher than 15 mg/day, Crane (1967) considered both parkinsonism and dystonia as dose-related manifestations. In variance with this are the observations that the incidence (as well as the severity) of extrapyramidal side effects are less frequent with a high than with a low dosage (Shader, 1970). Although haloperidol-induced extrapyramidal side effects can be controlled with anticholinergic drugs (e.g., diphenhydramine or amantidine) there are indications that some of the therapeutic effects of haloperidol are reversed by administration of the anticholinergic drug benztropine (Singh and Smith, 1973).

Oversedation, marked orthostatic hypotension, blood dyscrasias, and liver dysfunctions are less frequent with the butyrophenones than with the phenothiazines; and in view of the virtual absence of electrocardiographic changes, Pratt (1971) believes that the haloperidol-induced "tranquil state of twilight sleep" may be beneficial to patients during the immediate postinfarct period. While photosensitivity reactions may not have been associated with haloperidol administration, there is some evidence of elevated prolactin concentrations (Frantz, Kleinberg, and Noel, 1972) and suppressed gonadotropin secretion (Boris, Milmore, and Trmal, 1970) in patients receiving high doses of haloperidol over an extended period of time. Most important, however, are the findings that haloperidol, like reserpine, may induce severe depression. Because of this, a previous history of depression might be considered a contraindication for treatment with haloperidol.

Although eye and skin deposits have not been detected in the course of long-term maintenance therapy with haloperidol, there are indications that tardive (and withdrawal) dyskinesia may occur, in spite of the early negative reports (Jacobsen, Baldessarini, and Manschreck, 1974). Furthermore, although haloperidol has not been implicated in drug interactions with digitalis, diuretics, and antidiabetics, there are indications that it potentiates the activity of oral anticoagulants (Sigell and Flessa, 1970). There is sufficient evidence to indicate that haloperidol inhibits the metabolism of tricyclic antidepressants in man (Gram and Overø, 1972). Finally, Casier, DeSchaepdryner, Piette, Danechmand, and Hermans (1966) showed that blood alcohol levels are significantly lower with alcohol and haloperidol than when alcohol is taken alone.

CONCLUSIONS

Seventeen years have passed since the discovery of the first psychoactive butyrophenone preparation. During this interval the various actions of these drugs have been increasingly clarified, greatly contributing to the treatment as well as to the understanding of the pathological mechanisms involved in a number of psychiatric disorders. Although in his initial reports Janssen (1966) suggested that butyrophenones exert their therapeutic effect by occupying γ-aminobutyric acid receptors, or by their cell membrane permeability-decreasing effect, during the 1960s a positive relationship had been revealed between the postsynaptic dopamine receptor blockade and therapeutic effects in schizophrenia.

In view of the fact, however, that schizophrenia is not cured by the administration of haloperidol, probably more important than the therapeutic impact of the butyrophenones is the fact that studies with them have contributed to the changes in our thinking and understanding of psychopathological manifestations in psychiatric patients.

TREATMENT SUMMARY

Generic name	Trade name	Daily dosage range (mg)[a]
Haloperidol	Haldol	2–15

[a] Dosage range for the treatment of psychosis.

REFERENCES

Abuzzahab, F. S. (1973): Prescribing for patients with depression, anxiety and insomnia. *Am. Fam. Physician,* 8:116–121.

Ahlenius, S., and Engel, J. (1971): Behavioral effects of haloperidol after tyrosine hydroxylase inhibition. *Eur. J. Pharmacol.,* 15:187–192.

Ahlenius, S., and Engel, J. (1973): On the interaction between pimozide and α-methyltyrosine. *J. Pharm. Pharmacol.,* 25:172–174.

Angrist, B., Lee, H. K., and Gershon, S. (1974): The antagonism of amphetamine-induced symptomatology by a neuroleptic. *Am. J. Psychiatry,* 131:817–819.

Angyal, L. (1967): Clinical experiences with the application of haloperidol to mental patients. *Ther. Hung.,* 15:155–162.

Axley, J. (1972): Rheumatic chorea controlled with haloperidol. *J. Pediatr.,* 81:1216–1217.

Ayd, F. J. (1972): Comparative trial of low dose haloperidol and fluphenazine in office patients. *Dis. Nerv. Syst.,* 33:192–195.

Ayd, F. J. (1973): Rational pharmacotherapy once-a-day drug dosage. *Dis. Nerv. Syst.,* 34:371–373.

Ban, T. A. (1969): Treatment of acute and chronic psychoses with haloperidol: Review of clinical results. *Curr. Ther. Res.,* 11:284–288.

Ban T. A. (1973): Haloperidol and the butyrophenones. *Psychosomatics,* 14:286–297.

Ban, T. A., and Lehmann, H. E. (1967): Efficacy of haloperidol in drug refractory patients. *Int. J. Neuropsychiatry,* 3:78–86.

Ban, T. A., and Stonehill, E. (1964): Clinical observations on the differential effects of a butyrophenone (haloperidol) and a phenothiazine (fluphenazine). In: *The Butyrophenones in Psychiatry,* edited by H. E. Lehmann and T. A. Ban. Quebec Psychopharmacological Research Association, Montreal.

Bobon, J., and Collard, J. (1972): Present treatment of manic states. *Acta Psychiatr. Belg.,* 72:617–632.

Bobon, J., Pinchard, A., Collard, J., and Bobon, D. P. (1972): Clinical classification of neuroleptics, with special reference to their antimanic, antiautistic, and ataraxic properties. *Compr. Psychiatry,* 13:123–131.

Boris, A., Milmore, J., and Trmal, T. (1970): Some effects of haloperidol on reproductive organs in the female rat. Endocrinology, 86:429–431.

Braun, G. A., Kade, C. F., and Roscoe, E. L. (1967): Metabolism of haloperidol in the rat. *Int. J. Neuropsychiatry,* 3:(S)22–(S)25.

Candelise, L., and Faglioni, P., Spinnler, H., and Vignolo, L. A. (1973): Treatment of Huntington's chorea. *N. Engl. J. Med.,* 289:1201–1210.

Casier, H., DeSchaepdryner, A., Piette, Y., Danechmand, L., and Hermans, W. (1966): Blood alcohol levels and psychotropic drugs. Arzneim. Forsch., 16:1505–1507.

Challas, G., and Brauer, W. (1963): Tourette's disease: Relief of symptoms with R1625. *Am. J. Psychiatry,* 120:283–284.

Chouinard, G., Pinard, G., Prenoveau, Y., and Tetreault, L. (1973a): Alpha-methyldopa-chlorpromazine interactions in schizophrenic patients. *Curr. Ther. Res.,* 15:60–72.

Chouinard, G., Pinard, G., Prenoveau, Y., and Tetreault, L. (1973b): Potentiation of haloperidol by α-methyl-tyrosine in the treatment of schizophrenic patients. *Curr. Ther. Res.,* 15:473–483.

Claghorn, J. L. (1972): A double-blind comparison of haloperidol (Haldol) and thioridazine (Mellaril) in out-patient children. *Curr. Ther. Res.,* 14:785–789.

Cocito, E., Ambrosini, G., Arate, A., Berilacqua, P., and Tortora, E. (1970): Clinical evaluation in 112 psychiatric patients of a butyrophenone neuroleptic, dehydrobenzperidol (R4749): A controlled study in 45 patients of dehydrobenzperidol versus haloperidol. *Arzneim. Forsch.,* 20:1119–1125.

Cohen, W. J. and Cohen, N. H. (1974): Lithium carbonate, haloperidol, and irreversible brain damage. *J.A.M.A.,* 230:1283–1287.

Connell, P. H., Corbett, J. A., Horne, D. J., and Matthews, A. M. (1967): Drug treatment of adolescent tiqueurs. *Br. J. Psychiatry,* 113:375–381.

Cookson, I. B., and Wells, P. G. (1973): Haloperidol in the treatment of stutterers. *Br. J. Psychiatry,* 123:491.

Crane, G. E. (1967): A review of clinical literature on haloperidol. *Int. J. Neuropsychiatry,* 3:(S)110–(S)123.

Delay, J., Pichot, P., Lemperiere, T., and Elissalde, B. (1960): L'action du haloperidol dans les psychoses. *Acta Neurol. Psychiatr. Belg.,* 60:121–138.

DiMascio, A. (1972): The butyrophenones: an overview of their pharmacologic and metabolic properties. In: *Butyrophenones in Psychiatry,* edited by A. DiMascio and R. I. Shader. Raven Press, New York.

Divry, P., Bobon, J., and Collard, J. (1960): Rapport sur l'activité neuropsychopharmacologique de haloperidol (R1625). In: *Symposium International sur le Haloperidol (Beerse 1959).* Acta Medica Belgica, Bruxelles.

Donald, J. F. (1967): A study of a recognized antipsychotic agent as a tranquillizer in general practice. *Practitioner,* 203:684–687.

Donlon, P. T., and Tupin, J. P. (1974): Rapid "digitalization" of decompensated schizophrenic patients with antipsychotic agents. *Am. J. Psychiatry,* 131:310–312.

Engelhardt, D. M., Polizoes, P., Waizer, J., and Hoffman, S. P. (1973): A double-blind comparison of fluphenazine and haloperidol in out-patient schizophrenic children. *J. Autism Child. Schizo.,* 3:128–137.

Escalar, G., and Majeron, M. A. (1969): The use of butyrophenone preparations in Huntington's chorea. *Minerva Med.*, 60:2494–2496.

Faretra, G., Droher, L., and Dowling, J. (1970): Comparison of haloperidol and fluphenazine in disturbed children. *Am. J. Psychiatry*, 126:146–149.

Fedi, A. (1967): Clinical experience with the new antidystonic HP32 (haloperidol) and isopropamide iodide. *Gazz. Med. Ital.*, 126:42–45.

Ford, R. B., and Beyer, E. C. (1974): Tic de Gilles de la Tourette: Case report and brief discussion. *J. S. C. Med. Assoc.*, 70:1–3.

Frantz, A. G., Kleinberg, D. L., and Noel, G. L. (1972): Studies on prolactin in man. *Recent Prog. Horm. Res.*, 28:527–573.

Friedman, J. J., and Lecompt, G. (1972): No addictive drug (haloperidol) antagonism program community setting. Presented at the American Public Health Association, Atlantic City, N.J.

Friedman, J. J., and Lecompt, G. (1973): Haloperidol as a methadone substitute. Presented at the 2nd International Symposium on Drug Addiction, New Orleans, La.

Friel, P. B. (1973): Familial incidence of Gilles de la Tourette's disease, with observations on aetiology and treatment. *Br. J. Psychiatry*, 122:655–658.

Garriotti, J. C., and Stolman, A. (1971): Detection of some psychotherapeutic drugs and their metabolites in urine. *Clin. Toxicol.*, 4:225–243.

Gerle, B., Petersson, B., and Widmark, M. (1961): Clinical experience of Haldol (haloperidol "Janssen"). *Sven. Lakartidn.*, 58:415–422.

Giacobini, E., and Lassenius, B. (1961): Haloperidol vid behanding av delirium tremens. *Sven. Lakartidn.*, 58:1429–1433.

Gilbert, G. J. (1971): Spasmodic torticollis treated effectively by medical means. *N. Engl. J. Med.*, 284:896–898.

Gilbert, G. J. (1972): The medical treatment of spasmodic torticollis. *Arch. Neurol.*, 27:503–506.

Gilbert, M. M. (1969): Haloperidol in the treatment of anxiety-tension states. *Curr. Ther. Res.* 11:520–523.

Goforth, E. G. (1974): A single case study: Gilles de la Tourette's Syndrome, a 25-year follow-up study. *J. Nerv. Ment. Dis.*, 159:306–310.

Goldstein, B. J., Clyde, D. J., and Caldwell, J. M. (1968): Clinical efficacy of the butyrophenones as antipsychotic drugs. In: *Psychopharmacology*, edited by D. H. Efron. Public Health Service Publication No. 1836, Washington, D.C.

Grabowski, S. W. (1973): Safety and effectiveness of haloperidol for mentally retarded, behaviorally disordered and hyperneurotic patients. *Curr. Ther. Res.*, 15: 856–861.

Gram, L. F., and Overø, K. F. (1972): Drug interaction: Inhibitory effect of neuroleptics on metabolism of tricyclic antidepressants in man. *Br. Med. J.*, 1:463–465.

Greenberg, A. (1970): A double-blind comparison of low-dose haloperidol with chlordiazepoxide in anxiety-tension states. Presented at the Annual Meeting of the American Medical Association, Chicago, Ill.

Hall, W. B., Vestre, N. D., Schiele, B. C., and Zimmerman, R. A. (1968): A controlled comparison of haloperidol and fluphenazine in chronic treatment—resistant schizophrenic. *Dis. Nerv. Syst.*, 29:405–408.

Hanson, H., and Cimini, C. (1973): Effects of administration of haloperidol on morphine self administration in the rat. Presented at the 2nd International Symposium on Drug Addiction, New Orleans, La.

Heilman, K. M., Kohler, W. C., and LeMaster, P. C. (1971): Haloperidol treatment of chorea associated with systemic lupus erythematosus. *Neurology (Minneap.)*, 21:963–965.

Hollister, L. E. (1972): Treatment of chronic schizophrenia with butyrophenones. In: *Butyrophenones in Psychiatry*, edited by A. DiMascio and R. I. Shader. Raven Press, New York.

Hollister, L. E., Overall, J. E., Caffey, E., Bennett, J. L., Meyer, R., Kimbell, I., and Honingfeld, G. (1962): Controlled comparison of haloperidol with thiopropazate in newly admitted schizophrenics. *J. Nerv. Ment. Dis.*, 135:544–549.

Inose, T., Hirata, I., Kajiwara, A., Iwata, A., Tano, T., Takahashi, K., Seo, I., and Sakai, H. (1969): Depressive condition with electroencephalographic abnormalities:

Contribution to differential diagnosis of endogenous depression—with special references to haloperidol. *Psychiatr. Neurol. Jap.,* 71:764–775.

Jacobsen, G., Baldessarini, R. J., and Manschreck, T. (1974): Tardive and withdrawal dyskinesia associated with haloperidol. *Am. J. Psychiatry,* 131:910–913.

Janssen, P. A. J. (1966): The pharmacological and clinical mode of action of neuroleptic drugs. *Clin. Trials J.,* 2:370–379.

Janssen, P. A. J. (1970): The butyrophenone story. In: *Discoveries in Biological Psychiatry,* edited by F. J. Ayde and B. Blackwell. Lippincott, Philadelphia.

Janssen, P. A. J. (1972): Long-acting neuroleptics and other psychoactive drugs of the future. *Clin. Med.,* 79:12–14.

Janssen, P. A. J., and Allewijn, F. N. (1968): Distribution of butyrophenones; haloperidol, trifluperidol, neoperone and clofluperidol in rats and its relationship with their neuroleptic activity. *Arzneim. Forsch.,* 19:199–208.

Janssen, P. A. J., Niemegeers, C. J. E., and Schellekens, K. H. L. (1965): Is it possible to predict the clinical effects of neuroleptic drugs (major tranquilizers) for annual data? II. Neuroleptic activity spectra for drugs. *Arzeim. Forsch.,* 15:1196–1206.

Janssen, P. A. J., van de Westeringh, C., Jageneau, A. H. M., Demoen, P. J. A., Hermans, B. K. F., van Daele, G. H. P., Schellekens, K. H. L., van der Eycken, C. A. M., and Niemegeers, C. J. E. (1959): Chemistry and pharmacology of CNS depressants related to 4-(4-hydroxy-4-phenylpiperidino) butyrophenone. I. Synthesis and screening data in mice. *J. Med. Pharm. Chem.,* 1:281–297.

Johnson, P. C., Charalampous, K. D., and Braun, G. A. (1967): Absorption and excretion of tritiated haloperidol in man. *Int. J. Neuropsychiatry,* 3:(S)24–(S)25.

Karkalas, J., and Lal, H. (1971): A comparison of haloperidol with methadone in blocking heroin-withdrawal symptoms. *Int. Pharmacopsychiatry,* 8:248–251.

Kenway, A. K. (1973): A double-blind comparison of pimozide and haloperidol in the treatment of recurrent anxiety states. *Br. J. Clin. Pract.,* 27:67–68.

Kivalo, E., and Weckman, N. (1970): The effect of haloperidol on hyperkinetic syndromes. *Duodecim,* 86:129–132.

Klawans, H. L., and Ringel, S. P. (1972): Huntington's chorea: Survey of treatment. *Physician Drug Man.,* 4:60–62.

Korczyn, A. D. (1971): "Hiccup." *Br. Med. J.,* 2:590–591.

Landsberg, R. (1973): Use of haloperidol for heroin-withdrawal in a prison environment. Presented at the 2nd International Symposium on Drug Addiction, New Orleans, La.

Lanski, L. (1972): Treatment of Sydenham's chorea with haloperidol. *Neurology (Minneap.),* 22:418–419.

Lecoeur, J. L. J. (1965): Contribution to the study of haloperidol in the treatment of chorea. Thesis, Faculty of Medicine, University of Paris, France.

Lehmann, H. E., Ban, T. A., Matthews, V., and Garcia-Rill, T. (1964): The effects of haloperidol on acute schizophrenic patients: a comparative study of haloperidol, chlorpromazine and chlorprothixine. In: *The Butyrophenones in Psychiatry,* edited by H. E. Lehmann and T. A. Ban. Quebec Psychopharmacological Research Association, Montreal.

Leiman, P., and Nussbaum, E. (1974): Treatment with haloperidol in "maladie des tics" in children. *J. Isr. Med. Assoc.,* 86:10–11.

LeVann, L. J. (1969): Haloperidol in the treatment of behavioral disorders in children and adolescents. *Can. Psychiatr. Assoc. J.,* 14:217.

LeVann, L. J. (1971): Clinical comparison of haloperidol with chlorpromazine in mentally retarded children. *Am. J. Ment. Defic.,* 75:719–723.

Lewis, P. J. E., and James, N. (1973): Haloperidol and chlorpromazine: A double-blind cross-over trial and clinical study in children and adolescents. *Aust. N.Z. J. Psychiatry,* 7:59–65.

Lingi, F. A. (1973): Double-blind comparison of haloperidol and thioridazine in treatment resistant psychiatric out-patients. *Psychosomatics,* 14:235–240.

Lord, D. J., and Kidd, C. B. (1973): Haloperidol versus diazepam: A double-blind cross-over clinical trial. *Med. J. Aust.,* 1:586–588.

Mahler, M., and Rangell, L. (1943): A psychosomatic study of "maladie des tics." *Psychiatr. Q.,* 17:655–658.

Man, P. L. (1973): Long-term effects of haloperidol. *Dis. Nerv. Syst.,* 34:113–118.

Man, P. L., and Chen, C. H. (1973): Rapid tranquilization of acutely psychotic patients with intramuscular haloperidol and chlorpromazine. *Psychosomatics,* 14:59–63.
Messiha, F. S., Knoop, W., Vanecko, S., O'Brien, V., and Corson, S. A. (1971): Haloperidol therapy in Tourette's syndrome: Neurophysiological, biochemical and behavioral correlates. *Life Sci.,* 10:449–457.
Mones, R. J. (1972): The use of haloperidol in neurologic patients. In: *Butyrophenones in Psychiatry,* edited by A. DiMascio and R. I. Shader. Raven Press, New York.
Morgan, H. G. (1972): The incidence of depressive symptoms during recovery from hypomania. *Br. J. Psychiatry,* 120:537–539.
O'Brien, C. P., DiGiacomo, J. N., and Webb, W. (1974): Management of hostile, suspicious patients. *Dis. Nerv. Syst.,* 35:75–78.
Oldham, A. J., and Bott, M. (1971): The management of excitement in a general hospital psychiatric ward by high dosage haloperidol. *Acta Psychiatr. Scand.,* 47:369–376.
Oles, M. (1960): Behandlung von psychoser mit haloperidol. *Med. Monatsschr.,* 7:452–455.
Olsson, M. (1961): Klinisk provning av haldol. *Sven. Lakartidn,* 58:1433–1438.
O'Neil, D. P., Klawans, H. L., Jr., and Holmes, A. W. (1971): Treatment of choreo-athetotic movements in chronic liver disease with a dopamine-blocking agent. *Confin. Neurol.,* 33:258–270.
Palestine, M. L. (1973): Drug treatment of the alcohol withdrawal syndrome and delirium tremens: A comparison of haloperidol with mesoridazine and hydroxyzine. *Q. J. Stud. Alcohol,* 34:185–193.
Patlak, E. M. (1973): Use of haloperidol in methadone detoxification. Presented at the 2nd International Symposium on Drug Addiction, New Orleans, La.
Plotkin, D. A., Plotkin, D., and Okun, R. (1973): Haloperidol in the treatment of nausea and vomiting due to cytotoxic, drug administration. *Curr. Ther. Res.,* 15:599–602.
Pratt, I. T. (1971): Twilight sleep after infraction. *Br. Med. J.,* 3:475–476.
Prien, R. F., Caffey, E. M., and Klett, C. J. (1972): A comparison of lithium carbonate and chlorpromazine in the treatment of mania. *Arch. Gen. Psychiatry,* 26:146–153.
Puri, S. K., and Lal, H. (1974): Tolerance to the behavioral and neurochemical effects of haloperidol and morphine in rats chronically treated with morphine or haloperidol. *Naunyn Schmiedebergs Arch. Pharmacol.,* 282:155–170.
Quinn, P. T., and Peachey, C. (1973): Haloperidol in the treatment of stutterers. *Br. J. Psychiatry,* 123:247–248.
Reschke, R. W. (1974): Parenteral haloperidol for rapid control of severe, disruptive symptoms of acute schizophrenia. *Dis. Nerv. Syst.,* 35:112–115.
Ritter, R. M., and Davidson, D. E. (1971): Haloperidol for acute psychiatric emergencies: A double-blind comparison with perphenazine in acute alcoholic psychosis. *South. Med. J.,* 64:249–250.
Rogerson, R., and Butler, J. K. (1971): Assessment of low dosage haloperidol in anxiety states. *Br. J. Psychiatry,* 119:169–170.
Rossman, R., Moskowitz, M., Fleishman, P., Sheppard, C., and Merlis, S. (1970): The anti-anxiety effects of haloperidol and trifluoperazine in an out-patient neurotic population. *Clin. Basic Res.,* 31:130–133.
Rubin, R. (1971): A double-blind comparison of the onset of activity of haloperidol and trifluoperazine. *Ala. J. Med. Sci.,* 8:414–418.
Sangiovanni, F., Taylor, M. A., Abrams, R., and Gaztanagna, P. (1973): Rapid control of psychotic excitement states with intramuscular haloperidol. *Am. J. Psychiatry,* 130:1155–1156.
Schou, M. (1968): Lithium in psychiatry—a review. In: *Psychopharmacology,* edited by D. H. Efron. Public Health Service Publication No. 1836, Washington, D.C.
Seignot, J. N. (1961): Un cas de maladie des tics de Gilles de la Tourette gueri par le R1625. *Ann. Medicopsychol.,* 119:578–579.
Serrano, A. C., and Forbis, O. L. (1973): Haloperidol for psychiatric disorders in children. *Dis. Nerv. Syst.,* 34:226–231.
Shader, R. I. (1970): Antianxiety agents: A clinical perspective. In: *Clinical Handbook of Psychopharmacology,* edited by A. DiMascio and R. Shader. Science Press, New York.

Shapiro, A. K., Shapiro, E., and Wayne, H. (1973): Treatment of Tourette's syndrome with haloperidol: A review of 34 cases. *Arch. Gen. Psychiatry,* 28:92–97.

Shenker, D. M., Grossman, H. J., and Klawans, H. L. (1973): Treatment of Sydenham's chorea with haloperidol. *Dev. Med. Child Neurol.,* 15:19–24.

Shields, K. G., Ballinger, C. M., and Hathaway, B. N. (1971): Antiemetic effectiveness of haloperidol in human volunteers challenged with apomorphine. *Anesth. Analg. (Cleve.),* 50:1017–1027.

Siegel, G. J., and Mones, R. J. (1971): Modification of corresponding activity by haloperidol. *J.A.M.A.,* 216:675–676.

Sigell, L. T., and Flessa, H. C. (1970): Drug interaction with anticoagulants. *J.A.M.A.,* 214:2035–2038.

Singh, M. M., and Smith, J. M. (1973): Reversal of some therapeutic effects of an antipsychotic agent by an antiparkinsonism drug. *J. Nerv. Ment. Dis.,* 157:50–58.

Smith, S. G., and Davis, W. M. (1973): Haloperidol effects on morphine self-administration: Testing for pharmacological modification of the primary reinforcement mechanism. *Psychol. Rec.,* 23:209–221.

Snyder, S. H., Taylor, K. M., Coyle, J. T., and Meyerhoff, J. L. (1970): The role of brain dopamine in behavioral regulation and the actions of psychotropic drugs. *Am. J. Psychiatry,* 127:199–207.

Still, C. N., and Han, C. H. (1973): Vestavariant of Tourette's disease: Treatment with haloperidol. *South. Med. J.,* 66:1222–1225.

Stotsky, B. A. (1972): Haloperidol in the treatment of geriatric patients. In: *Butyrophenones in Psychiatry,* edited by A. DiMascio and R. I. Shader. Raven Press, New York.

Suarez, M. V. (1969): The butyrophenones in neurology. *Rev. Gharma,* 33:16–20.

Sugerman, A. A., Williams, B. H., and Adlerstein, A. M. (1964): Haloperidol in the psychiatric disorders of old age. *Am. J. Psychiatry,* 120:1190–1192.

Tapia, F. (1969): Haldol in the treatment of children with tics and stutterers and an incidental finding. *Behav. Neuropsychiatry,* 1:28–32.

Tewfik, G. I., Jain, V. K., Harcup, M., and Magowan, S. (1970): Effectiveness of various tranquilizers in the management of senile restlessness. *Gerontol. Clin. (Basel),* 12:351–359.

Tobin, J. M., Brousseau, E. R., and Lorenz, A. A. (1970): Clinical evaluation of haloperidol in geriatric patients. *Geriatrics,* 25:119–122.

Tornetta, F. J. (1972): Double-blind evaluation of haloperidol for antiemetic activity. *Anesth. Analg. (Cleve.),* 51:964–967.

Tsuang, M. M., Lu, L. M., Stotsky, B. A., and Cole, J. O. (1971): Haloperidol versus thioridazine for hospitalized psychogeriatric patients: Double-blind study. *J. Am. Geriatr. Soc.,* 19:593–600.

Ucer, E., and Kreger, K. C. (1969): A double-blind study comparing haloperidol with thioridazine in emotionally disturbed, mentally retarded children. *Curr. Ther. Res.,* 11:278–283.

Villeneuve, A., Dogan, K., Lachance, R., and Proulx, C. A. (1970): Controlled study of fluspirlene in chronic schizophrenia. Presented at the 7th Congress of the CINP, Prague, Czechoslovakia.

Volmat, R., and Allers, G. (1970): The contribution of currently used neuroleptics to the treatment of depressions. *Therapeutique,* 46:1017–1080.

Warnes, H., Lehmann, H. E., Ban, T. A., and Lee, H. (1966): Butaperazine and haloperidol: A comparative trial of two antipsychotic drugs. *Laval Med.,* 37:143–145.

Wells, P. G., and Malcolm, M. T. (1971): Controlled trial of the treatment of 36 stutterers. *Br. J. Psychiatry,* 119:603–604.

Weston, M. J., Bentley, R., Unwin, A., Morris, M., and Harper, M. A. (1973): A comparative trial of haloperidol and thioridazine management of chronic schizophrenia. *Aust. N.Z. J. Psychiatry,* 7:52–57.

Whanger, A. D. (1973): Paranoid syndromes of the senium. In: *Psychopharmacology and Aging,* edited by C. Eisdorfer and W. E. Fann. Plenum Press, New York.

Zingales, I. A. (1971): A gas chromatographic method for the determination of haloperidol in human plasma. *J. Chromatographr.,* 54:15–24.

Chapter 5

Diagnosis of Anxiety and Differential Use of Antianxiety Drugs

Donald F. Klein

DEFINITION OF ANXIETY

"Anxiety" is certainly one of the key words in psychiatry. It occupies this exalted state because it is used to refer to a heterogeneous collection of unpleasant negative affects and subjective sensations, and therefore frequently describes aspects of many different psychiatric syndromes. It also has a core conceptual role in both popular theories of psychopathogenesis, i.e., psychoanalysis and learning theory.

Anxiety is readily apprehended without the need for a complex detailed description, because as a subjective mood it is identical to the fearful feelings experienced under conditions of actual danger. Furthermore, normal people have similar feelings during the expectation of danger. Common parlance distinguishes between fear and anxiety. *Webster's New World Dictionary of the American Language* (1966) defines anxiety as a state of being "uneasy, apprehensive, or worried about what may happen." This definition points both to the subjective distress (i.e., "uneasy") and to anticipatory orientation (i.e., "what may happen") as opposed to fear, which implies a present danger.

The problem confronting psychiatrists is how to understand the professed feelings of the ubiquitous people who state that they feel anxious, or who make specific complaints compatible with anxiety but who have neither current reason for fear nor apparent reason to anticipate danger. It seems unlikely that such complaints always result from a common set of psychopathological antecedents. They may well come from a final common pathway stemming from a host of different pathogenic processes. It is conceivable that there are drugs that would nonspecifically damp such a final common pathway and therefore be of symptomatic utility to an etiologically heterogeneous group. The benzodiazepines and propanediols may fulfill this role. Other agents specifically effective at a more distal part of the causal chain might have more profound effects in multiple psychophysiological areas but be effective in fewer people. The antidepressants may fit this bill.

The history of the notion of anxiety in psychodynamic psychiatry is too complex to review here. It is well known that Freud went through a number of different stages in his conception of anxiety, finally coming very close to the common sense notion that anxiety is the result of the anticipation of danger.

However, psychoanalytic theory specifically posits an internal danger of which the patient is unaware—the release of a repressed unconscious wish.

Recently some psychiatrists, under the influence of learning theory, have argued that the anxiety of the psychiatric patient is entirely analogous to the anxiety of the normal person. The lack of apparent adequate psychological cause is simply due to the observer's misunderstanding of the intensity of the conditioning process in these patients. The patients are still reacting to a present stimulus signaling danger but have not discriminated the inciting stimulus pattern at a verbalizable level. Except for certain traumatic phobias, this theory is difficult to believe.

DRUG LABELS AND ANXIETY

Until recently it was standard to refer to the three major new classes of psychotropic drugs as the major tranquilizers, minor tranquilizers, and antidepressants. However, there has been an illuminating terminological shift that represents a growing comprehension of the relationship between drug effects and psychopathology. When chlorpromazine first appeared during the 1950s, it was considered a sedative antianxiety agent similar to the barbiturates but without their propensity for intoxication, ataxia, and medullary depression. It was immediately widely assumed that these powerful agents, so useful for psychoses, would be of value in the treatment of minor emotional disorders such as the neuroses. The minor tranquilizers, on the other hand, were simply considered to be less effective antianxiety agents—effective on the neuroses but not strong enough to affect the psychoses.

However, the major tranquilizers are currently called antipsychotic agents, and the minor tranquilizers are termed antianxiety agents. In fact, in a recent article Loffts and Demars (1974) vigorously pleaded for considering the phenothiazine thioridazine as a possible alternative to the standard antianxiety agents, the benzodiazepines! We return to the substance of this claim later, but a tremendous shift in viewpoint has clearly occurred. Originally the idea that a phenothiazine such as thioridazine possessed antianxiety activity would have seemed obvious. Now it is a notion requiring defense even for consideration. What has happened to our grasp of the action of these drugs?

Increasing experience, detailed by Klein and Davis (1969), has clearly shown that the minor tranquilizers are not simply lesser major tranquilizers. The major tranquilizers work well on the psychoses but have proved disappointing, or even deleterious, in the treatment of apparently lesser illnesses characterized by anxiety. Furthermore, in studies of the effects of major tranquilizers on psychotic symptomatology, the anxious symptomatology of the psychotic was among the most refractory aspects of the illness. It was difficult to maintain that the antipsychotic effect of the phenothiazines was secondary to their antianxiety effect, because retarded, withdrawn, perplexed, psychotic patients, upon cognitive improvement, often began to express many anxious paranoid concerns and somatic complaints. Similarly, the treatment of non-psychotic states marked by anxiety with "major tranquilizers" often led to a nontranquil patient (Klein and Fink, 1962). Not only did the symptomatology frequently worsen, but the patients often urgently rejected major tranquilizers in favor of minor tranquilizers.

This growing clinical experience has led to a revised drug terminology: The terms antipsychotic and antianxiety agents are replacing the terms major and minor tranquilizers, indicating a qualitative distinction in their targets and mode of action.

CONSCIOUS AND UNCONSCIOUS ANXIETY

The psychoanalytic theory of neurosis affirmed that "anxiety is the chief characteristic of the neuroses. It may be felt and expressed directly, or it may be controlled unconsciously and automatically by conversion, displacement, and various psychological mechanisms. Generally these mechanisms produce symptoms experienced as subjective distress from which the patient desires relief" (Committee, 1968). Showing that a person may be influenced by drives and goals of which he is not aware was one of Freud's salient contributions to our understanding of human personality and psychopathology.

Many neurotic symptoms can be understood as the effort of a patient to prevent the development of manifest anxiety. The situation seems quite analogous to conditioned escape studies with animals. For instance, a dog may be trained, on hearing a bell, to jump from an electric grid to avoid receiving a shock. After a brief period of training, the dog never receives any subsequent electric shocks because on signal it instantly removes itself from the potentially threatening situation. This behavior does not extinguish, becoming a smooth, automatic, unruffled performance. It is plain that the dog is responding to the anticipation of pain, but this thoroughly automatized process does not require emotional arousal to occur. Signs of affective arousal and autonomic discharge appear only when the dog is prevented from leaving the grid.

This behavior markedly resembles compulsive neurotic behavior in which certain rituals are performed smoothly and mechanically, anxiety occurring only if the ritual is blocked. Stating that the behavior results from unconscious anxiety implies the existence of a covert physiological process quite analogous to conscious anxiety that has somehow been kept out of awareness. Therefore the treatment of such patients with "antianxiety agents" (i.e., agents that ameliorate manifest anxiety) should diminish such compulsive rituals if they are dependent on the existence of covert concurrent unconscious anxiety.

In fact, such medications are routinely ineffective with either the conditioned animal or the human compulsive ritual that occurs in a calm setting.

Therefore the term "unconscious" in this context means predisposition. The effectiveness of the antianxiety agents occurs in the presence of overt, manifest anxiety, but the predisposition to anxiety is not affected.

Antianxiety agents may allow the subject to remain in a threatening field by lessening manifest anxiety. Then if the threat does not materialize, the anticipation of danger may decrease by learning. This leads to a decreased predisposition to anxiety via extinction, given corrective experience.

DIFFERENTIAL INDICATIONS

Can we then simply affirm that antipsychotic drugs should be restricted to patients with manifest psychoses and that antianxiety drugs be used for non-psychotic patients with manifest anxiety? Unfortunately this simple set of indications fails because of two clinical facts. First, there are some apparently anxious nonpsychotic patients who do benefit from antipsychotic agents (Klein, 1966). Second, there are anxious nonpsychotic patients who receive slight benefit from antianxiety drugs and for whom antidepressants—both monoamine oxidase (MAO) inhibitors and tricyclics—appear useful (Klein, 1964). Finally, to confuse the situation further, there are some patients, often considered to have a borderline psychosis related to schizophrenia, who respond reasonably well to antidepressant drugs and not so well to antipsychotic drugs (Klein, 1968, 1975; Hedberg, Houck, and Glueck, 1971).

NECESSITY FOR DIAGNOSIS

The surest route to therapeutic simplicity is via differential diagnosis. Simply because a psychopathological state is labeled anxiety does not ensure that it represents the same psychobiological process as another state labeled anxiety. Such resemblance may be due to overlapping final common pathways of distinct pathogenesis or even to fortuitous resemblances.

The target-symptom approach often implicitly promotes a mosaic view of psychopathology, considering each symptom independent of the others and assuming that each is identical in nature from patient to patient. Another approach is to see each symptom as a prominent aspect of an integrated disease syndrome. These symptoms cannot be abstracted from the symptom complex without leading to false equivalences with similar aspects of entirely different configurations. One must discriminate between anticipatory anxiety, panic anxiety, agitation in a depressive setting, anxiety in acute schizophrenic psychosis, expressive histrionics, etc. Therefore this viewpoint requires that diagnostic formulations be systematic, patterned, multivariate descriptions.

For instance, when panic occurs with auditory hallucinations, it is usually alleviated by chlorpromazine. However, in the presence of agoraphobia, panic is made worse by this drug. Thus the two panic states are vastly different. $Panic_1$ is simply not the same as $Panic_2$, and identical coding of these two phenomenologically similar behaviors does violence to the possibility of determining their relationships correctly.

Formulating such complexities where the meaning of a behavior can be derived only from its behavioral context requires interaction terms that are not part of the usual additive multivariate approach. Furthermore, these terms are very difficult if not impossible to establish on a statistical inductive basis. They require stipulation derived from clinical experience, which in turn requires a new level of creative interaction between clinicians and statisticians. In any case, the clinician is still faced with the necessity of a detailed diagnostic exploration prior to prescription.

SYMPTOMATOLOGY OF ANXIETY

There have been many investigations wherein psychiatric patients express their symptomatology. Various statistical procedures are then applied (notably factor analysis) in an attempt to see which symptoms hang together. A close look at the variety of features frequently endured by anxious people indicates that they can be subgrouped into a number of conceptual unities, e.g., motor tension, autonomic hyperactivity, panic, phobic avoidance, apprehensive expectation, vigilance, and scanning.

The diagnostician is primarily dependent on both the patient's verbal report and his behavior when investigating anxiety, although they do not invariably corroborate each other. Both sources of information require attention. Testimony from other informed sources can be invaluable.

Manifestations of Motor Tension

Shaky, jittery, jumpy, trembling, tense, keyed-up, muscular aches, easily fatigued, and unable to relax are frequent verbal reports by the patient with motor tension. Concomitant behavior may be eyelid twitch, shaking, furrowed brow, strained face, fidgeting, restlessness, jumpiness, and easy startle. The common underlying feature is increased striated muscle tone. This may also be associated with sighing respirations perhaps due to diaphragmatic spasm restricting diaphragmatic excursion, with compensatory sighing intercostal respiration.

These motor manifestations must be distinguished from states of agitation where the patient is in manifest gross motor movement including pacing, hand wringing, and agonized gestures, sometimes accompanied by pleading and shouting as well as reports of severe intrapsychic pain. The agitated person is tense and anxious, but the tense person is not necessarily agitated.

Autonomic Hyperactivity

A wide variety of somatic complaints seem directly due to individually different patterns of hyperactivity in the sympathetic and parasympathetic nervous systems. Verbal complaints include sweating, heart pounding or racing, cold clammy hands, dry mouth, dizziness, light-headedness, tingling feelings in hands or feet, upset stomach, hot or cold spells, frequent urination or defecation, diarrhea, discomfort at the pit of the stomach, lump in the throat, flushing, pallor, and high resting pulse and respiration rate. The common feature seems to be a potpourri of smooth-muscle and glandular hyper- and hypofunction. All of these verbal complaints may be verified by observable bodily signs, i.e., diarrhea, sweating, etc.

Panic

The patient states that he suddenly develops extremely fearful feelings or terror accompanied by cardiorespiratory distress. What differentiates this state from chronic anxiety is the sudden exacerbation of distress, often associated with feelings of impending doom. Feighner and co-workers present diagnostic criteria for a panic attack (Feighner, Robins, Guze, Woodruff, Winokur, and Munoz, 1972). Four of the following symptoms should be present during the majority of attacks associated with apprehension, fearfulness, and a sense of impending doom: dyspnea, palpitations, chest pain or discomfort, choking or smothering sensation, dizziness, paresthesias.

Pitts and McClure (1967) define an anxiety attack as an acute episode of extreme fearfulness, feeling of impending doom, fear of insanity, or fear of "having a heart attack" or of some other serious affliction, in addition to the occurrence of five or more of the following symptoms, with a minimum of two in the first group and three in the second group: (1) dyspnea or awareness of difficulty breathing ("can't get full breath"), "smothering" or choking or struggling to breathe, sighing, chest discomfort or chest pain, lump in throat; and (2) dizziness or giddiness, faintness, weakness, fatigue, inward shakiness, tremor, paresthesias, vascular throbbing, palpitation. These symptoms seem almost entirely autonomic. It is noteworthy that symptoms related to avoidance and vigilance are conspicuously lacking.

Phobic Avoidance

The patient complains (and acts consonantly) that there are certain things or situations that must be avoided on pain of severe distress (e.g., being left alone; traveling on buses, subways, or trains; traveling alone).

Apprehensive Expectation

The patient is generally apprehensive and continually worries, ruminates, and anticipates something bad happening either to himself (e.g., fear of fainting, losing control, dying) or valued others (e.g., close relatives may become ill, injured in an accident). Such patients self-label, stating that they are anxious, frightened, scared, fearful, etc.

Vigilance and Scanning

Anxious expectation may result in sentry-like behavior such that the patient is on edge, impatient, or irritable; he complains of distractability and finds it hard to keep his mind on a task. This arousal is often associated with insomnia, difficulty in falling asleep, broken sleep, unsatisfying sleep, and fatigue on waking.

SYNDROMES WITH ANXIETY COMPONENTS

The following nine syndromes, often considered anxious, must be diagnostically dissected before rational pharmacotherapy can be prescribed:
1. Reactive anxiety,
2. Phobic neurosis associated with spontaneous panic attacks,
3. Phobic neurosis associated with specific objects or situations,
4. Anxiety neurosis,
5. Obsessive-compulsive neurosis,
6. Depersonalization neurosis,
7. Hypochondriacal neurosis,
8. Agitated depression, and
9. Schizophrenia.

Reactive Anxiety

Reactive anxiety appears to be simply a quantitative variant of normal apprehension. It is the typical anxious symptomatology of the person facing a severe danger associated with marked uncertainty, e.g., being drafted, getting divorced, taking a new job. Rickels (1972) indicated that short duration, acute, anxious states of a reactive nature respond as well to placebo as to medication. There are anecdotal reports concerning the utility of benzodiazepines in facing specific dangers such as occur in bullfighting and going to the dentist. Simple reactive anxiety needs little more than support. The use of medication is questionable, except perhaps small doses of an antianxiety agent, primarily for placebo value. Certainly antipsychotic or antidepressant agents seem unwarranted.

Phobic Neurosis Associated with Spontaneous Panic Attacks

Certain patients present massive and diffuse anxiety with prominent autonomic and tension symptoms complicated by phobic avoidance and panic attacks. Phobic avoidance usually relates to being alone or traveling alone;

it may misleadingly be referred to as agoraphobia. However, recently we found that phobic patients with spontaneous panic attacks may have many different situational avoidances but similar medication-response patterns.

The outstanding characteristic of this syndrome is that the panic attack precedes development of the massive free-floating tension—anxiety. Chronic anxiety represents the anticipation of recurrent panic attacks. The panic attack is the proximal inciting cause of the chronic anxiety state, which then leads to the variety of phobic avoidances used by the patient, who hopes to prevent a recurrence of the panic or at least guarantee easy, quick acccess to help and safety if he becomes panicked.

Such panic can be blocked through the use of both tricyclic antidepressants and MAO inhibitors (Klein, 1964; Lipsedge, Hajioff, Huggins, Napier, Pearce, Pike, and Rich, 1973; Tyrer, Candy, and Kelly, 1973; Zitrin, Klein, Lindemann, Tobak, Rock, Kaplan, and Ganz, 1975). Although the panics respond within a few weeks or even earlier, the chronic tensional expectant anxiety requires a subsequent period of extinction prior to the cessation of avoidance maneuvers.

Interestingly, the benzodiazepines, meprobamate-like drugs, alcohol, and barbiturates are all useful in decreasing the chronic anticipatory anxiety but are of no value in the panic attacks. Antidepressant drugs stop the panic attacks but are of no value for chronic anxiety. This clearly indicates that these are two markedly different processes; the panic attacks are not simply the quantitative extension of chronic anxiety. Furthermore, panic anxiety, so defined, is refractory to antipsychotics and may be exacerbated by them. Because alcohol and barbiturates decrease chronic anxiety, patients frequently become addicted as they continually raise the self-administered dosage in the hope that their panics will also be relieved (Quitkin, Rifkin, Kaplan, and Klein, 1972).

Phobic Neurosis Associated with Specific Objects or Situations

A large number of patients feel relatively normal except when exposed to a specific phobic object or situation (e.g., elevators, cats, public speaking); they do not have spontaneous panic attacks. I hypothesized some time ago that since the specific psychopathology which responds to antidepressants is the panic, the nonpanicking anxious patient should not respond to antidepressants. A recent placebo-controlled double-blind trial indicates that imipramine is not better than placebo in the treatment of such patients (Zitrin et al., 1975). Therefore imipramine does not have a nonspecific antianxiety effect but does have an extremely specific effect related to the appearance of spontaneous panic.

One diagnostic headache is that patients often deny spontaneous panics, especially if they have figured out some reason for them. They therefore do not consider the attacks as coming out of the blue, but as due to some specific interpersonal or intrafamilial problem. One must persist in asking the patient to list all recent panic attacks. Frequently the patient denies spontaneous panic attacks, but on being pressed for examples describes situations in which the attack was completely startling, with no apparent stimulus. Such reports actually indicate the sort of anxiety process that responds to antidepressants.

It is unclear if the situation-bound phobias respond to antianxiety agents, e.g., benzodiazepines. It seems quite reasonable that treatment with benzodiazepines might allow an expansion of behavior into the avoided areas, resulting in decreased apprehension leading to extinction. There have been reports of using intravenous diazepam in such a context.

Anxiety Neurosis

Such patients seem simply to have a chronic free-floating anxiety without either panic attacks or phobic avoidance. I have actually seen very few people who come close to this description. I believe that many such patients actually have panic attacks which go unrecognized and for some reason have not led to phobic behavior. My guess is that such patients would respond to antidepressants if they are having panic attacks, or to antianxiety agents if they are not. Since panic attacks are periodic phenomena, it is possible that a patient may have a self-limited series of panic attacks, develop expectant anxiety, have the panic attacks cease during the natural course of the illness, and be left with a chronic tensional state that does not respond to antidepressants but instead requires antianxiety agents. Phenothiazines and other antipsychotic agents are ineffective or even deleterious in purely anxious patients. Claims that they are effective are usually due to inclusion of mild agitated depressives in the study sample.

Obsessive-Compulsive Neurosis

The obsessive-compulsive neurotic does not primarily complain about anxiety but rather about his obsessions and compulsions. Anxiety becomes manifest only if his rituals are interfered with. I have found only minor benefits from antianxiety agents, and none from phenothiazines. Occasionally the patient has an unrecognized depressive component that exacerbated his obsessive-compulsive symptomatology and presents as a ruminative tension state. These patients are usually agitated depressives and respond to treatment for agitated depression, as described below, by a return to their obsessional baseline.

Depersonalization Neurosis

Depersonalization neurosis is a difficult syndrome, both diagnostically and therapeutically, in which the primary experience seems to be that of depersonalization and/or derealization. Secondary to this there is marked reactive anxiety. However, it is possible that the depersonalization is secondary to the anxiety, since depersonalization is frequently reported as a concomitant of the panic attack in the so-called phobic anxiety depersonalization syndrome.

If the patient is not having panic attacks the depersonalization and secondary anxiety is quite refractory to any of our usual treatments. Sargant and Slater (1972) suggest using intravenous methamphetamine.

Hypochondriacal Neurosis

Hypochondriacs are patients without manifest depression who are anxious and overconcerned with the possibility of being ill and thus require much reassurance. Sedative agents are apparently well accepted by this group, and so diazepam may be more beneficial than chlordiazepoxide (Rickels, 1972).

Agitated Depression

A very important differential diagnosis is that between anxiety and agitation. Agitated patients are regularly tense and anxious, but tense-anxious patients are not regularly agitated. The differential diagnosis revolves about the fact that the agitated depressive almost always has a massive pervasive inability to experience pleasure and interest in usually rewarding areas. This may occur without experiencing sadness or mood change; nonetheless, this defines agitation as an aspect of depression. Since such patients are often misleadingly called anxious depressives, a distinction must be made between anxiety and agitation.

The anxious patient has the symptomatology described above. The agitated patient manifests both anxious symptomatology and marked motor facilitation. He paces, wrings his hands, and pleads in a loud, vociferous fashion. One possibility is that depressive patients suffer from inhibition of their pleasure evaluative center.

Whereas the anxious patient responds to the anticipation of pain, the agitated patient acts as if in actual pain and complains of severe psychic distress. It is well known that the pain experience is a combination of the afferent pain sensation and the central evaluative reaction (often called distress). Morphine, for instance, does not affect the pain threshhold but markedly benefits the distress reaction to pain. One might hypothesize that agitated depressives should respond poorly to an injection of benzodiazepine but well to an injection of morphine, whereas patients with an anxiety state should respond well to both agents. Conversely, the distress of patients with chronic pain may be relieved by antidepressants. Controlled trials in this area would be most valuable.

The treatment of agitated depression depends on the life circumstances of the patient. If his illness can be contained and tolerated, a tricyclic antidepressant is usually quite effective within 2 to 3 weeks. Phenothiazines are also effective but incur certain risks, e.g., the faint possibility of tardive dyskinesia; nonetheless, they are very useful in maintenance of the outpatient who does not accept hospitalization, as they quickly reduce agitation and insomnia. The antianxiety agents are not effective, and have a role only as sedatives. If a sedative is needed, one should bear in mind that certain tricyclic drugs (e.g., amitryptyline) have soporific activity.

Schizophrenia

It is well recognized that the agitation and anxiety of schizophrenic psychosis is refractory to antianxiety agents. The agitation is handled well by the antipsychotics, the anxiety less well. Antidepressants do not seem useful in this context.

CONCLUSION

The term anxiety can interfere with observing and describing patients, as well as prescribing for them. A wide variety of patients, all considered anxious, may require different psychopharmacological interventions. This clearly indicates that the term anxiety is being applied to a wide variety of pathophysiologies, as well as normal adaptive mechanisms. The distinctions between anxiety, agitation, and panic are particularly crucial; such distinctions facilitate rational drug therapy of the patient.

TREATMENT SUMMARY

Syndromes with anxiety aspects	Suggested treatment
Reactive anxiety	No drug needed. Small doses of antianxiety drug may be prescribed for placebo purposes.
Phobic neurosis associated with spontaneous panic attacks	Tricyclic antidepressants or MAO inhibitors.
Phobic neurosis associated with specific objects or situations	Benzodiazepines or propanediols?
Anxiety neurosis	With panic attacks: antidepressants. Without panic attacks: antianxiety agents.
Obsessive-compulsive neurosis	Minor benefit from antianxiety agents. Some patients are agitated depressives and should be treated as such.
Depersonalization neurosis	Refractory to usual treatments.
Hypochondriacal neurosis	Diazepam.
Agitated depression	Tricyclic antidepressants; antipsychotic agents.
Schizophrenia	Refractory to antianxiety agents. Antipsychotic agents are useful for entire syndrome but not particularly for anxiety.

REFERENCES

Committee on Nomenclature and Statistics of the American Psychiatric Association (1968): *Diagnostic and Statistical Manual of Mental Disorders,* Ed. 2. American Psychiatric Association, Washington, D. C.

Feighner, J. P., Robins, E., Guze, S. B., Woodruff, R. A., Jr., Winokur, G., and Munoz, R. (1972): Diagnostic criteria for use in psychiatric research. *Arch. Gen. Psychiatry,* 26:57–63.

Hedberg, D. F., Houck, J. H., and Glueck, B. C. (1971): Tranylcypromine-trifluoperazine combination in the treatment of schizophrenia. *Am. J. Psychiatry,* 127:1144–1146.

Klein, D. F. (1964): Delineation of two drug-responsive anxiety syndromes. *Psychopharmacologia,* 5:397–408.

Klein, D. F. (1966): Chlorpromazine-procyclidine combination, imipramine and placebo in depressive disorders. *Can. Psychiatr. Assoc. J.,* 11:S146–S149.

Klein, D. F. (1968): Psychiatric diagnosis and typology of clinical drug effects *Psychopharmacologia,* 13:359–386.

Klein, D. F. (1975): Psychopharmacology and the borderline patient. *Psychiatr. Semin. (in press).*

Klein, D. F., and Davis, J. M. (1969): *Diagnosis and Drug Treatment of Psychiatric Disorders.* Williams & Wilkins, Baltimore.

Klein, D. F., and Fink, M. (1962): Behavioral reaction pattern with phenothiazines. *Arch. Gen. Psychiatry,* 7:449–459.

Lipsedge, M. S., Hajioff, J., Huggins, P., Napier, L., Pearce, J., Pike, D. J., and Rich, M. (1973): The management of severe agoraphobia: A comparison of iproniazid and systematic desensitization. *Psychopharmacologia,* 32:67–80.

Lofft, J. G., and Demars, J. P. (1974): A chemotherapeutic alternative to the antianxiety agents for the extended treatment of psychoneuroses. *Dis. Nerv. Syst.,* 35:409–415.

Pitts, F. N., Jr., and McClure, J. N., Jr. (1967): Lactate metabolism in anxiety neurosis. *N. Engl. J. Med.,* 277:1329–1336.

Quitkin, F., Rifkin, A., Kaplan, J., and Klein, D. F. (1972): Phobic anxiety syndrome complicated by drug dependence and addiction. *Arch. Gen. Psychiatry,* 27:159–161.

Rickels, K. (1972): Predictors of response to benzodiazepines in anxious outpatients. In: *The Benzodiazepines,* edited by S. Garattini, E. Mussini, and L. O. Randall, pp. 257–281. Raven Press, New York.

Sargant, W. W., and Slater, E. (1972): *An Introduction to Special Methods of Treatment in Psychiatry.* Science House, New York.

Tyrer, P., Candy, J., and Kelly, D. (1973): A study of the clinical effects of phenelzine and placebo in the treatment of phobic anxiety. *Psychopharmacologia,* 32:237–254.

Webster's New World Dictionary of the American Language (1966): Edited by D. B. Guralnik and J. H. Friend, p. 66. World Publishing, New York.

Zitrin, C. M., Klein, D. F., Lindemann, C., Tobak, P., Rock, M., Kaplan, J., and Ganz, V. H. (1975): Comparison of short-term treatment regimens in phobic patients: a preliminary report. In: *Proceedings, American Psychopathological Association.* APA, Boston *(in press).*

Chapter 6

Therapeutic Uses of the Benzodiazepines

Phillip H. Bookman and Lowell O. Randall

Development of the benzodiazepines stands as a major landmark in the history of modern psychopharmacology. The usefulness of this group of compounds is attributable to a broad spectrum of unique pharmacological qualities that members of this group possess. Their widest application is in the treatment of emotional illness.

Sternbach, who synthesized the first benzodiazepine during the mid-1950s, recognized that its chemical structure was not that of a group of pharmacologically inert compounds he had been working with. In the hands of Randall, who did the initial animal studies, its unique pharmacological properties were revealed in 1957. This entirely new compound, whose molecular structure was later to be correctly identified as a 1,4-benzodiazepine, was found to calm and relax cats.

Clinical trials by psychiatrists throughout the United States and abroad demonstrated that the drug was effective in controlling anxiety and tension in neurotic patients, and that the beneficial results could be sustained with a minimum of side effects. By the end of 1959 the accumulated clinical experience was sufficient to warrant review by the Food and Drug Administration (FDA). In 1960 chlordiazepoxide hydrochloride was introduced in the United States as Librium, and was followed in 1963 by the second member of this class, diazepam (Valium). Another analogue to receive FDA approval in 1965 was oxazepam, marketed in the United States as Serax. At the present time five benzodiazepine compounds (chlordiazepoxide, diazepam, oxazepam, clorazepate, flurazepam) are available to the practicing physician in the United States, and several others (e.g., nitrazepam, medazepam) are marketed in Europe. Their chemical structures are shown in Fig. 1. A number of other members of the series are under intensive clinical investigation, including bromazepam, clonazepam, flunitrazepam, and lorazepam. New derivatives continue to be tested for a possible high degree of specificity and minimum likelihood of producing side effects.

BASIC PHARMACOLOGY

The chief pharmacological characteristics of the benzodiazepine class are taming, antiaggressive, sedative, muscle relaxant, and anticonvulsant activi-

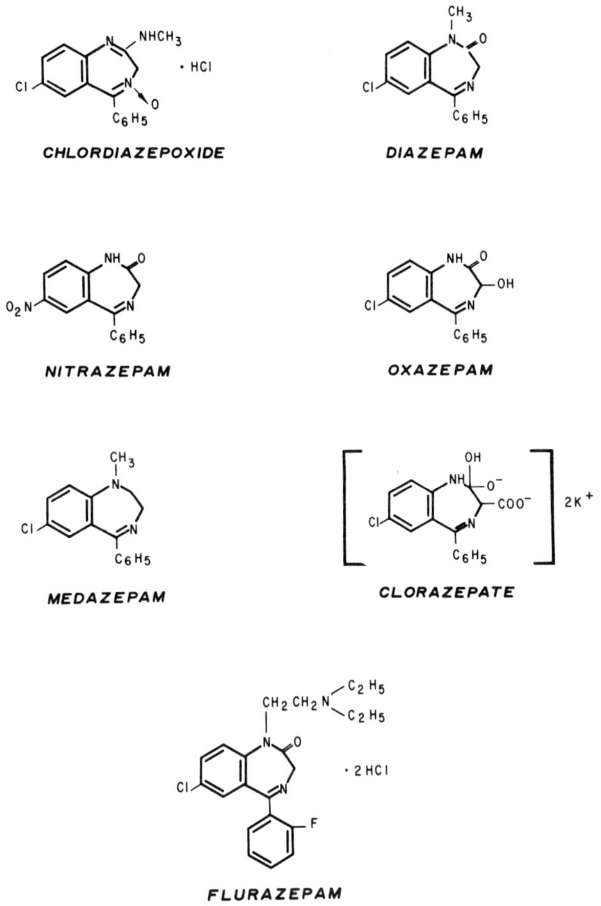

FIG. 1. Chemical structures of the major benzodiazepines.

ties, as demonstrated in mice, rats, cats, and cynomolgous and squirrel monkeys. Although there is some overlap of pharmacological activity between benzodiazepines and other tranquilizers, hypnotics, and muscle relaxants, they have been differentiated by a series of screening tests. These same tests have demonstrated significant qualitative as well as potency differences among the derivatives in the benzodiazepine series. Thus flurazepam is an effective nighttime sedative; oxazepam is an antianxiety agent; and diazepam, which is widely accepted as an antianxiety agent, is also effective as a muscle relaxant and an anticonvulsant. By using these drugs differentially, animals can be restrained, their muscles relaxed, and convulsions prevented. Certainly in the animal model there are apparent differences in pharmacological effects (Randall and Kappell, 1973).

Psychosedative Effects

The striking antianxiety effect of chlordiazepoxide was first discovered clinically. Since there is no specific counterpart of human anxiety in animals, efforts were made to devise appropriate tests to study analogous behavioral manifestations in animals, e.g., fear or aggression. A combination of tests have become useful to profile individual members of the benzodiazepine series, as well as to differentiate them from other psychotropic drugs. In addition to taming laboratory or wild animals and modifying elicited aggressive behavior, drugs were tested for their effects on experimentally induced conflict and conditioned behavior.

Conflict behavior is induced in animals by presenting them simultaneously with food and with a shock to the foot when the animal reaches for the food. The hungry animal normally approaches food rapidly, but if the approach is punished by a foot shock the animal's speed and frequency of approaches are reduced. In this conflict situation the frequency of approaches is increased by benzodiazepines, presumably because the drugs attenuate the conflict by decreasing fear of the punishing stimulus. By this test chlordiazepoxide and oxazepam were about equal in conflict-reducing properties, while diazepam was the most potent of the three in attenuating the conflict.

In an operant procedure squirrel monkeys were trained to press levers in Skinner boxes to avoid a foot shock. Drugs of the benzodiazepine class increase the number of shocks taken by the animals, even with doses well below those which produce significant central nervous system (CNS) depression. This could be due to decreased fear—the result of the "antianxiety" effect of the drug. In an operant procedure for assessing avoidance (of shock) behavior, Gluckman (1965) reported oxazepam equal to chlordiazepoxide in reducing avoidance.

Chlordiazepoxide effectively blocked isolation-induced aggression in mice, electrically induced fighting in mice, vicious behavior produced by lesions in the brains of rats, and the spontaneous aggressiveness of killer cats and vicious monkeys. These effects occurred at doses below the sedation level, showing a degree of specificity not observed with some other classes of CNS depressants, e.g., barbiturates.

Muscle-Relaxant Activity

Based on direct observations of relaxation in animals, other types of pharmacological tests were used to reveal the muscle-relaxant properties of the benzodiazepines. It is speculated that the major locus for the muscle-relaxant effects of diazepam is central—the brainstem reticular formation. Muscle-relaxant effects also occur at the spinal level, where presynaptic inhibition is enhanced (Schallek, Schlosser, and Randall, 1972).

Anticonvulsant Activity

Anticonvulsant activity in animals is demonstrated by the ability of benzodiazepines to antagonize convulsions induced by standard convulsant agents, and by changes in electroencephalographic (EEG) patterns. For example, the drugs are potent in antagonizing pentylenetetrazol (Metrazol)-induced seizures in mice, rats, and rabbits. Some of the compounds are 400 times more potent than trimethadione in certain seizure tests.

SITES OF ACTION

A variety of techniques have been employed to determine the areas in the brain where the benzodiazepines selectively act. Evidence indicating that the psychosedative effects of benzodiazepines may be mediated through the limbic system was provided by several procedures: (1) changes in spontaneous electrical activity; (2) effect on the "septal rat" (rats with lesions in the septal area become extremely vicious); and (3) evoked potentials in the limbic system. Further insight into areas in the brain that are selectively affected by these drugs has been obtained by electrophysiological, behavioral, and radiochemical studies (Schallek et al., 1972).

Evidence for selective action in the hippocampus by chlordiazepoxide and diazepam was provided by studies reviewed by Schallek et al. (1972). These investigators tested the effects of the drugs on spontaneous electrical activity in seven subcortical areas of the immobilized cat: the caudate nucleus, basolateral amygdala, posterior hippocampus, septum, lateral hypothalamus, medial hypothalamus, and mesencephalic reticular formation. The largest changes were in the hippocampus; in contrast, chlorpromazine acted on all brain areas except the hippocampus.

CLINICAL APPLICATIONS

The indications for which the benzodiazepines are prescribed can be classified into five major areas: (1) psychiatric states and organic diseases in which anxiety is a major component or a contributing factor in the etiology; (2) neuromuscular disorders; (3) convulsive disorders; (4) acute alcohol withdrawal; and (5) insomnia. It should be noted, however, that not all of the marketed benzodiazepines are approved for all the above indications; for example, flurazepam is indicated only for insomnia.

(1) Anxiety, tension, nervousness, apprehension, and agitation are among the most frequently observed signs and symptoms in psychoneurotic disorders, and to some degree are present in other forms of mental illness or are associated with many underlying organic diseases. Anxiety is also a component of psychosomatic disorders, e.g., gastric ulcers, ulcerative colitis, neuroderma-

titis, asthma, and hyperventilation syndrome. Many of these conditions respond favorably to benzodiazepines.

(2) Neuromuscular disorders in which skeletal muscle spasm may be associated with local pathology, cerebral palsy, athetosis, stiff-man syndrome, and tetanus are among the indications for some benzodiazepines.

(3) Oral benzodiazepines may be used adjunctively in convulsive disorders. Intravenous diazepam is notably effective in status epilepticus and is considered by most clinicians to be the drug of choice.

(4) Acute alcohol withdrawal is an accepted indication for benzodiazepines, affording symptomatic relief or prevention of the acute agitation, tremor, and impending delirium that may be part of the syndrome.

(5) Although all the benzodiazepines may promote sleep in certain clinical states, flurazepam is specifically indicated as a hypnotic agent.

The earliest reports by psychiatrists, internists, and general practitioners dealt with the use of chlordiazepoxide in anxious nonpsychotic patients; meaningful improvement was obtained in over 70% of patients in largely uncontrolled trials covering some 1,100 patients (Greenblatt and Shader, 1974). However, over the span of a decade and a half, the clinical studies paralleling the pharmacological and pharmacokinetic research reached a high level of sophistication both as to approach and techniques employed, e.g., comparative trials with other classes of drugs and placebos by double-blind randomized procedures. Furthermore, new congeners were developed during this period that proved useful for additional indications. Today the benzodiazepines are the most frequently prescribed antianxiety agents. This broad clinical acceptance is based on their well-established efficacy and unusual degree of safety.

Guidelines for Optimal Antianxiety Therapy

A precept that applies to all psychotherapeutic drugs, but especially to antianxiety agents, was recently stated by Hollister (1973a): "Use of drugs, at least in our present understanding, should be considered no more than symptomatic, adjunctive treatment." He additionally states that since "anxiety is often episodic, waxing and waning with changes in one's life," drugs should be used only when the symptoms are disabling or at least discomforting, but not indefinitely. Some patients truly have chronic anxiety; Hollister contends that these patients often do well by being maintained with small doses of an antianxiety agent.

When drugs for the treatment of anxiety are indicated, one should differentiate those drugs that have a primary antianxiety effect from drugs such as antihistamines, hypnotics, antipsychotics, and antidepressant agents whose antianxiety effect, if present, is secondary. Benzodiazepines are predominantly antianxiety compounds (Cazzullo, 1969).

In addition to knowing when to use antianxiety drugs, one must also know whom to treat and the factors that may be expected to influence the response. Some clinicians believe that most patients can handle the ordinary tensions of daily life such as those associated with an ailing spouse, decreased income, separation from grown children, and being widowed and alone. For those patients who can manage to overcome an anxiety state without medication, the experience supports self-esteem. In fact, the use of drugs to alleviate stress may actually be harmful in some instances if it prevents the patient from understanding the source of the problem (Kiev, 1972). If the patient is confident he can master even the most severe anxiety and is familiar with some technique for reducing it, he is not likely to be incapacitated by it. Only when his functioning is impaired is he likely to seek help. The physician must decide on the basis of knowledge of his patient and his problem whether reassurance, drugs, or both are necessary (Katz, 1972). In any case, tranquilizers should not be used as placebos, merely to "do something" for the patient (Cohen, 1965).

A benzodiazepine may be a valuable adjunct at certain times during psychotherapy. During the initial stages relief of anxiety may facilitate contact and communication with the patient (Cazzullo, 1969). The drug may also be helpful during the probing phase when insights can precipitate acute emotional responses. Finally, there may be a resurgence of anxiety near the termination phase of psychotherapy, with the patient having an awareness of soon being on his own; treatment with an antianxiety agent at this time may provide a less traumatic transition.

The way in which a patient responds to the selected drug varies for many reasons. The patient's personality may contribute to his response. For example, extroverted and physically active patients, whom Hollister (1973b) characterizes as "doers," tend to respond to antianxiety drugs with increased anxiety. Presumably the drug interferes with their will to achieve, making things worse. The "thinkers," on the other hand, who are more passive and esthetically or intellectually inclined, are more likely to benefit from the drugs.

Kiev (1972) finds that the following type of patient probably benefits most from drug therapy: one who has faith in the physician, has had previous successful experience with drug treatment, has a supportive environment, possesses a well-integrated and well-organized ego, shows no tendency toward hypochondriasis or gratification from being sick, and whose symptoms are of acute onset and recent occurrence. Moreover, he is likely to remain in treatment until a positive therapeutic response occurs. Patients with chronic anxiety who derive secondary gains from the symptoms are more likely to have a poorer prognosis than patients who come for treatment because of an acute situational anxiety.

It is well known to psychiatrists that anxiety is rarely encountered without some concomitant depressive symptomatology, just as nonpsychotic depression without anxiety is rare (Detre and Jarecki, 1971; Hollister, Overall, Pokorny, and Shelton, 1971; Kiev, 1972). Benzodiazepines such as diazepam are frequently of therapeutic value in patients with "anxious depressions." Anxiety and depressive mood are the primary target symptoms of this neurotic complex. In most, the principal symptom is anxiety, which is likely to respond to treatment with a benzodiazepine; the associated depressive symptoms also often are improved concurrently. Hollister et al. (1971) documented these beneficial effects in a study in which diazepam was compared with a phenothiazine without concurrent administration of an antidepressant.

Detre and Jarecki (1971) also recognized that the benzodiazepines have a place in the treatment of anxious patients with depressed moods. Their approach differs in that they recommend concurrent administration of either a monoamine oxidase inhibitor or a tricyclic antidepressant with the benzodiazepine. Their rationale is that since benzodiazepines act promptly, they afford temporary relief of certain symptoms (e.g., agitation, insomnia, anorexia) thus making the patient more comfortable for a few weeks until the antidepressant takes effect. Rickels (*personal communication,* 1974) believes that benzodiazepines help patients to tolerate tricyclic antidepressants better.

The response to therapy is influenced also by the physician's sensitivity. Apart from his sympathetic understanding, and reassuring attitude, his familiarity with the use of a particular drug and general confidence in its efficacy compared with other modalities may well affect the patient's salutary response. In a study by Uhlenhuth, Rickels, Fisher, Park, Lipman, and Mock (1966), an active drug was compared with a placebo in a double-blind manner. There was an additional variable in this trial: two physicians did the prescribing. One took a "therapeutic" stance, had confidence in the treatment, and was generally supportive and sympathetic; the other assumed the "experimental" stance. The difference in response between drug and placebo was significant in the hands of the first prescribing physician but not in the hands of the second. Commenting on this, Hollister (1973*a*) states: "The moral is clear: If you are going to prescribe these drugs, at least try to work up some enthusiasm for them and try to communicate it to your patients."

The "doctor variable" as a nonspecific or nondrug factor was evaluated in a collaborative double-blind clinical trial organized by the Psychopharmacology Research Branch of the National Institute of Mental Health (Rickels, Lipman, Park, Covi, Uhlenhuth, and Mock, 1971); it involved participating clinics at Johns Hopkins Hospital, Philadelphia General Hospital, and Hospital of the University of Pennsylvania. The study population comprised 485 anxious neurotic outpatients. The drugs under comparison were chlordiazepoxide, meprobamate, and placebo. Of the three possible main effects, only "doctor warmth" and "drug," but not "clinic," significantly influenced the improvement rate. Several main drug effects, present only at 2 weeks, indicated that chlordiazepoxide produced significantly more improvement than either meprobamate or placebo. The warmth effects, present only at 4 weeks, showed that patients who rated their physicians at the initial visit as warm improved significantly more than patients rating their physicians as nonwarm.

Furthermore, the drug and warmth effects were particularly marked in initially sicker patients.

Assuming that the diagnosis is correct and that the dosage is titrated optimally, some patients still fail to respond to a particular benzodiazepine and are often referred to as problem patients. Granting that some are genuinely refractory, there is the possibility that the patient will respond to another of the benzodiazepine series or to a propanediol.

Some patients are simply reluctant to continue medication for reasons other than side effects. The physician who becomes irritated with a patient's unwillingness to cooperate and "gives up on them" must recognize that the personality patterns and defenses of that patient may involve cycles of rejection, guilt, and anxiety as part of a dependency behavior pattern. Kiev (1972) suggests that these patients may find it easier to endure their original distress than to endure the fear of losing control over events or the fear of accepting responsibility for their behavior, which drug therapy may promote; he advises prescribing medication in very low doses for these patients.

Choice of Appropriate Antianxiety Drug

Based on differential pharmacological properties (e.g., antianxiety/sedative ratio, duration of action, tolerance, dependence), Hollister (1973b) described the positive and negative attributes of available drugs used to treat anxiety. Perhaps the most important attribute of the benzodiazepines is that they are "virtually suicide-proof" (Hollister, 1973b), probably because they depress the neurogenic respiratory function less than other sedative-hypnotic drugs. Greenblatt and Shader (1972) stated that "benzodiazepines provide a marked increment of safety in that fatal overdoses seldom if ever occur."

Dosage and Dosage Schedule

Recommended dosages for the treatment of anxiety must be used with the utmost flexibility within the limits of the range for each of the benzodiazepines. Dosages for both geriatric patients and children are somewhat lower. In addition to dosage differences, the recommendation for use in children at various ages differs from drug to drug.

Katz (1972) pointed out that the difference in dosage requirements by two patients for a particular drug may be as much as 10-fold. Therefore the dosage should be titrated to the patient's need for relief of symptoms in accordance with initial severity, waxing and waning of the anxiety, and occurrence of side effects. The dosage schedule should also be flexible; for example, traditional divided dosage may be inconvenient and not in consonance with the rather long plasma half-lives (12 to 30 hr) of benzodiazepines. Giving the major portion of the daytime dose at bedtime optimizes the hypnotic effect. This is important when insomnia is a component of the anxiety state (Hollister, 1973a). As a general principle, the schedule should be designed to maximize symptomatic relief and minimize daytime oversedation.

Certain pharmacokinetic differences between the various benzodiazepines must be kept in mind because they may have a bearing on dosage schedule. For example, unlike diazepam, in which both diazepam itself and its pharmacologically active metabolite desmethyldiazepam accumulate, oxazepam has a relatively short half-life and no active metabolites. One implication is that diazepam can be given in decreasing doses, whereas with oxazepam the established dosage must be maintained (Greenblatt and Shader, 1974).

If a patient is encouraged to adjust the dosage according to his subjective need but within prescribed upper limits, it cuts down unnecessary use and promotes a feeling of control by the patient (Winstead, Anderson, Eilers, Blackwell, and Zaremba, 1974). A novel study illustrating this point was conducted at the Cincinnati General Hospital on a 16-bed ward where 100 patients were admitted during a 6-month period. These psychiatric patients were allowed to seek diazepam on demand. There were three very interesting findings to emerge from the study. First, patients tended to seek drugs for the right reasons; in other words, diazepam was sought mainly for relief of anxiety. Second, patients did not use drugs excessively; on the contrary, they tended to discontinue drug use when it was not therapeutically essential. Finally, there was no evidence that patients became dependent on diazepam.

Predicting Response

There are many nonspecific factors that can influence the response to benzodiazepines. Many of these factors (e.g., patient demographic background, patient attitude, physician attitudes and expectations, illness history, treatment setting, presenting symptomatology, prognosis) have been studied (Rickels, 1973). Although there may be factors that can serve as predictors of drug response in some populations, predictors of widespread applicability have yet to be identified (Greenblatt and Shader, 1974).

Side Effects

Most side effects encountered during benzodiazepine therapy are extensions of expected pharmacological effects. CNS depression manifested primarily by drowsiness is the most frequently reported side effect.

In a study by the Boston Collaborative Drug Surveillance Program (Greenblatt and Shader, 1974), unwanted reactions were recorded for 2,086 hospitalized medical patients given chlordiazepoxide and 2,623 patients given diazepam. Apart from drowsiness (8.7% for chlordiazepoxide, 5.7% for diazepam), all other adverse effects—e.g., confusion, excitement, agitation, hypotension, vertigo, drug fever, gastrointestinal disturbances—had an incidence of less than 1.0% (range 0.2 to 0.7%). The six deaths reported occurred in patients with advanced or terminal disease.

In a subsequent study by the same group (Boston Collaborative Drug Surveillance Program, 1973), drowsiness was related to drug dosage and patient age. In both drug groups this side effect was more common with increasing daily doses. The frequency among older patients was also greater, although they did not receive higher doses. These findings further emphasize the need for careful titration of dose, especially in older patients.

Svenson and Hamilton (1966) reviewed the literature through 1965 dealing with clinical studies of chlordiazepoxide; there were 17,935 patients, the vast majority having been anxious neurotic outpatients. The findings were somewhat different in that the incidence of drowsiness was 3.9% and of ataxia 1.7%. The type of setting and of patients probably accounts for the difference in the percentage of these side effects. The incidence of all other side effects was negligible, occurring in less than 1%.

Unlike most psychotic patients, neurotics are highly sensitive to unwanted effects. These can usually be managed by simple expedients: (1) temporarily reducing the dosage; (2) adjusting the schedule to provide a higher dose at bedtime; (3) attempting to have the patient accept and live with the inconveniences for the duration of treatment; (4) eliminating or suspending use of the drug, but only if side effects do not disappear or wane with continued administration. The latter alternative is rarely necessary.

The cardinal manifestations of overdosage with the benzodiazepines are degrees of CNS depression, ranging from somnolence to coma. Minimal effects on respiration, pulse, and blood pressure are likely to be encountered unless overdosage is extreme or the patient has ingested another CNS-depressing drug. Treatment is nonspecific and supportive, e.g., gastric lavage, intravenous fluids, monitoring vital signs, maintenance of airway. CNS stimulants (e.g., caffeine sodium benzoate) may be given but are not generally recommended. Dialysis appears to be of very limited value. Generally with simple support the patient shows a gradual lessening of the CNS depression and recovers uneventfully. Occasionally there may be a temporary period of stimulation and hyperactivity during the recovery phase; barbiturates should not be used if this excitation occurs.

Hostility and Assertiveness

Whether hostility is an effect of chlordiazepoxide therapy has been under discussion for several years (Gardos, DiMascio, Salzman, and Shader, 1968; DiMascio, Shader, and Harmatz, 1969; Salzman, DiMascio, Shader, and Harmatz, 1969). In double-blind, placebo-controlled studies, the effects of chlordiazepoxide and oxazepam on feelings of hostility were compared. These studies, which emanated from the Psychopharmacology Research Laboratory of the Massachusetts Mental Health Center, were carried out in healthy male college student volunteers who were stratified for levels of anxiety according to their scores on the Taylor Manifest Anxiety Scale. Chlordiazepoxide administration for 1 week increased hostility in the high- and medium-anxious subjects, as judged by changes in scores on the Buss-Durkee Inventory. Oxazepam did not have this effect.

DiMascio (1973), who subscribes to the idea that chlordiazepoxide may increase aggressive behavior, believes that this may also be viewed as a form of self-assertiveness, which may be therapeutically beneficial. He states that this may be "considered part of the overall therapeutic movement rather than as a drug-induced behavior with adverse or negative features."

On the premise that the answer to the question of drug-released hostility should be sought not in "normal" subjects with anxiety but in anxious neurotic outpatients, Rickels and Downing (1974) analyzed data on 120 chlordiazepoxide-treated and 105 placebo-treated patients from three clinical settings: a hospital psychiatric clinic, a private general practice, and a private psychiatric practice. The daily drug regimen for 4 weeks of treatment was chlordiazepoxide 40 mg or placebo capsules. The results were evaluated (1) by physician measures (rated on a seven-point scale) of anxiety, irritability, and hostility; and (2) on patient symptom checklist ratings (on a four-point scale) of fear-anxiety and anger-hostility, e.g., "suddenly scared for no reason," "easily annoyed or irritated."

Chlordiazepoxide was significantly better than placebo in reducing hostile, irritable, and anxious symptomatology. They found no evidence that chlordiazepoxide induced or released clinical hostility in their patients and concluded that "there seems little justification for avoiding the use of chlordiazepoxide by anxious outpatients suffering from concomitant symptoms of irritability and hostility."

Anxiety in Nonpsychiatric Patients

Nonpsychiatric patients under stressful situations such as the interval prior to surgery, cardioversion, or endoscopic procedures frequently exhibit a high degree of anxiety and tension. The highly anxious preoperative patient may require excessively high doses of anesthetic agents with correspondingly increased risk. Narcotics and barbiturates as preanesthetic agents have the disadvantage of causing a profound effect on respiration and circulation and of potentiating the depressant action of anesthesia.

Steen and Hahl (1969) administered diazepam to 800 patients who underwent a variety of miscellaneous surgical procedures. Comparing the results in those receiving diazepam with those on placebo, they observed significant salutary effects on restlessness, apprehension, sedation, induction, and 24-hr recall. Changes in vital signs were not significantly different in the two groups.

Both chlordiazepoxide and diazepam are effective preanesthetic agents for reducing preoperative anxiety as well as postsurgical excitement and restlessness (Tornetta, 1965; Crawford, 1973). Diazepam is the more widely used of the two. Ease of administration, antianxiety action, a tendency to produce amnesia, and minimal effects on cardiorespiratory indices enhance its value as a preanesthetic.

A rather novel use of diazepam was reported by McClish, Andrew, and Tetreault (1968) in controlling the psychiatric reactions frequently exhibited by patients following cardiac surgery. The incidence of these complications—which may include severe anxiety, nervous tension, disorientation, confusion, depression, hostility, and even hallucinations—ranges from 3 to 46% in closed-heart surgery, 20 to 57% in open-heart operations, and 80 to 90% in cases of valve replacement. In this controlled study in consecutive, un-selected patients undergoing open-heart surgery with extracorporeal circulation, diazepam was effective in preventing and terminating postoperative psychiatric reactions. In the control group of 37 patients, 13 (35.1%) had postoperative psychiatric reactions, eight of which were minor and five major. Among the 42 diazepam-treated patients, only two (4.7%) had minor reactions; this group had received diazepam, 2.5 to 5.0 mg i.v. every 4 hr, in addition to the usual postoperative analgesic medications. These patients were also noted to be calm, relaxed, cooperative, conversant, and slightly drowsy during the postoperative period. Prolonged intubation with respiratory assistance, when needed, was well tolerated for 48 to 72 hr. There was no need for muscle relaxants or large doses of narcotics, and insomnia was no longer a problem. The investigators stated: "Above all, intravenous diazepam produced very good amnesia," with patients rarely recalling their stay in the intensive care unit. The drug also was effective in terminating the psychiatric reactions which occurred in the control group.

Intravenous diazepam may be a useful adjunct in endoscopic procedures (e.g., bronchoscopy, cystoscopy, peritoneoscopy). It may afford relief of apprehension and anxiety, promote cooperation of the patient, and reduce or eliminate the need for narcotics (Ticktin and Trujillo, 1968; Akdamar, Lilly, Mary, and Maumus, 1971).

Cardioversion by precordial direct-current countershock for the termination of arrhythmias is uncomfortable to the conscious patient. Anesthesia presents a hazard that cannot be minimized in patients with heart disease. In addition to relieving anxiety and tension and reducing recall of the procedure, an intravenous injection of diazepam circumvents some practical problems: the need for an anesthesiologist, medical preparation of the patient, and scheduling of the operating room (Nutter and Massumi, 1965; Roth, Ferando, Sr. Maureen Patricia, Chrystal, Shields, and Pierce, 1968; Lebowitz, 1969; Lown, 1969).

Acute Alcohol Withdrawal

For some time now the benzodiazepines have commonly replaced many medications (e.g., phenothiazines, barbiturates, meprobamate, paraldehyde) as adjunctive treatment in the management of acute alcohol withdrawal. For at least a decade Kaim, Klett, and Rothfeld (1969) and Kissin and Gross (1968) have used chlordiazepoxide as the standard drug in treatment of the acute withdrawal syndrome. In the majority of cases, intramuscular chlordiazepoxide, 50 to 100 mg initially and every few hours as needed, produced satisfactory sedation by itself, although supportive measures were provided concurrently (Becker and Scott, 1972). After initial intramuscular administration, most clinicians give smaller doses by mouth.

Several investigators (Spenader and Schwamberger, 1971; Brown, Moggey, and Shane, 1972; Becker and Scott, 1972) have favored the use of diazepam. Although the results in general have been comparable to those with chlordiazepoxide, according to Brown et al. (1972), diazepam has a more rapid onset of action in the treatment of delirium tremens, provides greater control over restlessness and agitation, and affords better sleep. The dosage is more precise and predictable than with chlordiazepoxide. The fact that it has a greater anticonvulsant effect may also be an advantage.

Benzodiazepines and Sleep

Certain benzodiazepines are effective hypnotic agents and affect sleep patterns in a number of ways. They can lengthen total sleep time, shorten the onset of sleep, reduce the number of awakenings, and improve the subjective quality of sleep. When there is continuous administration over a period of time, these drugs tend to reduce sleep stages 3 and 4 (Oswald, Lewis, Tagney, Firth, and Haider, 1973). They produce little alteration in rapid eye movement (REM) sleep and in particular do not cause REM rebound following drug withdrawal (Kales and Scharf, 1973). In contrast, most nonbenzodiazepine hypnotics consistently depress REM sleep and produce rebound following withdrawal (Greenblatt and Shader, 1974).

In the United States flurazepam is the benzodiazepine prescribed for its hypnotic properties only. It is useful in all types of insomnia: difficulty in falling asleep, frequent nocturnal awakenings, early morning awakenings. Dement and co-workers noted that with flurazepam there appeared to be a carryover effect of both subjective and objective improvement in sleep parameters for at least one night after the active drug was replaced by placebo (Dement, Zarcone, Hoddes, Smythe, and Carskadon, 1973). They also noted that the carryover was not associated with a hangover during the day. These investigators observed that although flurazepam significantly reduces slow-wave sleep, it does not have a profoundly suppressive effect on REM sleep, in contrast to many hypnotics.

A major advantage of a benzodiazepine hypnotic like flurazepam is its relative safety (Koch-Weser and Greenblatt, 1974). The risk resulting from barbiturate overdosage is well known; this has not been shown to be the case with flurazepam. On the basis of risk as well as other factors—REM suppression and rebound, enzyme induction, and propensity to dependence—

Koch-Weser and Greenblatt (1974) concluded that barbiturates should not be used as hypnotics.

On the basis that diazepam suppresses stage 4 sleep, Fisher and co-workers administered the drug to a small group of patients suffering from night terrors, which are known to arise from stage 4 sleep (Fisher, Kahn, Edwards, and Davis, 1973). The night terrors were markedly reduced or eliminated within a week or two by the administration of 5 to 20 mg diazepam at bedtime. The suppressing effect was roughly dose-related, and the drug remained effective over a prolonged period.

INTERACTIONS WITH OTHER DRUGS

Drug interactions that modify pharmacological responsiveness in man are attributed to a variety of factors, e.g., alteration in the rate of drug metabolism or excretion, interference with absorption from the gastrointestinal tract, displacement from protein binding sites (Solomon, Barakat, and Ashley, 1971).

Benzodiazepines potentiate the depressant effect of ethyl alcohol in man; and in animals they potentiate the central depressant properties of barbiturates and other hypnotic agents. In view of this, patients should be cautioned about possible combined effects of benzodiazepines plus alcohol and other CNS depressants.

Enzyme induction, a property of many chemicals, notably phenobarbital, may affect the metabolism of other drugs such as coumarin anticoagulants. The interference of barbiturates with oral anticoagulant therapy has created some serious problems in medical management (Koch-Weser and Sellers, 1971). There is little evidence that benzodiazepines cause clinically significant enzyme induction in man (Greenblatt and Shader, 1974), making them especially useful as antianxiety agents in coronary care patients, who frequently receive anticoagulants.

DRUG DEPENDENCY

Tolerance—the need for increasing doses of a drug to obtain the same pharmacological effect—is a major factor in the development of addiction. Tolerance is much less of a problem with the benzodiazepines than with phenobarbital or meprobamate. This relative lack of tolerance coupled with a long duration of action makes the benzodiazepines unlikely to produce physical dependence (Hollister, 1973a).

Even if physical dependence on the benzodiazepines is virtually nonexistent, does psychological dependence develop leading to overuse or abuse? Factors favoring the development of psychic dependence on a drug include rapid onset of action, euphoriant effect, and absence of unpleasant side effects. Although the benzodiazepines have a relatively rapid onset of action, they are generally not considered to produce euphoria and at higher doses cause ataxia, an unpleasant side effect.

Studying patterns of abuse of and dependence on drugs, Glatt (1968) found from his experience in terms of chlordiazepoxide that occasional "unstable personalities" who take any CNS drug in excess find to their disgust that the drug in high doses fails to provide a desirable experience. Ayd (1972) noted similar characteristics in the "infinitesimally few abusers" of the minor tranquilizers. His findings were that almost invariably the abusers were "unstable, inadequate personalities with histories of prior abuse of alcohol and/or drugs." Accordingly, the benzodiazepines should be administered to dependent-prone individuals with special caution.

One investigational approach to drug dependency involves observations of the differential effects of drugs (stimulants and depressants) on REM sleep (Kales, 1969). As noted above, nonbenzodiazepine hypnotics decrease the amount of REM sleep, and REM rebound follows their withdrawal. Marked clinical disturbances, including unpleasant dreams, nightmares, and insomnia, are associated with these rebound increases in REM sleep time. To avoid these unpleasant rebound phenomena, patients resume and continue to take the drugs. Kales believes that this vicious circle appears to be an important factor in the development of drug dependency. If, as has been speculated, the unpleasant physiological changes after drug withdrawal are crucial factors in the development of drug dependency, it appears by the above criteria that this phenomenon would not occur with the benzodiazepines.

In 1961 Hollister, Motzenbecker, and Degan administered chlordiazepoxide in daily doses of 300 to 600 mg to schizophrenic patients for 2 to 6 months and then abruptly discontinued the drug. They noted definite withdrawal symptoms, which developed more slowly and were less acute than those with barbiturates or meprobamate. However, a decade later Hollister stated that physical dependence to chlordiazepoxide occurs only with excessive doses over prolonged periods, as in the 1961 study. Furthermore, he wrote: "Over the years, it has been difficult to find well-documented cases of withdrawal reaction associated with clinical use of benzodiazepines" (Hollister, 1973a).

It is worth mentioning that some clinicians postulate that what might be interpreted as withdrawal phenomena in certain instances is in reality a reemergence of symptoms (Covi, Lipman, Pattison, Derogatis, and Uhlenhuth, 1973). Pretreatment symptoms controlled by the drug may return on discontinuance of therapy.

The consensus appears to be that dependency on the benzodiazepines is unlikely within the recommended therapeutic doses; the risk seems to be associated with excessive doses given for extended periods of time. Actual addiction to them appears to be a rare possibility, despite the large number of patients taking benzodiazepines throughout the world.

TREATMENT SUMMARY

Generic name	Trade name	Daily dosage range (mg)
Diazepam	Valium	4–40[a]
Clorazepate	Tranxene	15–60[a]
Chlordiazepoxide	Librium	15–100[a]
Oxazepam	Serax	30–120[a]
Flurazepam	Dalmane	15–30[b]

[a] Dosage range for treatment of anxiety.
[b] Dosage range for treatment of insomnia.

REFERENCES

Akdamar, K., Lilly, J. O., Mary, C. C., and Maumus, L. (1971): Peritoneoscopy facilitated by premedication with diazepam. *South. Med. J.,* 64:891–893.

Ayd, F. J., Jr. (1972): Patterns, range and effects of misused psychotropic substances in North America today. *World Med. J.,* 19:9–13.

Becker, C. D., and Scott, R. (1972): The treatment of alcoholism. *Ration. Drug Ther.,* 6:1–8.

Boston Collaborative Drug Surveillance Program (1973): Clinical depression of the central nervous system due to diazepam and chlordiazepoxide in relation to cigarette smoking and age. *N. Engl. J. Med.,* 288:277–280.

Brown, J. H., Moggey, D. E., and Shane, F. H. (1972): Delirium tremens: A comparison of intravenous treatment with diazepam and chlordiazepoxide. *Scott. Med. J.,* 17:9–12.

Cazzullo, C. L. (1969): Drug treatment of anxiety. In: *Studies of Anxiety,* edited by M. H. Lader. Headley Brothers, Ashford, Kent, Great Britain.

Cohen, S. (1965): *Modern Treatment.* Harper & Row, New York.

Covi, L., Lipman, R. S., Pattison, J. H., Derogatis, L. R., and Uhlenhuth, E. H. (1973): Length of treatment with anxiolytic sedatives and response to their sudden withdrawal. *Acta Psychiatr. Scand.,* 49:51–64.

Crawford, T. I. (1973): Preanesthetic medication in elective surgery: Comparison of intravenous diazepam with meperidine. *Curr. Ther. Res.,* 15:441–448.

Dement, W. C., Zarcone, V. P., Hoddes, E., Smythe, H., and Carskadon, M. (1973): Sleep laboratory and clinical studies with flurazepam. In: *The Benzodiazepines,* edited by S. Garattini, E. Mussini, and L. O. Randall. Raven Press, New York.

Detre, T. P., and Jarecki, H. G. (1971): *Modern Psychiatric Treatment.* Lippincott, Philadelphia.

DiMascio, A. (1973): The effects of benzodiazepines on aggression: Reduced or increased? *Psychopharmacologia,* 30:95–102.

DiMascio, A., Shader, R. I., and Harmatz, J. S. (1969): Psychotropic drugs and induced hostility. *Psychosomatics,* 10:46–47.

Fisher, C., Kahn, E., Edwards, A., and Davis, D. (1973): A psychophysiological study of nightmares and night terrors. *Arch. Gen. Psychiatry,* 28:252–259.

Gardos, G., DiMascio, A., Salzman, C., and Shader, R. I. (1968): Differential actions of chlordiazepoxide and oxazepam on hostility. *Arch. Gen. Psychiatry,* 18:757–760.

Glatt, M. M. (1968): Recent patterns of abuse of and dependence on drugs. *Br. J. Addict.,* 63:111–128.

Gluckman, M. I. (1965): Pharmacology of oxazepam (Serax), a new antianxiety agent. *Curr. Ther. Res.,* 7:721–740.

Greenblatt, D. J., and Shader, R. I. (1972): The clinical choice of sedative-hypnotics. *Ann. Intern. Med.,* 77:91–100.

Greenblatt, D. J., and Shader, R. I. (1974): *Benzodiazepines in Clinical Practice.* Raven Press, New York.

Hollister, L. E. (1973a): *Clinical Use of Psychotherapeutic Drugs.* Charles C Thomas, Springfield, Ill.

Hollister, L. E. (1973b): Uses of psychotherapeutic drugs. *Ann. Intern. Med.,* 79:88–98.

Hollister, L. E., Motzenbecker, F. P., and Degan, R. O. (1961): Withdrawal reactions from chlordiazepoxide ('Librium'). *Psychopharmacologia,* 2:63–68.

Hollister, L. E., Overall, J. E., Pokorny, A. D., and Shelton, J. (1971): Acetophenazine and diazepam in anxious depressions. *Arch. Gen. Psychiatry,* 24:273–278.

Kaim, S. C., Klett, C. J., and Rothfeld, B. (1969): Treatment of the acute alcohol withdrawal state: A comparison of four drugs. *Am. J. Psychiatry,* 125:1640–1646.

Kales, A. (1969): Drug dependency: Investigations of stimulants and depressants. *Ann. Intern. Med.,* 70:591–614.

Kales, A., and Scharf, M. B. (1973): Sleep laboratory and clinical studies of the effects of benzodiazepines on sleep: flurazepam, diazepam, chlordiazepoxide, and Ro 5–4200. In: *The Benzodiazepines,* edited by S. Garattini, E. Mussini, and L. O. Randall. Raven Press, New York.

Katz, R. L. (1972): Drug therapy: Sedatives and tranquilizers. *N. Engl. J. Med.,* 286:757–760.

Kiev, A. (1972): Minor tranquilizers: Perceptive management of the anxious patient. *Drug Ther.,* 2:105–116.

Kissin, B., and Gross, M. M. (1968): Drug therapy in alcoholism. *Am. J. Psychiatry,* 125:31–41.

Koch-Weser, J., and Greenblatt, D. J. (1974): The archaic barbiturate hypnotics. *N. Engl. J. Med.,* 291:790–791.

Koch-Weser, J., and Sellers, E. M. (1971): Drug interactions with coumarin anticoagulants. *N. Engl. J. Med.,* 285:487–498, 547–558.

Lebowitz, W. B. (1969): Electrical conversion of arrhythmias under diazepam sedation. *Conn. Med.,* 33:173–174.

Lown, B. (1969): Cardioversion. *S.D. J. Med.,* 22:21–23.

McClish, A., Andrew, D., and Tetreault, L. (1968): Intravenous diazepam for psychiatric reactions following open-heart surgery. *Can. Anaesth. Soc. J.,* 15:63–79.

Nutter, D. O., and Massumi, R. A. (1965): Brief recording: Diazepam in cardioversion. *N. Engl. J. Med.,* 273:650.

Oswald, I., Lewis, S. A., Tagney, J., Firth, H., and Haider, I. (1973): Benzodiazepines and human sleep. In: *The Benzodiazepines,* edited by S. Garattini, E. Mussini, and L. O. Randall. Raven Press, New York.

Randall, L. O., and Kappell, B. (1973): Pharmacological activity of some benzodiazepines and their metabolites. In: *The Benzodiazepines,* edited by S. Garattini, E. Mussini, and L. O. Randall. Raven Press, New York.

Rickels, K. (1973): Predictors of response to benzodiazepines in anxious outpatients. In: *The Benzodiazepines,* edited by S. Grattini, E. Mussini, and L. O. Randall. Raven Press, New York.

Rickels, K., and Downing, R. W. (1974): Chlordiazepoxide and hostility in anxious outpatients. *Am. J. Psychiatry,* 131:442–444.

Rickels, K., Lipman, R. S., Park, L. C., Covi, L., Uhlenhuth, E. H., and Mock, J. E. (1971): Drug, doctor warmth, and clinic setting in the symptomatic response to minor tranquilizers. *Psychopharmacologia,* 20:128–152.

Roth, O., Ferando, L., Sr. Maureen Patricia, Chrystal, L., Shields, M., and Pierce, J. (1968): Organization of a four-bed coronary care unit at the Hospital of St. Raphael. *Conn. Med.,* 32:214–220.

Salzman, C., DiMascio, A., Shader, R. I., and Harmatz, J. S. (1969): Chlordiazepoxide, expectation and hostility. *Psychopharmacologia,* 14:38–45.

Schallek, W., Schlosser, W., and Randall, L. O. (1972): Recent developments in the pharmacology of the benzodiazepines. In: *Adv. Pharmacol. Chemother.,* 10:121–128.

Solomon, H. M., Barakat, M. J., and Ashley, C. J. (1971): Mechanisms of drug interaction. *J.A.M.A.,* 216:1997–1999.

Spenader, W. F., and Schwamberger, B. V. (1971): The treatment of acute alcoholism in a small rural hospital. *Ill. Med. J.,* 140:508, 530–531.

Steen, S. N., and Hahl, D. (1969): Controlled evaluation of parenteral diazepam as preanesthetic medication: A statistical study. *Anesth. Analg. (Cleve.),* 48:549–554.

Svenson, S. E., and Hamilton, R. G. (1966): A critique of overemphasis on side effects with the psychotropic drugs: An analysis of 18,000 chlordiazepoxide-treated cases. *Curr. Ther. Res.,* 8:455–464.

Ticktin, H. E., and Trujillo, N. P. (1968): Further experience with diazepam for pre-endoscopic medication. *Gastrointest. Endosc.,* 15:91–92.

Tornetta, F. J. (1965): Diazepam as preanesthetic medication. *Anesth. Analg. (Cleve.),* 44:449–452.

Uhlenhuth, E. H., Rickels, K., Fisher, S., Park, L. C., Lipman, R. S., and Mock, J. (1966): Drug, doctor's verbal attitude and clinic setting in the symptomatic response to pharmacotherapy. *Psychopharmacologia,* 9:392–418.

Winstead, D. K., Anderson, A., Eilers, M. K., Blackwell, B., and Zaremba, A. L. (1974): Diazepam on demand: Drug-seeking behavior in psychiatric inpatients. *Arch. Gen. Psychiatry,* 30:349–351.

Chapter 7

Therapeutic Uses of Meprobamate and the Propanediols

F. M. Berger

The propanediol derivatives were among the first psychotropic agents successfully used in the treatment of psychoneurotic patients (Fig. 1). Since their introduction during the late 1940s, numerous other drugs for the treatment of psychoneurotic patients have been developed. Among these, meprobamate,

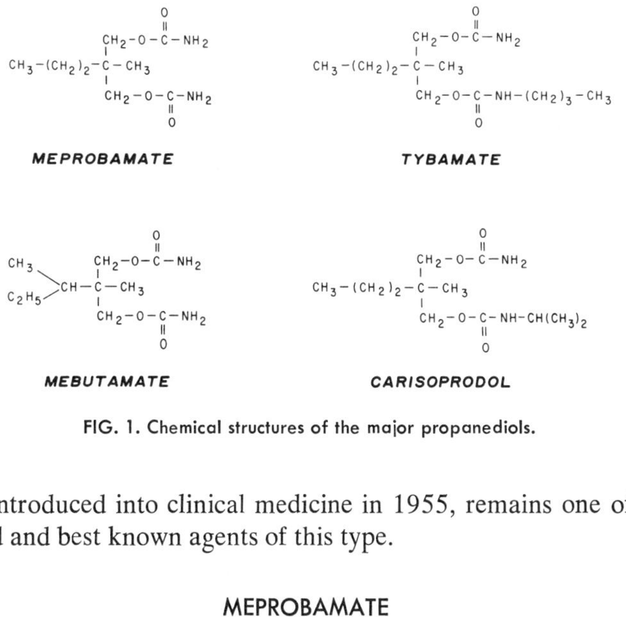

FIG. 1. Chemical structures of the major propanediols.

originally introduced into clinical medicine in 1955, remains one of the most widely used and best known agents of this type.

MEPROBAMATE

Pharmacological Basis for Clinical Use of Meprobamate

The clinical use of meprobamate, or any other drug for that matter, should be based on the pharmacological properties of the drug. The sites and structures in the central nervous system (CNS) that are preferentially affected by the drug and the manner in which the drug affects these sites should be taken into consideration.

The structural units of the CNS that appear selectively affected by meprobamate are the interneurons (Berger, 1954). The interneurons comprise a network of neurons within the CNS that connect the sensory input lines with the outgoing connections leading to the effector organs. Meprobamate selectively depresses conductivity of the interneuron. The drug is particularly effective in this respect when the interneurons are in a state of hyperexcitability. Under these conditions, incoming stimuli reverberate for long periods of time along the interneuronal circuits. These reverberations may constitute the neurological modality responsible for the irritability, emotional overreactivity, and psychological rigidity so characteristic of the psychoneurotic state. Anxiety itself, which is known to be associated with increased reactivity of specific areas of the brain, may be due to the hyperexcitability of the interneurons located in the thalamus and limbic system (Berger, 1970).

The two sites in the brain characteristically affected by meprobamate are the thalamus and the limbic system (Berger, 1968). Both structures, which form a functional unit, are very rich in interneurons and are closely interconnected through them. The limbic system is considered the seat of emotional life, while the thalamus is the area through which emotional stimuli enter consciousness.

Short electrical stimulation of a part of the limbic system produces long-lasting seizure discharges that continue long after cessation of the stimulation that induced them. The seizure discharges remain confined to the limbic system and do not spread to the cortex. Meprobamate, in a characteristic and specific manner, either prevents the occurrence of these discharges or greatly shortens their duration (Kletzkin and Berger, 1959). It is of particular interest that antidepressants such as imipramine or amitriptyline possess a similar action on seizure discharges induced by stimulation of limbic structures (Berger, Kletzkin, and Margolin, 1967). It may well be that this phenomenon represents the common physical basis for the action of meprobamate and related tranquilizers, and of the antidepressant drugs. The effect of meprobamate on limbic seizure discharges may be the mechanism responsible for the antidepressant activity of this drug.

Meprobamate induces characteristic changes in the spontaneous electrical activity of the thalamus (Hendly, Lynes, and Berger, 1957). These changes consist of a synchronization of electrical activity and thus could also be interpreted as decreasing and counteracting the state of hyperreactivity that may be the basis of psychoneurotic disease and anxiety states.

Meprobamate has little or no effect on the cortex. Unlike barbiturates, it does not elevate the threshold of stimulation for motor responses (Berger, 1968) and does not produce excitation prior to inhibition in animals (Read, Cutting, and Furst, 1960). Similarly, meprobamate produces no disinhibition of higher cortical processes in humans (Lehmann, 1968).

The effectiveness of meprobamate in psychosomatic conditions may be based on the ability of the drug to counteract the autonomic concomitants of conditioned reflexes. The classical conditioned reflex is always accompanied by autonomic responses—e.g., increase in heart rate, blood pressure, and respiration; inhibition of urine secretion; or alteration of the electrocardiogram (Gantt, 1960). The autonomic concomitants of conditioning may represent a response to a stressful situation. They develop rapidly and persist even after the classical conditioned reflex has disappeared. In contrast to drugs such as chlorpromazine and reserpine, meprobamate markedly diminishes the cardiac component of the conditional reflex while leaving the motor component intact (Gantt, 1964). It is also effective in counteracting the conditioned antidiuretic response in dogs (Corson, O'Leary, Dykman, Peters, Reese, and Seager, 1962).

Use of Meprobamate in Medicine

Apart from its antianxiety effect, meprobamate also has a relaxant action on skeletal muscles and an anticonvulsant activity. For this reason it has been recommended in the past for the treatment of certain musculoskeletal disorders in which muscle spasm was a factor, and in the treatment of certain petit mal and related minor epilepsies. More effective and specific remedies for the treatment of the latter two conditions have now become available (e.g., the benzodiazepines). At the present time meprobamate and related propanediols are being found useful in the treatment of psychoneurotic disease, insomnia, certain depressive states, and psychosomatic conditions. The rationale for the use of the drug in these conditions is as follows.

Psychoneurotic Disease

Freud considered anxiety the fundamental and central problem of the psychoneurotic state. As a result of this attitude, "psychoneurotic disease" is no longer mentioned in some textbooks of psychiatry, having been replaced by the "anxiety state." Although anxiety, particularly when occurring in acute attacks, is an important symptom of psychoneurosis, it is not the only manifestation of the psychoneurotic state. Other psychological, primarily subjective symptoms (e.g., restlessness, irritability, hyperexcitability, psychological rigidity, fatigue, insatiability) may be of equal or greater importance in individual cases. Psychoneurosis is also accompanied by objectively assessable symptoms that can be considered physiological concomitants of anxiety, e.g., breathlessness, increased muscular tension, sweating, trembling, broken sleep. Meprobamate appears effective in relieving all these symptoms, as long as they are due to the underlying psychoneurotic disease.

Meprobamate and many other "minor" tranquilizers (e.g., the benzodiazepines) are often classified as "anxiolytics." This term has a limited usefulness for two reasons. First, it implies that these drugs are effective only in the treatment of anxiety; and second, that they are capable of relieving anxiety irrespective of its etiology. Both these assumptions are incorrect. Like many other drugs of this class, meprobamate, while possessing a powerful antianxiety action, is equally effective in relieving many other symptoms of psychoneurosis. These drugs, however, possess an anxiolytic action only when the anxiety is a manifestation of psychoneurotic disease. Thus meprobamate is of little value in the control of anxiety due to schizophrenia. Similarly, it does not affect anxiety resulting from a fear of punishment (Pronko and Kenyon, 1959), does not counteract fatigue (Holliday and Devery, 1962), and does not facilitate the encounter with unanticipated "socially taboo" words (Peterson, Haun, and Upton, 1962).

Meprobamate is rapidly absorbed after oral administration, and the peak concentration in plasma is attained within 1 hr. For this reason the drug is particularly well suited for treating acute attacks of anxiety and restlessness, as well as insomnia. In addition, meprobamate exerts its antianxiety effect immediately on absorption and does not require metabolic conversion to a more potent compound, as is the case with some of the benzodiazepines. Because of these considerations meprobamate appears to be the treatment of choice in acute attacks of anxiety and restlessness.

Insomnia

The effectiveness of meprobamate in insomnia, particularly when this condition is due to physical and emotional tension, is well documented. In a double-blind study of chronically ill hospitalized patients, Lasagna (1956) found meprobamate to be about as effective in relieving insomnia as phenobarbital, in regard to both time of onset and duration of effect. Keller and Vogt (1958), in a placebo-controlled study of patients suffering from severe neuroses, reactive depression, and headaches, found the drug effective in relieving insomnia without producing nightmares, drowsiness, or a slowed-down feeling.

In outpatients suffering from psychoneurosis, Rickels and co-workers found meprobamate consistently and significantly more effective in relieving insomnia than amobarbital or prochlorperazine (Rickels, Clark, Ewing, Klingensmith, and Morris, 1959). The beneficial effect of meprobamate on insomnia could not be attributed primarily to a sedative effect alone, since very little clinical sedation occurred. The best results were achieved when the patient took meprobamate regularly during the day and not just at night.

In a double-blind crossover study in geriatric inpatients with insomnia, flurazepam (7.5 mg) was in most cases equivalent to meprobamate (200 mg). Flurazepam, however, produced a greater incidence of unwanted side effects, especially skin reactions and nightmares. The authors of the study concluded that meprobamate is still the hypnotic of choice among the aged (Keston and Brocklehurst, 1974). The greater acceptance of meprobamate over flurazepam may be due to the fact that meprobamate does not interfere with the high-voltage, slow-wave stage 4 sleep (Freemon, Agnew, and Williams, 1965), whereas pentobarbital, chlordiazepoxide, diazepam, and flurazepam significantly decrease the duration of this sleep stage (Kales, Scharf, Ling-Tan, Kales, Allen, and Malmstrom, 1969).

Oswald and Priest (1965) pointed out that the brain processes underlying normal sleep may be disturbed by a barbiturate or a benzodiazepine drug, and that return to normal may take several weeks. This long-lasting effect may be due to the slow rate at which these drugs are metabolized and eliminated from the body. Meprobamate, which is degraded and eliminated more rapidly, would not be expected to cause such long-lasting disturbances of the brain wave patterns.

Depression

It is well recognized that anxiety and depression are closely related and interlocked forms of emotional response. Nevertheless, there is solid evidence indicating that there are two distinct syndromes corresponding to anxiety and depression (Roth, Gurney, Garside, and Kerr, 1972). This finding does not conflict with the presence of isolated depressive symptoms in patients suffering from anxiety states and anxiety symptoms in patients with depression. However, symptoms of anxiety and depression coexist in most patients. Among 365 neurotic outpatients consecutively referred to a psychopharmcology research clinic located in a large municipal hospital, only 16% were diagnosed as purely anxious and only 5% as purely depressed (Rickels, Downing, Raab, and Hesbacker, 1967a).

Meprobamate has been found of greatest value in reactive depressions and in those cases in which anxiety was a prominent symptom (Phillips, 1956; Tucker, 1957). Hollister and co-workers found meprobamate helpful in all types of depression, and noted that those who had failed to benefit had been on relatively low doses (Hollister, Elkins, Hiler, and St. Pierre, 1957). They recommended that with the exception of critical situations, a brief, intensive course of meprobamate be tried before a decision is made to use shock therapy.

The antidepressant action of meprobamate also became apparent during a clinical evaluation of tranquilizing drugs in medical outpatients (Rickels et al., 1959). These investigators, in a double-blind, well-controlled study, found meprobamate markedly and significantly superior to amobarbital and prochlorperazine in the treatment of depression and irritability, confirming previously reported studies (West and da Fonseca, 1956; Ruchwarger, 1959). In the treatment of anxiety symptoms, amobarbital and meprobamate were similarly superior to placebo and prochlorperazide.

Subsequently the effect of protriptyline, meprobamate, and the combination of the two drugs was studied in depressed neurotic patients (Rickels, Raab, DeSilverio, and Etemad, 1967b). After 2 weeks of treatment, only patients treated with meprobamate and the combination, but not with protriptyline alone, improved significantly more than those given placebo. At this time the effect of the drug combination and of meprobamate were indistinguishable from each other. After 4 weeks of treatment, protriptyline displayed significant antidepressant activity which was equal to but not greater than that of meprobamate given alone. Thus protriptyline, although no more effective than meprobamate in this population, displayed a slower onset of action. It was clinically most effective in low-anxiety patients but was ineffective in high-anxiety, depressed patients. Meprobamate and a combination of meprobamate with protriptyline produced significant improvement in both high- and low-anxiety, depressed patients.

Imipramine is primarily effective in the treatment of endogenous depression and ineffective in neurotic depression (Kiloh and Garnside, 1963). Meprobamate, on the other hand, was clinically most effective in depressed patients with high concomitant anxiety and hypochondriacal features, as well as in depressed patients who tend to express their symptoms as somatic manifestations (Rickels, Ward, and Schut, 1964).

Psychosomatic Conditions

Depending on one's outlook and orientation, anxiety and depression can be considered either as underlying causes or as symptoms of disease. Perhaps they can be both. If they are considered to be the underlying causes of a disease, we call the disease psychosomatic. In this case life stresses greater than can be handled by an individual can lead to structural changes in organs that may be life-threatening. In psychosomatic conditions the physical symptoms dominate the clinical picture, although emotional factors play a causative or contributory role. Conditions that may have a psychosomatic origin are headache, backache, bronchial spasm, hypertension, peptic ulcer, irritable colon, various skin conditions, and many others. The psychosomatic conditions (sometimes also called psychophysiological, autonomic, and visceral disorders) can be differentiated from psychoneurotic disease and depression by a tendency to a predominant and persistent involvement of a single organ system and the relative absence of anxiety and depressive symptoms. Meprobamate is of value in the treatment of many psychosomatic conditions (e.g., headaches, gastrointestinal and cardiovascular disorders), as a useful adjunct in the treatment of gynecological disorders (e.g., premenstrual tension, menopause), and in the treatment of dermatological conditions, particularly when a strong emotional component is present.

In a controlled study Friedman (1957) found meprobamate superior to chlorpromazine, reserpine, and placebo in the preventive treatment of headache. Bodi (1969) demonstrated that short-term therapy with large doses of meprobamate produced favorable therapeutic effects in hospitalized patients with intractable peptic ulcers. Relief of pain and other symptoms was prompt, within 1 to 3 days, and there was complete healing in most cases within 8 to 12 days. Meprobamate and other tranquilizers also proved useful in the management of geriatric patients with functional bowel distress (Sklar, 1970). Numerous clinical reports indicated that antianxiety drugs are useful adjuncts in the treatment of heart disease. Meprobamate was effective in relieving anxiety in cardiac neuroses and in easing the patient's adjustment to his condition.

Differences Between Meprobamate and the Benzodiazepines

Diazepam and chlordiazepoxide, the two most important members of the benzodiazepine series, and meprobamate, the principal representative of the propanediols, share many pharmacological properties. Both classes of drugs possess skeletal muscle relaxant, anticonvulsant, and antianxiety properties; have a depressant effect on interneurons; and affect primarily the structures of the limbic system. The only important differences between the two classes of drugs lie in the area of metabolism. Meprobamate has a relatively short duration of action and is rapidly eliminated from the body in the form of pharmacologically inactive, highly water-soluble metabolites. In contrast, the benzodiazepines are long-acting; their metabolites are sometimes as potent or more potent than the parent compound; and they persist in the body for several days before being completely eliminated.

Absorption and Distribution

Propanediols and benzodiazepines after oral absorption easily pass the blood-brain barrier and are present in similar concentrations in all tissues of the body. There is little or no evidence to indicate selective accumulation of these compounds in any particular part of the brain. Thus blood or plasma levels of these drugs and of their pharmacologically active metabolites in individuals not habituated to these agents correlate well with the observed clinical effectiveness of these drugs.

With meprobamate, peak blood levels occur 1 to 2 hr after oral administration. A steady decline in concentration occurs thereafter, with a half-life of approximately 10 hr (Hollister and Levy, 1964; Ludwig and Potterfield, 1971). Benzodiazepines and barbiturates remain in the blood for longer periods of time. Single oral doses of diazepam (10 mg) produced blood levels with a half-life of 27.5 hr (de Silva, Koechlin, and Basler, 1966). With a single oral dose of chlordiazepoxide (15 mg), the blood level half-life was 2.5 days (Koechlin and d'Arconte, 1963). Secobarbital was also cleared slowly from blood with a half-life of 28.9 hr (Clifford, Cookson, and Wickham, 1974).

Biotransformation and Excretion

The most abundant metabolite of meprobamate is the hydroxylated derivative 2-(p-hydroxypropyl)-2-methyl-1,3-propanediol dicarbamate (Ludwig, Douglas, Powell, Meyer, and Berger, 1961). This compound proved to be a true detoxification product of meprobamate in that it was very highly water soluble and pharmacologically inert. The rest of the ingested meprobamate is excreted in the urine in the form of a glucuronide of unaltered meprobamate (Berger, 1954). Both metabolites are rapidly eliminated from the body; most appear in the urine within 24 hr, and all are eliminated within 48 hr.

Many benzodiazepines share the same metabolic pathways, and in some instances the metabolites seem to be as clinically effective as the parent compound (Tyrer, 1974). Benzodiazepines are metabolized in the body by N-demethylation and hydroxylation. The metabolites are eliminated more slowly in man than are the parent drugs, are pharmacologically active, and contribute significantly to the therapeutic effect of the drug (Randall and Kappell, 1973). The biotransformation of diazepam, the most widely used and most thoroughly studied benzodiazepine, proceeds in several stages (Garattini, Mussini, Marcucci, and Guaitani, 1973). Diazepam undergoes a process of N-demethylation to nordiazepam (desmethyldiazepam) and a process of C3-hydroxylation to form N1-methyloxazepam. These two metabolites are then further N1-demethylated and C3-hydroxylated to form a common metabolite, oxazepam. Repeated administration of diazepam leads to nordiazepam blood levels that are even higher than those of the parent drug, because nordiazepam persists in blood longer than diazepam itself. It also appears that the various pharmacological properties of these drugs (e.g., anticonvulsant, muscle relaxant, antiaggressive action) that can be demonstrated after administration of benzodiazepines may depend on the blood levels of specific metabolites as well as on the blood level of the parent compound. Metabolites of benzodiazepines are present in urine for about 2 weeks after the administration of these drugs (Koechlin and d'Arconte, 1963; Randall and Kappell, 1973).

The duration of action of barbiturates is longer than is generally assumed. These compounds and their metabolites always persist in the body much longer than meprobamate. Pentobarbital, one of the most rapidly metabolized barbiturates, has a biotransformation half-time of approximately 50 hr after its distribution throughout the body is complete (Smith, Dittert, Griffen, and Doluisio, 1973). It takes 4 to 5 days before 50% of a single dose of pentobarbital or amobarbital is eliminated in the urine (Maynert, 1965).

Clinical Indications for Meprobamate

Although the propanediols and benzodiazepines share many pharmacological actions, they also differ in several important respects. These have to do with the metabolic transformation of these drugs in the body and the speed of excretion of these substances.

Meprobamate is rapidly absorbed and exerts its antianxiety and antidepressant actions in its unchanged form within an hour after ingestion and long before the drug has been metabolized. Diazepam (and some other benzodiazepines), on the other hand, cannot exert their full antianxiety effect until some time has elapsed. This results from two facts. First, the benzodiazepines are not absorbed as rapidly as meprobamate; and second, both the parent compound (e.g., diazepam) and its metabolites (e.g., nordiazepam) possess antianxiety activity. Time must elapse before significant amounts of the metabolite can accumulate. Because of this the full antianxiety action of benzodiazepines may not become apparent until the drugs have been administered over a period of time (Curry, 1974).

Another important difference between meprobamate and the benzodiazepines is their rate of elimination from the body. Meprobamate is rapidly eliminated in the urine, most within 24 hr and almost all within 48 hr. The benzodiazepines disappear from the body very gradually, and metabolites of these drugs may be present in the urine for as long as 2 weeks after administration has been discontinued. Because of the rapid elimination of meprobamate from the body, the drug is not likely, when given in clinically useful doses, to interfere significantly with activities of everyday living (Berger and Potterfield, 1969). Barbiturates (e.g., secobarbital), presumably because of their slow excretion, may cause impairment of performance even after a single dose (Kornetsky, Vates, and Kessler, 1959; McKensie and Elliot, 1965).

The rapid onset of action, relatively short duration of action, and rapid elimination from the body make meprobamate the drug of choice in acute anxiety states, whereas the benzodiazepines, with their more sustained action (which is slower in onset but of much longer duration), are more suited for the treatment of chronic anxiety states.

Adverse Reactions to Meprobamate

Widespread use of both the benzodiazepines and the propanediols has been associated with a low incidence of adverse reactions. Nevertheless, there are two potential sources of concern that merit attention: drug interactions and drug dependence.

Meprobamate can interact adversely with other CNS depressants. The cumulative effect of meprobamate and another depressant may be greater than would be predicted on the basis of a simple additive effect. Therefore patients should be advised not to use meprobamate together with other CNS depressants, e.g., alcohol.

Meprobamate also has a dependence liability. In other words, if the drug were to be used at high doses over an extended period of time, a patient (or a drug abuser) might become dependent on it. This dependence would manifest itself as a withdrawal syndrome when usage of the drug is abruptly discontinued. This may represent a problem for those persons who, because of personality disorders, are prone to use antianxiety drugs excessively. By contrast, the dependence liability of meprobamate is minimal in the average patient. In patients in whom problems are anticipated, meprobamate should not be used and in patients that have used the drug in excessive amounts, discontinuance of the drug should not be abrupt.

MEBUTAMATE

Mebutamate, chemically closely related to meprobamate, was originally developed in an effort to obtain a drug with a stronger depressant effect on the vasomotor centers of the brainstem than the parent compound (Berger, Douglas, Kletzkin, Ludwig, and Margolin, 1961). The blood pressure-lowering effect of mebutamate has been demonstrated in animals but was obscured in man by the hypnotic action of the drug (Bodi, Levy, Nodine, and Moyer, 1960; Morin, Turmel, Grantham, and Fortier, 1963).

Mebutamate is rapidly absorbed and rapidly eliminated after oral ingestion in adults. Maximum blood concentrations are achieved within 1 to 2 hr. Metabolic transformation leads to hydroxymebutamate, the primary metabolite; like hydroxymeprobamate, this metabolite is of unusually low toxicity and devoid of discernible pharmacological properties. The secondary metabolites are the glucuronide conjugates of mebutamate and of hydroxybutamate, both of which are rapidly eliminated in the urine (Douglas, Ludwig, Ginberg, and Berger, 1962).

Tetreault, Richer, and Bordeleau (1967) demonstrated that mebutamate was an effective hypnotic in psychiatric patients. The hypnotic efficacy of mebutamate in elderly institutionalized "insomniac" patients was further documented by Morgan, Wardell, Lasagna, Mazzullo, Weintraub, Mudholkar, and Mietlowski (1973). Mebutamate was an effective hypnotic in this population with a potency slightly greater than that of secobarbital sodium. Mebutamate (300 mg) also showed hypnotic activity which was clearly greater than placebo, whereas secobarbital sodium (100 mg) never had significantly greater activity than placebo.

In normal, noninsomniac males, mebutamate, like other hypnotics, altered the electroencephalographic (EEG) sleep profile. There was a significant reduction in REM sleep, which was seen only during the first half of the night, however. During the "withdrawal" nights there was no REM rebound, in contrast to the withdrawal REM rebound reported following REM suppression with glutethimide, pentobarbital, secobarbital, and methyprylon (Whitsett, Hoyt, Gzerwinski, and Clark, 1974). It is of particular interest that secobarbital, at a dose with a hypnotic activity no greater than placebo, had a marked effect on REM rebound, while mebutamate, which has marked hypnotic action, did not affect REM rebound. Subjects who have been taking drugs causing REM rebound and who discontinue use of the drugs usually experience nightmares, insomnia, and a feeling of having slept poorly. The absence of these complaints after administration of mebutamate may be related to the absence of REM rebound.

It is of importance and great interest that mebutamate markedly increased the stage 4 sleep (Whitsett et al., 1974). Stage 4 sleep, characterized in the EEG by large amounts of high-amplitude, slow-wave activity, is believed to be related to the physical restfulness experienced after a "good night's sleep." Many hypnotics and anxiolytics (e.g., flurazepam, pentobarbital, chlordiazepoxide, diazepam), in contrast to mebutamate, decrease the duration of stage 4 sleep (Kales et al., 1969). Meprobamate does not affect the slow-wave stage 4 sleep (Freemon et al., 1965).

Gresham, Agnew, and Williams (1965) and Mendels and Hawkins (1967) observed that stage 4 sleep is markedly short in depressed patients. A shorter duration of stage 4 sleep was also noted in patients suffering from chronic brain syndrome (Feinberg, Koresko, and Keller, 1967). Because of its unique ability to increase the deep-sleep stage 4, mebutamate may be particularly useful as a hypnotic in these conditions. It would also be the preferred hypnotic for subjects complaining of shallow sleep. Mebutamate may be preferable to barbiturates and benzodiazepines as a hypnotic because of its relatively short duration of action and rapid elimination from the body.

TYBAMATE

Tybamate is obtained from meprobamate by replacing a hydrogen on one of the carbamyl nitrogens with an N-butyl group. The drug shares many pharmacological properties with meprobamate. It differs from the parent compound in being able to counteract the lysergic acid diethylamide (LSD)-induced activation of the EEG and in counteracting the pressor responses produced by serotonin (Berger, Kletzkin, and Margolin, 1964). It is not known if these properties are clinically significant.

Tybamate is rapidly absorbed, and peak blood concentrations are reached within approximately 1 hr. The drug is rapidly transformed to hydroxytybamate, the chief metabolite, and is completely eliminated from the body within 24 hr (Douglas, Ludwig, Schlosser, and Edelson, 1966). The plasma half-life of tybamate is approximately 4 hr (Shelton and Hollister, 1967).

A double-blind evaluation of tybamate in anxious, neurotic medical clinic patients of low socioeconomic level demonstrated that the drug was primarily indicated for patients exhibiting a high degree of anxious neurotic symptomatology with somatic and hypochondriacal complaints. The drug appeared less effective in mildly anxious patients and in those showing high awareness of their autonomic functions (Raab, Rickels, and Moore, 1964). Tybamate was ineffective in controlling symptoms in schizophrenic patients (Fransway, Wells, and Chen, 1967; Meshel and Denber, 1968) but provided some relief of delusions, hallucinations, and depressive symptoms in drug-resistant hospitalized patients with chronic psychoses (Lapolla, 1965).

Rickels' group found tybamate a perplexing drug (Rickels, Hesbacher, Vandervort, Phillips, Hutchison, Sablosky, and Lavan, 1968). In private practice patients suffering from anxiety, tension, or mild depression, tybamate proved most effective in improving somatic and, to a lesser extent, phobic-obsessive-compulsive symptoms. Tybamate did not appear to act generally against neurotic symptoms or "free anxiety." Barsa and Saunders (1963) found tybamate less sedative than meprobamate in chronically ill psychotic patients. In 172 comparisons with meprobamate, tybamate was superior to meprobamate in 21, equal to it in 72, and inferior in 79. The drug has been shown effective in the treatment of depressive and anxiety states in penitentiary inmates (Brick, Doub, and Perdue, 1966) and in geriatric patients (Chesrow, Kaplitz, Sabatini, Vetra, and Marquardt, 1965; Goldstein, 1967). In a double-blind study Chieffi (1965) found tybamate superior to meprobamate in the treatment of acute and chronic anxiety and functional complaints, and Hollister (1966) found the two drugs to possess similar properties in healthy volunteers.

In a double-blind study in elderly patients, tybamate relieved agitation more effectively than chlordiazepoxide. The two drugs were almost equivalent in improving depressed mood and insomnia, but chlordiazepoxide was more effective in relieving anxiety. Hesbacher, Rickels, and Weiss (1968) found tybamate more effective in neurotic patients with primarily somatic symptoms, whereas diazepam was more effective in neurotics with primarily psychological symptoms. Splitter (1964), in a double-blind, controlled clinical trial, showed that tybamate produced greater relief of anxiety and other symptoms than chlordiazepoxide or placebo.

It is particularly interesting that it has been impossible to produce habituation to tybamate in animals or humans. Chronic intoxication in dogs given massive doses of tybamate several times daily for 6 months did not produce physical dependence or abstinence signs on abrupt withdrawal (Margolin, Pleks, and Berger, 1965). No tolerance or withdrawal symptoms occurred in hospitalized psychotic patients given high doses of tybamate for 4 to 12 weeks followed by abrupt substitution with placebo (Feldman and Mulinos, 1966). Similarly, abrupt discontinuation of large doses of tybamate in healthy males did not cause withdrawal symptoms or dependence. In this respect tybamate is unlike meprobamate and similar to carisoprodol (Colmore and Moore, 1967). Shelton and Hollister (1967) found that prolonged use of large doses of tybamate failed to produce withdrawal reactions in anxious or depressed patients who were likely to become habituated to drugs. The authors believe that the short half-life of tybamate (approximately 4 hr) is a factor that may account for the lack of withdrawal symptoms.

The area of clinical usefulness of tybamate appears narrower than that of meprobamate. Tybamate is primarily indicated for treating psychoneurotic conditions in which somatic and hypochondriacal symptoms predominate. Because of the lack of a habituation and/or dependence liability of the drug, tybamate is particularly suited for the treatment of anxiety, tension, and depression in alcoholics and other patients prone to drug abuse. The drug is less likely to produce drowsiness than meprobamate or mebutamate and is thus less suitable for use as a hypnotic.

CARISOPRODOL

Carisoprodol is obtained by replacing a hydrogen on one of the carbamyl nitrogens of meprobamate with an isopropyl group. This compound, in spite of its close chemical relationship to meprobamate, possesses little or no antianxiety action. It is primarily a centrally acting muscle relaxant, and this action is not only much more intense but also qualitatively different from that of meprobamate. In addition, carisoprodol differs from meprobamate in having analgesic action in certain types of pain and an atropine-like effect on the CNS (Berger, Kletzkin, Ludwig, Margolin, and Powell, 1959).

Clinically carisoprodol is used in conditions where skeletal muscle spasm and pain (e.g., low back pain) are factors (Kestler, 1960) and a variety of acute and chronic rheumatic and traumatic musculoskeletal disorders (Kolodny, 1960; Cole, 1964). The drug also reduced muscular tension and significantly increased cooperation in a controlled trial when it was administered as dental premedication to handicapped children suffering from cerebral palsy, mental retardation, and emotional problems (Joyce and Swallow, 1964).

MEPROBAMATE-LIKE COMPOUNDS

There are several compounds chemically related to meprobamate that have been introduced for the treatment of anxiety and tension (Berger and Ludwig, 1964). Most of these compounds appear to be of limited clinical usefulness and are no longer in wide use. A complete listing of all these compounds is found in Usdin and Efron (1972).

MEPHENESIN AND RELATED DRUGS

Mephenesin was the first modern psychopharmacological agent introduced into medicine, long before the discovery of chlorpromazine, reserpine, or meprobamate (Berger and Bradley, 1946). The pharmacological properties and clinical actions of mephenesin and related drugs were reviewed by Berger (1949). Mephenesin is no longer used in the treatment of psychiatric disorders. A few chemically related compounds are occasionally used in the treatment of anxiety and tension states (Usdin and Efron, 1972).

TREATMENT SUMMARY

Generic name	Trade name	Daily dosage range (mg)
Meprobamate	Equanil, Miltown	400–1,200[a]
Tybamate	Solacen, Tybatran	750–1,500[a]
Mebutamate	Dormate	600[b]

[a] Dosage range for treatment of anxiety.
[b] Dosage range for treatment of insomnia.

REFERENCES

Barsa, J. A., and Saunders, J. C. (1963): Tybamate, a new tranquilizer. *Am. J. Psychiatry,* 120:492–493.

Berger, F. M. (1949): Spinal cord depressant drugs. *Pharmacol. Rev.,* 1:243–278.

Berger, F. M. (1954): The pharmacological properties of 2-methyl-2-n-propyl-1,3-propanediol dicarbamate (Miltown), a new interneuronal blocking agent. *J. Pharmacol. Exp. Ther.,* 112:413–423.

Berger, F. M. (1968): The relations between the pharmacological properties of meprobamate and the clinical usefulness of the drug. In: *Psychopharmacology,* edited by D. H. Efron, pp. 139–152. Superintendent of Documents, Washington, D.C.

Berger, F. M. (1970): Anxiety and the discovery of the tranquilizers. In: *Discoveries in Biological Psychiatry,* edited by F. J. Ayd and B. Blockwell, pp. 115–129. Lippincott, Philadelphia.

Berger, F. M., and Bradley, W. (1946): The pharmacological properties of alpha-beta-dihydroxy-gamma-(2-methylphenyloxy)-propane (Myanesin). *Br. J. Pharmacol.,* 1:265–272.

Berger, F. M., Douglas, J. F., Kletzkin, M., Ludwig, B. J., and Margolin, S. (1961): The pharmacological properties of 2-methyl-2-secbutyl-1,3-propanediol dicarbamate (mebutamate, W-583), a new centrally acting blood pressure lowering agent. *J. Pharmacol. Exp. Ther.,* 134:356–365.

Berger, F. M., Kletzkin, M., Ludwig, B. J., Margolin, S., and Powell, L. S. (1959): Unusual muscle relaxant and analgesic properties of N-isopropyl-2-methyl-2-propyl-1,3-propanediol dicarbamate (corisoprodol). *J. Pharmacol. Exp. Ther.,* 127:66–73.

Berger, F. M., Kletzkin, M., and Margolin, S. (1964): Pharmacologic properties of a new tranquilizing agent 2-methyl-2-propyltrimethylene butycorbamate corbamate (Tybamate). *Med. Exp.,* 10:327–344.

Berger, F. M., Kletzkin, M., and Margolin, S. (1967): The action of certain tranquilizers, antidepressants and anticholinergic drugs on hippocampal after-discharges. In: *Antidepressant Drugs, Proceedings of the First International Symposium,* edited by S. Garattini and M. N. G. Dukes, pp. 241–246. Excerpta Medica, New York.

Berger, F. M., and Ludwig, B. J. (1964): Meprobamate and related compounds. In: *Psychopharmacological Agents,* Vol. 1, pp. 103–135. Academic Press, New York.

Berger, F. M., and Potterfield, J. (1969): The effect of antianxiety tranquilizers on the behavior of normal persons. In: *The Psychopharmacology of the Normal Human,* edited by W. O. Evans and N. S. Kline, pp. 38–113. Charles C Thomas, Springfield, Ill.

Bodi, T. (1969): Use of meprobamate for control of stress associated with "intractable" peptic ulcer. *Curr. Ther. Res.,* 11:216–226.

Bodi, T., Levy, H. A., Nodine, J. H., and Moyer, J. H. (1960): The hypnotic effect of a new propanediol dicarbamate, W583 (a double blind, double dose study) *Am. J. Med. Sci.,* 239:207–212.

Brick, H., Doub, W. H., Jr., and Perdue, W. C. (1966): Effects of tybamate on depressive and anxiety state in penitentiary inmates: A preliminary report. *Int. J. Neuropsychiatry,* 2:637–644.

Chesrow, E. J., Kaplitz, S. E., Sabatini, R., Vetra, H., and Marquardt, G. H. (1965): A new psychotherapeutic agent effective in the management of geriatric anxiety, depression, and behavioral reactions. *J. Am. Geriatr. Soc.,* 13:449–454.

Chieffi, M. (1965): A two-part, double-blind study of the anti-neurotic action of tybamate. *Dis. Nerv. Syst.,* 26:369–374.

Clifford, J. M., Cookson, J. H., and Wickham, P. E. (1974): Absorption and clearance of secobarbital, heptabarbital, methaqualone, and ethinamate. *Clin. Pharmacol. Ther.,* 16:376–389.

Cole, W. V. (1964): A double-blind evaluation of corisoprodol as a muscle relaxant and analgesic. *D.O.* 4:86–88.

Colmore, J. P., and Moore, J. D. (1967): Lack of dependence and withdrawal symptoms in healthy volunteers given high doses of tybamate. *J. Clin. Pharmacol.,* 7:319–323.

Corson, S. A., O'Leary, C., Dykman, E., Peters, J. E., Reese, W. G., and Seager, L. D. (1962): The nature of conditioned anti-diuretic and electrolyte retention responses. *Activ. Nerv. Syst.,* 4:359–382.

Curry, S. H. (1974): Concentration-effect relationships with major and minor tranquilizers. *Clin. Pharmacol. Ther.,* 16:192–197.

de Silva, J. A., Koechlin, B. A., and Basler, G. (1966): Blood level distribution patterns of diazepam and its major metabolite in man. *J. Pharm. Sci.,* 55:692–702.

Douglas, J. F., Ludwig, B. J., Ginberg, T., and Berger, F. M. (1962): The metabolic fate of mebutamate (Capla). *J. Pharmacol. Exp. Ther.,* 136:5–9.

Douglas, J. F., Ludwig, B. J., Schlosser, A., and Edelson, J. (1966): The metabolic fate of tybamate in the rat and dog. *Biochem. Pharmacol.,* 15:2087–2095.

Feinberg, I., Koresko, R. L., and Keller, N. (1967): EEG sleep patterns as a function of normal and pathological aging in man. *J. Psychiatr. Res.,* 5:107–144.

Feldman, H. S., and Mulinos, M. G. (1966): Lack of addiction from high doses of tybamate. *J. New Drugs,* 6:354–360.

Fransway, R. L., Wells, M. L., and Chen, C. H. (1967): Tybamate in the treatment of chronic mental patients. *Curr. Ther. Res.,* 9:42–45.

Freemon, F. R., Agnew, H. W., Jr., and Williams, R. L. (1965): An electroencephalographic study of the effects of meprobamate on human sleep. *Clin. Pharmacol. Ther.,* 6:172–176.

Friedman, A. P. (1957): The treatment of chronic headache with meprobamate. *Ann. N.Y. Acad. Sci.,* 67:822–826.

Gantt, W. H. (1960): Cardiovascular component of the conditional reflex to pain, food, and other stimuli. *Physiol. Rev. (Suppl.),* 40:266–291.

Gantt, W. H. (1964): Experimental studies in animals of the effects of drugs on cardiac stress symptoms. *J. Neuropsychiatry,* 5:472–474.

Garattini, S., Mussini, E., Marcucci, F., and Guaitani, A. (1973): Metabolic studies on benzodiazepines in various animal species. In: *The Benzodiazepines,* edited by S. Garattini, E. Mussini, and L. O. Randell, pp. 75–97. Raven Press, New York.

Goldstein, B. J. (1967): Double-blind comparison of tybamate and chlordiazepoxide in geriatric patients. *Psychosomatics,* 8:334–337.

Gresham, S. C., Agnew, H. W., and Williams, R. L. (1965): The sleep of depressed patients. *Arch. Gen. Psychiatry,* 13:503–507.

Hendley, C. D., Lynes, T. E., and Berger, F. M. (1957): Effect of meprobamate on electrical activity of thalamus and other subcortical areas. In: *Tranquilizing Drugs,* edited by H. E. Himwich, p. 35. American Association for the Advancement of Science, Washington, D.C.

Hesbacher, P. T., Rickels, K., and Weise, C. (1968): Target symptoms a promising improvement criterion in psychiatric drug research. *Arch. Gen. Psychiatry,* 18:595–600.

Holliday, A. R., and Devery, W. J. (1962): Effects of drugs on the performance of a task by fatigued subjects. *Clin. Pharmacol. Ther.,* 3:5–15.

Hollister, L. E. (1966): A comparison of primetine with amphetamine and of tybamate with meprobamate. *J. New Drugs,* 6:339–344.

Hollister, L. E., Elkins, H., Hiler, E. G., and St. Pierre, R. (1957): Meprobamate in chronic psychiatric patients. *Ann. N.Y. Acad. Sci.,* 67:789–798.

Hollister, L. E., and Levy, G. (1964): Kinetics of meprobamate elimination in humans. *Chemotherapia*, 9:20–24.

Joyce, C. R. B., and Swallow, J. N. (1964): The controlled trial in dental surgery: Premedication of handicapped children with corisoprodol. *Dent. Pract.*, 15:44–47.

Kales, A., Scharf, M., Ling-Tan, T., Kales, J., Allen, C., and Malmstrom, E. (1969): Sleep patterns with short term drug use. *Psychophysiology*, 6:262–263.

Keller, H., and Vogt, L. (1958): Restenil (meprobamate) in the treatment of vegetative, neurotic and reactive disorders. *Dtsch. Med. Wochenschr.*, 83:1483–1485.

Kestler, O. (1960): Conservative management of low back syndrome. *J.A.M.A.*, 172: 2039–2043.

Keston, M., and Brocklehurst, J. C. (1974): Flurazepam and meprobamate—a clinical trial. *Age Aging*, 3:54–58.

Kiloh, L. G., and Garnside, R. F. (1963): The independence of neurotic depression and endogenous depression. *Br. J. Psychiatry*, 109:451–463.

Kletzkin, M., and Berger, F. M. (1959): Effect of meprobamate on limbic system of the brain. *Proc. Soc. Exp. Biol. Med.*, 100:681–683.

Koechlin, B. A., and d'Arconte, L. (1963): Determination of chlordiazepoxide (Librium) and of a metabolite of loctam character in plasma of humans, dogs, and rats by a specific spectrofluorometric micro method. *Anal. Biochem.*, 5:195–207.

Kolodny, A. L. (1960): Corisoprodol as a muscle relaxant and analgesic in rheumatic and traumatic conditions: Controlled placebo study. *Curr. Ther. Res.*, 2:436–441.

Kornetsky, C., Vates, T. S., and Kessler, E. K. (1959): A comparison of hypnotic and residual psychological effects of single doses of chlorpromazine and secobarbital in man. *J. Pharmacol Exp. Ther.*, 127:51–54.

Lapolla, A. (1965): A controlled pilot study of tybamate in therapy of psychotic patients with chronic anxiety and psychoneurotic reaction. *Int. J. Neuropsychiatry*, 1:125–130.

Lasagna, L. (1956): A study of hypnotic drugs in patients with chronic diseases. *J. Chronic Dis.*, 3:122–133.

Lehmann, H. E. (1968): Tranquilizers: clinical insufficiencies and needs. In: *The Present Status of Psychotropic Drugs*, pp. 168–175. International Congress Series No. 180. Excerpta Medica, Amsterdam.

Ludwig, B. J., Douglas, J. F., Powell, L. S., Meyer, M., and Berger, F. M. (1961): Structures of the major metabolites of meprobamate. *J. Med. Pharmacol. Chem.*, 3:53–64.

Ludwig, B. J., and Potterfield, J. R. (1971): The pharmacology of propanediol carbamates. *Adv. Pharmacol. Chemother.*, 9:173–240.

Margolin, S., Pleks, O. J., and Berger, F. M. (1965): Failure of chronic tybamate intoxication to induce withdrawal convulsions in dogs. *Pharmacologist*, 7:143.

Maynert, E. W. (1965): The alcoholic metabolites of pentobarbital and amobarbital in man. *J. Pharmacol. Exp. Ther.*, 150:118–121.

McKensie, R. E., and Elliot, L. E. (1965): The effect of secobarbitol and d-amphetamine on performance during a simulated air mission. *Aerospace Med.*, 36:774–779.

Mendels, J., and Hawkins, D. R. (1967): Sleep and depression, a controlled EEG study. *Arch. Gen. Psychiatry*, 16:344–354.

Meshel, E., and Denber, H. C. B. (1968): The use of tybamate in psychotic patients: A further double-blind study. *Dis. Nerv. Syst.*, 29:243–245.

Morgan, J. P., Wardell, W., Lasagna, L., Mazzullo, J. M., Weintraub, M., Mudholkar, G. S., and Mietlowski, W. (1973): Mebutamate as a hypnotic: Clinical trial and statistical considerations. *Clin. Pharmacol. Ther.*, 14:1001–1012.

Mornin, Y., Turmel, L., Grantham, H., and Fortier, J. (1963): Observations on the antihypertensive and sedative effects of mebutamate and reserpine. *Can. Med. Assoc. J.*, 89:980–982.

Oswald, I., and Priest, R. G. (1965): Five weeks to escape the sleeping-pill habit. *Br. Med. J.*, 2:1093–1095.

Peterson, E. A., Haun, K., and Upton, M. (1962): The effect of meprobamate, D-amphetamine and placebo on disjunctive reaction time to taboo and nontaboo words. *Psychopharmacologia*, 3:173–187.

Phillips, R. E. (1956): Use of meprobamate (Miltown) for the treatment of emotional disorders. *Am. Pract.,* 7:1573–1579.

Pronko, N. H., and Kenyon, G. Y. (1959): Meprobamate and laboratory induced anxiety. *Psychol. Rep.,* 5:217–238.

Raab, E., Rickels, K., and Moore, E. (1964): A double blind evaluation of tybamate in anxious neurotic medical clinic patients. *Am. J. Psychiatry,* 120:1005–1007.

Randall, L. O., and Kappell, B. (1973): Pharmacological activity of some benzodiazepines and their metabolites. In: *The Benzodiazepines,* edited by S. Garattini, E. Mussini, and L. O. Randall, pp. 27–51. Raven Press, New York.

Read, G. W., Cutting, W., and Furst, A. (1960): Comparison of excited phases after sedatives and tranquilizers. *Psychopharmacologia,* 1:346–350.

Rickels, K., Clark, T. W., Ewing, J. H., Klingensmith, W. C., and Morris, H. M. (1959): Evolution of tranquilizing drugs in medical outpatients. *J.A.M.A.,* 171:1649–1656.

Rickels, K., Downing, R. W., Raab, E., and Hesbacher, P. (1967a): Non-specific factors, with emphasis on symptomatology, and drug therapy outcome. In: *Neuropsycho-Pharmacology,* edited by H. Brill, pp. 717–721. Excerpta Medica, Amsterdam.

Rickels, K., Hesbacher, P., Vandervort, W., Phillips, F., Hutchison, J., Sablosky, L., and Lavan, D. (1968): Tybamate—a perplexing drug. *Am. J. Psychiatry,* 125:320–326.

Rickels, K., Raab, E., DeSilverio, R., and Etemad, B. (1967b): Drug treatment in depression. *J.A.M.A.,* 201:675–681.

Rickels, K., Ward, C. H., and Schut, L. (1964): Different populations, different drug responses. *Am. J. Med. Sci.,* 247:328–335.

Roth, M., Gurney, C., Garside, R. F., and Kerr, T. A. (1972): Studies in the classification of affective disorders. *Br. J. Psychiatry,* 121:147–161.

Ruchwarger, A. (1959): Use of Deprol (meprobamate combined with benactyzine hydrochloride) in the office treatment of depression. *Med. Ann. D.C.,* 28:438–441.

Shelton, J., and Hollister, L. E. (1967): Simulated abuse of tybamate in man: Failure to demonstrate withdrawal reactions. *J.A.M.A.,* 199:338–340.

Sklar, M. (1970): Functional gastrointestinal disease in the aged. *Am. J. Gastroenterol.,* 53:570–575.

Smith, R. B., Dittert, L. W., Griffen, W. O., Jr., and Doluisio, J. T. (1973): Pharmacokinetics of pentobarbital after intravenous and oral administration. *J. Pharmacokinet. Biopharm.,* 1:5–16.

Splitter, S. R. (1964): A new psychotropic drug: Evaluation of tybamate in the treatment of anxiety and tension states. *Psychosomatics,* 5:292–294.

Tetreault, L., Richer, P., and Bordeleau, J. (1967): Hypnotic properties of mebutamate: A comparative study of mebutamate, secobarbital, and placebo in psychiatric patients. *Can. Med. Assoc. J.,* 97:395–398.

Tucker, W. I. (1957): The place of Miltown in general practice. *South. Med. J.,* 50:1111–1114.

Tyrer, P. (1974): The benzodiazepine bonanza. *Lancet,* 2:709–710.

Usdin, E., and Efron, D. H. (1972): Psychotropic drugs and related compounds, Ed. 2. HEW Publication No. (HSM) 72–9074. Government Printing Office, Washington, D.C.

West, E. D., and da Fonseca, A. F. (1956): Controlled trial of meprobamate. *Br. Med. J.,* 5003:1206–1209.

Whitsett, T. L., Hoyt, H. J., Gzerwinski, A. W., and Clark, M. L. (1974): Effects of mebutamate on the electroencephalographic sleep profile. *Clin. Pharmacol. Ther.,* 15:51–58.

Chapter 8

Neuropharmacology of Depression

Dennis L. Murphy

The affective disorders, depression and mania, are multifaceted behavioral syndromes. Psychoactive drugs are often used in their treatment, with generally beneficial results. Individual, group, family, and milieu-oriented psychotherapy may also contribute to clinical improvement.

The occurrence during depression of changes in mood, activity, behavior, sleep, sex, and neuroendocrine and other functions thought to be mediated by brain neurotransmitters, especially the biogenic amines, has led to suggestions that brain biochemical alterations may contribute to depressive psychopathology. Direct measurement of neurotransmitters and their metabolites in cerebrospinal fluid, urine, and tissues as well as indirect data from pharmacological and neuroendocrine investigations have provided evidence that changes in neurotransmitter systems may occur in some depressed individuals. However, there are no unequivocal, replicated demonstrations of a specific change universally associated with clinical depression. Differences between subtypes of depressed patients and the contribution of various biological changes occurring in response to changes in activity, sleep, diet, and nonspecific stress during depressive episodes complicate interpretation of these studies.

Although therapeutic change in response to biogenic amine-affecting drugs like the tricyclic and monoamine oxidase (MAO)-inhibiting antidepressants has been considered as evidence supporting dysfunction in the amine neurotransmitter systems during depression, these data can be considered only as suggestive evidence and not validating proof. Many therapeutic agents in other areas of medicine have symptomatic effects without directly antagonizing an etiological pathophysiological process. Nonetheless, detailed study of the mechanism of action of drugs affecting mood, activity, and other depression-related behavior may illuminate some aspects of the normal regulators of these functions and their possible alterations in depression.

This chapter surveys several aspects of recently accumulated information concerning drug actions in depression. Clinical features affecting responses to antidepressant drugs are considered first because it is now apparent that there are great individual differences in the efficacy of these drugs. An overview of developments in the understanding of the mechanism of action of antidepressant drugs is then presented. More detailed discussion of the specific drugs used in the treatment of depression, their clinical efficacy, and their mode of action are presented in subsequent chapters. Other monographs and reviews (Schildkraut and Kety, 1967; Klein and Davis, 1969; Murphy, Goodwin, and Bunney, 1971*b*; Hollister, 1973; Schildkraut, 1974, 1975; Murphy and Redmond, 1975) also provide comprehensive information on various aspects of the neuropharmacology of depression.

SUBGROUPS OF DEPRESSED PATIENTS AND ANTIDEPRESSANT DRUG RESPONSES

Conceptualizations of depression and of the modes of action of the antidepressant drugs have grown more complex during the last several years. It is now well recognized that depression is not a single entity, and that depression as a temporary mood state (normal depression, grief states) must be differentiated from the depression accompanying other psychiatric or medical disorders (secondary depression) and from the full-blown, persistent syndrome of depression (primary depression or melancholia), which can be identified on the basis of a characteristic group of symptoms (Woodruff, Goodwin, and Guze, 1974). Furthermore, important differences in clinical phenomena, biological correlates, family history data, and pharmacological responses between unipolar and bipolar patients with recurrent primary de-

TABLE 1. *Characteristics of bipolar compared to unipolar depressed patients*

Clinical features of bipolar patients

History of mania (definitional characteristic)
Earlier average age of onset of affective symptoms
Different personality characteristics on MMPI, Maudsley personality inventory, and Nyman-Marke scale
Different symptomatology during depressive episodes
Higher incidence of postpartum affective episodes
Higher educational achievement and occupational level
Higher mortality from all causes

Family history ("genetic") features of bipolar patients

Higher frequency of bipolar affective symptomatology in close relatives
Overall higher prevalence of affective disorders in close relatives
Males and females equally affected (unlike preponderance of females among unipolar patients)

Biological features of bipolar patients

Lower sedation and flicker thresholds, with some EEG pattern differences
Greater rates of increase in average cortical evoked response amplitude ("augmentation") with increasing stimulus intensity
Lower urinary 17-hydroxycorticosteroid excretion during depression
In females, higher catechol-O-methyl-transferase (COMT) activity in red cells (but, like unipolar patients, lower COMT activity compared to normal controls)
Reduced MAO activity in blood platelets
Higher octopamine levels in platelets and greater urinary tryptamine excretion during depression
Greater formation of urinary dopamine from L-DOPA during depression

pressions (Table 1) suggest that the history of a characteristic manic episode requiring specific treatment (as found in bipolar depressed patients) must be utilized to separate bipolar and unipolar subgroups among patients with primary depressions (Murphy, Goodwin, and Bunney, 1975). Criteria for establishing these diagnoses have been described (Woodruff et al., 1974).

Even among groups of patients with primary depressions, heterogeneity beyond the unipolar/bipolar dichotomy is suggested by studies using factor analysis, discriminant function analysis, and other techniques to identify clinical correlates in patients responding to different antidepressant drugs. Research efforts to find identifying characteristics capable of predicting which patient might respond to a specific antidepressant drug have been stimulated by the increasing costs of hospitalization, limited insurance coverage for psychiatric hospitalization generally available, and delayed onset of anti-depressant drug effects, with improvement often occurring only after 2 to 4 weeks of treatment. In addition, improved prediction of response to anti-depressant drugs would not only contribute to reducing the social and eco-nomic consequences of depression but also help avoid the possible risks from side effects of unnecessary chronic drug treatment in some individuals.

Pharmacological Response Differences Between Bipolar and Unipolar Depressed Patients

In addition to the clinical, genetic, and psychologic differences summarized in Table 1, a proclivity for the bipolar patient subgroup to respond to tricyclic and MAO-inhibiting antidepressants with manic episodes (Table 2) has been reported (Bunney, Goodwin, Murphy, House, and Gordon, 1972). Whether antidepressant responses to the tricyclic drugs occur as frequently in bipolar patients as in unipolar patients has been questioned on the basis of a retrospective review (Bunney, Brodie, Murphy, and Goodwin, 1970), al-though a randomized, controlled study of this issue has not yet been com-pleted. An investigation of the prophylactic effects of imipramine in bipolar versus unipolar patients indicated that imipramine was inferior to lithium in bipolar patients, chiefly because of the frequent occurrence of manic episodes during the tricyclic drug treatment period (Prien, Klett, and Caffey, 1974).

Antidepressant responses to lithium carbonate have also been reported more frequently in bipolar than unipolar patients (Goodwin, Murphy, Dun-ner, and Bunney, 1972). In addition, relatives of bipolar patients appear more likely to have successful prophylactic responses to lithium carbonate

TABLE 2. *Responses to psychoactive drugs in bipolar compared to unipolar depressed patients*

More frequent episodes of hypomania during L-DOPA administration and mania during treatment with tricyclic and MAO-inhibiting antidepressants
More frequent prophylactic and antidepressant responses to lithium carbonate
More frequent antidepressant responses to L-tryptophan

than patients without such family histories (Mendlewicz, Fieve, and Stallone, 1972). Of special interest are the reports that the amino acids L-tryptophan and L-DOPA, which are metabolic precursors of brain neurotransmitters serotonin and the catecholamines, respectively, yield differential responses in bipolar and unipolar patients (Goodwin, Murphy, Brodie, and Bunney, 1970; Murphy, Brodie, Goodwin, and Bunney, 1971; Murphy, Baker, Goodwin, Miller, Kotin, and Bunney, 1974a). L-Tryptophan has been reported to have antidepressant properties in some studies but not in others of mixed populations of depressed patients, and to have some antimanic effects as well (Carroll, 1971; Murphy, et al., 1974a; Prange, Wilson, Lynn, Alltop, and Stikeleather, 1974). The one study comparing antidepressant responses in bipolar versus unipolar patients found a significantly greater response rate in the bipolar patients (Murphy, et al., 1974a). Although L-DOPA treatment was not associated with significant antidepressant effects, the few patients who did improve were among the unipolar patients with psychomotor retardation symptoms (Goodwin et al., 1970). L-DOPA treatment did lead to brief hypomanic episodes in almost all (eight of nine) of the bipolar patients but in only one of 12 of the unipolar patients studied (Murphy et al., 1971a). A possible difference in the metabolism of DOPA was also observed in the patients developing hypomania compared to those who did not "switch" into hypomania (Murphy, Goodwin, Brodie, and Bunney, 1973).

Pharmacological Response Differences in Other Depressed Patient Subgroups

Because traditional dichotomies of depressed patients (e.g., psychotic versus neurotic, endogenous versus reactive) generally have not correlated uniformly with antidepressant drug responses, some interesting attempts at better defining subgroups of depressed patients in relation to clinical variables have been explored. These approaches have utilized a variety of statistical procedures (e.g., factor analysis, discriminant function analysis, multivariate symptom analysis, and cluster analysis) to identify specific groups of characteristics of the individuals who did or did not respond to various drugs. Although different patient populations included in the various studies apparently contributed to the lack of replicability in defining patient subgroups by these methods—e.g., in Paykel's, (1972) attempted replication of the studies of Overall, Hollister, and associates (Overall, Hollister, Johnson, and Pennington, 1966; Hollister, Overall, Shelton, Pennington, Kimbell, and Johnson, 1967)—some general similarities emerged and are summarized in Table 3 (Overall et al., 1966; Hollister et al., 1967; Raskin, Schulterbrandt, Reatig, and McKeon, 1970; Paykel, 1972; Raskin, 1974). There is some agreement in these data to suggest that withdrawn, retarded ("endogenous," "psychotic") depressed patients might respond best to imipramine or amitriptyline, whereas anxious and hostile patients may respond less well to the tricyclic drugs. The original papers must be consulted to obtain the exact

TABLE 3. *Pharmacological response differences in patient subgroups identified by factor analysis or multivariate cluster analysis*

Patient group	Effective drug	Reference
Psychotic depression	Imipramine > placebo	Raskin et al., 1970
Withdrawn-retarded depression	Imipramine > thioridazine	Overall et al., 1966
Anergic-retarded depression	Imipramine > chlorpromazine	Raskin et al., 1970
Anxious depression	Thioridazine, chlorpromazine, or imipramine > placebo	Hollister et al., 1967; Raskin et al., 1970
	Diazepam > phenelzine or placebo	Raskin, 1974
Hostile depression	Placebo > imipramine, chlorpromazine, or diazepam	Raskin et al., 1970, 1974 Overall et al., 1966
Depressed patients with sleep disturbances	Imipramine, chlorpromazine, and diazepam > placebo or phenelzine	Raskin et al., 1970, 1974
Retarded > anxious depression	Amitriptyline	Overall et al., 1966
Psychotic > hostile > anxious depression	Amitriptyline	Paykel, 1972

procedures used to identify such patient characteristics as anxiety and hostility; these derived factors may or may not agree with global clinical estimates of such symptoms.

Pharmacological Response Differences Related to Biological Differences Between Patients

There are several indications that some biogenic amine-related characteristics of depressed patients may predict individual responses to the tricyclic drugs or to lithium carbonate. In addition, it is now possible to measure in individual patients the amount of biogenic amine uptake inhibition in the case of the tricyclic antidepressants, and the amount of MAO inhibition in the case of MAO-inhibiting drugs (Murphy, Colburn, Davis, and Bunney, 1970; Murphy, Brand, Baker, van Kammen, and Gordon, 1974). Although these drug effects may not constitute the direct mechanism of antidepressant action (*vide infra*), their measurement provides a means to estimate the effective concentrations of drugs on relevant cellular processes for comparisons between responding and nonresponding patients.

Some of the biological differences that correlate with antidepressant drug responses are outlined in Table 4 (Fawcett, Maas, and Dekirmenjian, 1972; Maas, Fawcett, and Dekirmenjian, 1972; Asberg, Bertilsson, Tuck, Cronholm, and Sjöqvist, 1973; Goodwin, Post, Dunner, and Gordon, 1973; Schildkraut, 1973; Schildkraut, Keeler, Grab, and Kantrowich, 1973; Rosenblatt and Chanley, 1974). Most of these differences have been observed in small groups of depressed patients not classified according to clinical characteristics. One additional study (Beckmann and Goodwin, 1975) has confirmed the urinary 3-methoxy-4-hydroxyphenylglycol (MHPG) findings, with unipolar depressed

TABLE 4. *Some experimental measures reported to correlate with antidepressant drug response*

Experimental measure correlating with drug response	Antidepressant drug	Reference
Reduction in psychiatrist's "depressed mood" rating (Clyde scale) following 30 mg d-amphetamine	Imipramine or desipramine	Fawcett et al., 1972
Lower urinary MHPG[a] excretion pretreatment and higher MHPG and normetanephrine excretion during treatment	Imipramine or desipramine	Maas et al., 1972
Higher urinary MHPG, normetanephrine and VMA[b] excretion	Amitriptyline	Schildkraut, 1973
Lower CSF[c] homovanillic acid and 5-HIAA[d] levels following probenecid	Lithium	Goodwin et al., 1973
Higher CSF 5-HIAA levels	Nortriptyline	Asberg et al., 1973

[a] 3-Methoxy-4-hydroxyphenylglycol.
[b] Vanillylmandelic acid.
[c] Cerebrospinal fluid.
[d] 5-Hydroxyindoleacetic acid.

patient responders to imipramine having lower pretreatment urinary MHPG excretion and amitriptyline responders higher levels. However, cerebrospinal fluid MHPG levels did not correlate with tricyclic drug response in a prior study by this same group (Post and Goodwin, 1973).

Pharmacological Response Differences Related to Individual Variations in Antidepressant Drug Metabolism

Among the many variables that may influence the final behavioral response to a psychoactive drug, the first requirement is attaining effective plasma and tissue concentrations required for a drug to produce its cellular effects. Recent data indicate that there may be quite large individual differences (10-fold and higher) in the plasma levels of the tricyclic antidepressants and some of the MAO-inhibiting antidepressants (Hammer and Sjöqvist, 1967; Alexanderson, Sjöqvist, and Price Evans, 1969; Asberg, Crönholm, Sjöqvist, and Tuck, 1971). Some of the variables demonstrated to affect antidepressant drug plasma levels include genetic factors (Alexanderson et al., 1969), prior exposure to drugs that affect drug-metabolizing enzymes (Alexanderson et al., 1969), and concurrent treatment with such drugs (Hammer and Sjöqvist, 1967; Moody, Tait, and Todrick, 1967; Asberg et al., 1971; Burrows and Davies, 1971; Wharton, Perel, Dayton, and Malitz, 1971; Zeidenberg, Perel, Kanzler, Wharton, and Malitz, 1971; Gram and Overø, 1972).

Some correlations of antidepressant responses with tricyclic plasma levels have been reported, with responders to the drugs having higher plasma levels in the case of imipramine (Wharton et al., 1971) and amitriptyline (Braithwaite, Goulding, Theano, Bailey, and Coppen, 1972). One study reported no relationship between nortriptyline plasma levels and response in a mixed group of depressed patients (Burrows, Davies, and Scoggins, 1972), whereas an inverted U-shaped curve was found in other studies, with good responders having midrange levels (50 to 140 ng/ml) and poor responders either higher or lower levels (Asberg et al., 1971; Kragh-Sørensen, Eggert-Hansen, and Asberg, 1975). The occurrence of side effects correlated positively with nortriptyline plasma levels but not with dosage in one study which compared side effects prior to and during treatment (Asberg et al., 1971). In two other studies of nortriptyline and amitriptyline that did not examine pretreatment side-effect-like symptoms, there were no significant correlations between apparent side effects and tricyclic plasma levels (Braithwaite et al., 1972; Burrows et al., 1972).

Although plasma levels of MAO-inhibiting antidepressants have not yet been measured, differences in the metabolism of these drugs may influence their clinical efficacy. Phenelzine, isoniazid, and other hydrazine MAO-inhibiting antidepressants are metabolized via acetylation. Drug acetylation is genetically influenced, with 50% of Caucasian populations exhibiting a rapid acetylation and 50% a slow acetylation phenotype. Severe adverse effects during phenelzine treatment occurred preferentially in the slow acetylators in one study (Price Evans, Davison, and Pratt, 1964) but not in another (Johnstone and Marsh, 1973). Conversely, improvement was observed more frequently in slow acetylators in one of these studies (Johnstone and Marsh, 1973) but not in the other (Price Evans et al., 1964).

These studies of blood levels and the metabolism of tricyclic antidepressants and MAO inhibitors require further clarification, with specific attention to the identification of possible patient subgroups. The available data clearly indicate the potential of these measurements for quantitatively evaluating some factors affecting individual differences in antidepressant drug responses.

MECHANISM OF ACTION OF ANTIDEPRESSANT DRUGS

Catecholamine and Indoleamine Hypotheses

Early attempts to relate the behavioral effects of the tricyclic and MAO-inhibiting antidepressants to their biochemical actions were focused on the possibility that the behavioral changes observed were mediated by changes in catecholamine metabolism. These drugs were known to increase catecholamine function at synapses by either directly inhibiting catecholamine degradation (the MAO inhibitors) or inhibiting catecholamine uptake from the synaptic cleft (the tricyclics). Data from animal studies on the synaptic effects of the antidepressants plus observations from animals and man indicating that reserpine depletes catecholamine stores and produces a sedated, "depressed" state in animals and apparent clinical depression in man were combined to suggest the "catecholamine hypothesis of depression," as outlined in Table 5 (Bunney and Davis, 1965; Schildkraut, 1965; Schildkraut and Kety, 1967).

On the basis that these same drugs have similar effects on serotonin uptake, metabolism, and storage in the brain, an "indoleamine hypothesis" was also suggested for depression (Lapin and Oxenkrug, 1969). This was supported by reports of the antidepressant efficacy of tryptophan, the brain serotonin precursor, although not all studies demonstrated improvement in depressed patients (Carroll, 1971; Murphy et al., 1974a). More recently

TABLE 5. *Original catecholamine hypothesis*

Norepinephrine concentration	Clinical state	Pharmacological correlate
High ↑ ı ↓ Intermediate ↑ ı ↓ Low	Mania ↑ ı ↓ Normality ↑ ı ↓ Depression	Tricyclic and MAO- inhibiting anti- depressants Reserpine

findings of reduced levels of brain serotonin and of reduced 5-hydroxyindoleacetic acid (5-HIAA) in cerebrospinal fluid from both depressed and manic patients further supported the existence of a serotonin deficit in patients with affective disorders. However, the persistence of reduced 5-HIAA levels in recovered patients and following drug and electroconvulsive treatment (ECT) is not consistent with a primary relationship between the depressed state, antidepressant drug effects, and serotonin depletion (Goodwin and Murphy, 1974). A "permissive hypothesis" for the role of indoleamines in the affective disorders was suggested as a possible way to understand combined serotonin and catecholamine alterations in these states (Wilson and Prange, 1972; Prange et al., 1974).

Other Transmitters Implicated in the Affective Disorders

Additional studies using the central cholinesterase-inhibiting drug physostigmine in conjunction with methyl scopolamine as an inhibitor of peripheral cholinergic function suggested a possible role for cholinergic changes contributing to the symptomatology of the affective disorders (Janowsky, El-Yousef, Davis, Hubbard, and Sekerke, 1972). Cholinergic effects may also be relevant to tricyclic antidepressant drug effects, since these agents have some anticholinergic properties. Furthermore, the evidence that some depressed patients became worse during treatment with L-DOPA and that the phenothiazines, which have catecholamine receptor-blocking properties, may have antidepressant effects in some depressed patients also suggested that dopamine function may contribute to manic-depressive symptomatology along the psychomotor retardation-activation axis (Murphy et al., 1975). Several other amines have also been recently suggested as being of some possible relevance to affective disorder states, including phenethylamine, tryptamine, epinephrine, and octopamine (Fischer, Spatz, Saavedra, Reggiani, Miro, and Heller, 1972; Murphy, 1972; Schildkraut, 1975).

TABLE 6. Models for depression, mania, and "normality"

Bipolar model	Continuum model	Separate bipolar and unipolar depression models
Mania ↑↓ Normality ↑↓ Depression	Mania ↑↓ Depression ↑↓ Normality	Mania ↗↖ Depression type I ⟷ "Normality" Depression type II or I ⟷ "Normality"

Because of the need to distinguish between depressions in bipolar and unipolar patients, neither of the conventional schema, the "bipolar model" or the "continuum model" (Table 6), seems adequate as a conceptual base for the affective disorders. For this reason a less-constraining triangular model (Table 6) for bipolar patients seems to be preferred, with a separate model required for unipolar patients. Following some of the lines of argument for patient differentiation in response to antidepressant drugs reviewed above, as well as some evidence presented elsewhere (Murphy and Redmond, 1975), it may be necessary to consider two subtypes of unipolar depression (Table 6): one with many characteristics of the bipolar depression, including psychomotor retardation and withdrawal (type I), and one with more marked anxiety and agitation features (type II).

A multitransmitter, multisubgroup summary of published information on the suggested biologic substratum of individuals with affective disorders is presented in Table 7. It should be emphasized that replicated biochemical evidence from brain and cerebrospinal fluid studies to support this schema is available only for serotonin in depression and mania, and perhaps for norepinephrine in depression. The other changes postulated are primarily based on inferences from drug effects and are speculative. This summary does

TABLE 7. *Postulated neuromediator alterations in mania and two major clinical subtypes of depression*

Neuromediator[a]	Mania	Type I depression[b]	Type II depression[c]
Dopamine	↑	↓	↑
Norepinephrine	↑ or ↓	↓	↓ or ↑
Serotonin	↓	↓	↓
Acetylcholine	— or ↓ (?)	↑ (?)	↑ (?)

[a] Other possible neuromediators involved in affective disorders: octopamine, β-phenethylamine, tryptamine, and epinephrine.

[b] "Endogenous" depression, as in bipolar and some unipolar patients.

[c] Anxious, agitated depression, as in many unipolar patients.

indicate, however, the complexity of present thinking in this area. It also suggests why it is no longer possible to postulate a simple mechanism of action for the various antidepressant drugs.

MECHANISMS OF ACTION OF ANTIDEPRESSANT DRUGS: RECONSIDERATION OF THEIR EFFECTS ON NEUROTRANSMITTER FUNCTION

Additional complexity in understanding the effects of the antidepressant drugs has resulted from new knowledge of synaptic mechanisms. Not only is it necessary to consider other neurotransmitter systems besides norepinephrine in seeking to correlate biochemical events with behavioral changes, it is also necessary to re-evaluate the effects of antidepressant drugs on newly discovered adaptational processes in all of the neurotransmitter systems.

Although it initially appeared that the antidepressant effects of the tricyclic drugs could be related to their amine uptake-inhibiting effects, and of the MAO inhibitors to the consequences of reduced MAO activity (Schildkraut and Kety, 1967), these changes represent acute effects of these drugs given in high dosages to animals. Recent studies of these drugs given chronically to animals in dosages closer to those utilized clinically, together with direct studies of some of their effects in patients receiving ordinary clinical dosages, suggest that additional biochemical processes may contribute to the behavioral effects of these antidepressant agents.

Tricyclic Antidepressants: Amine Uptake Inhibition Versus Other Synaptic Changes Possibly Contributing to Their Behavioral Effects

Imipramine, amitriptyline, nortriptyline, desipramine, protriptyline, and similar tricyclic agents are all extremely effective inhibitors of the amine reuptake process (Glowinski and Axelrod, 1964; Gyermek, 1966). Other structurally similar drugs—such as the antipsychotic phenothiazines like chlorpromazine—require 10-fold higher concentrations to reduce amine uptake (Glowinski and Axelrod, 1964; Gyermek, 1966). This amine transport process is principally responsible for the inactivation of neurotransmitter amines released at synapses. It was originally suggested that the tricyclics produce their behavioral effects in animals and their antidepressant effects in man via amine uptake inhibition, resulting in prolongation of the effects of the neurotransmitters—principally norepinephrine and serotonin, as dopamine uptake is much less sensitive to their effects and acetylcholine is inactivated enzymatically (Schildkraut and Kety, 1967).

Two recent series of studies complicated this predominant interpretation relating the clinical antidepressant efficacy of the tricyclic drugs to their uptake-inhibiting capacity. First, several clinical studies demonstrated that some phenothiazines (thioridazine and chlorpromazine) have equal antidepressant effects when compared directly to the tricyclic drugs (Overall, Hollister, Meyer, Kimbell, and Shelton, 1964). In addition, various newer drugs with some structural similarities to the tricyclics (e.g., iprindole) have also been reported to possess antidepressant efficacy equivalent to that of the tricyclics (Carlsson, Fuxe, Hamberger, and Malmfors, 1969; Fann, Davis, Janowsky, Kaufman, Griffith, and Oates, 1972). These drugs, like the phenothiazines, are markedly less effective amine uptake-inhibitors than the tricyclics (Fann et al., 1972). Despite this difference, they share with the tricyclics some of the behavioral activation effects that had been thought to be related to uptake inhibition, e.g., enhancement of motor activity in rodents (Carlsson et al., 1969; Fann et al., 1972).

A second group of studies that argue against uptake inhibition as the mechanism of action for antidepressant effects are those having to do with the synaptic effects of lithium carbonate. This drug enhances norepinephrine uptake in brain synaptosomes (Colburn, Goodwin, Bunney, and Davis, 1967) and serotonin uptake in platelets (Murphy et al., 1970). Enhanced amine uptake was considered as possibly relevant to its most dramatic clinical effects as an antimanic drug. However, recent studies have demonstrated that lithium also has antidepressant effects (Goodwin et al., 1972). Thus clinical antidepressant activity appears to be associated not only with drugs like the tricyclics, which inhibit amine uptake, but also with other drugs like iprindole and lithium, which either do not inhibit uptake or actually enhance it. Furthermore, even among the prototypical tricyclic drugs, the correlation between uptake inhibition and clinical efficacy is not high. Desipramine is the most effective inhibitor of brain norepinephrine uptake, but it is somewhat less useful clinically than amitriptyline and imipramine, which have less norepinephrine uptake-inhibiting potency (Carlsson, 1970; Lahti and Maickel, 1971; Kannengiesser, Hunt, and Raynaud, 1973). While drugs like imipramine and chlorimipramine, which have relatively greater serotonin-inhibiting capacity, have been reported to be among the most clinically effective antidepressant drugs, the single most effective tricyclic, amitriptyline, appears to have relatively less serotonin uptake-inhibiting effects in man (Murphy and Costa, 1975). Taken together, these data suggest that a single cause-effect relationship between amine uptake inhibition and clinical antidepressant efficacy is no longer tenable.

The tricyclic antidepressants affect biogenic amine synthesis, storage, release, metabolism, and receptor functions (Schanberg, Schildkraut, and Kopin, 1967; Reid, Stefano, Kurzepa, and Brodie, 1969; Mandell, Segal, Kuczenski, and Knapp, 1972; Murphy and Kopin, 1972) in addition to their effects on amine uptake. Although clinical antidepressant effects often do not become apparent for 2 to 3 weeks, the tricyclic drug effects on uptake occur rapidly, within the first several days of treatment. Similarly, the drug levels in plasma and brain plateau within the first few days of treatment. Although other plausible explanations (e.g., a psychological lag period) have been suggested, it may well be that there are some slower effects of the drugs or some compensatory, adaptive changes in amine synthesis or receptor function such as those demonstrated with other psychoactive drugs given chronically (Mandell et al., 1972). In particular, it might easily be hypothesized that the antidepressant efficacy of the tricyclic drugs in patients with the more agitated, anxious forms of depression might be dependent on receptor adaptations or synthesis-related mechanisms. This may be the case with other drugs that also alter amine receptor function, e.g., the phenothiazines.

Monoamine Oxidase Inhibitors

The activating effects of iproniazid led to the first clinical studies identifying this drug (and others that are inhibitors of biogenic amine degradation via oxidative deamination) as antidepressant agents. The increased levels of norepinephrine and serotonin in the brain following MAO inhibition suggested that these changes might account for the drugs' antidepressant effects. However, more comprehensive clinical studies during the past decade demonstrated that these drugs are not especially effective in the more severely depressed patients who require hospitalization (Medical Research Council, 1965; Murphy et al., 1974b). Although an "atypical" group of depressed patients was later suggested to constitute a subgroup of responsive patients (West and Dally, 1959; Pare, Rees, and Sainsbury, 1962), recent studies have been successful in identifying phobic, anxious patients as the psychiatric patients most likely to respond to the MAO-inhibiting drugs (Tyrer, Candy, and Kelly, 1973).

These clinical studies of MAO-inhibiting drugs lessen the potential importance of utilizing the drugs' biochemical effects to further our understanding of depressive symptomatology. In addition, these drugs have a number of cellular effects besides their capacity to inhibit MAO (Costa and Sandler, 1972; Weiner and Bjur, 1972). They do not increase brain levels of all the neurotransmitters equally; and, as with the uptake effects of the tricyclics, their MAO-inhibiting effects occur much more rapidly than do their clinical behavioral effects. It thus appears unlikely that their clinical effects can be simply understood as an immediate consequence of their MAO-inhibiting effects.

Taken together, this newer information on the mechanism of action of the antidepressants is in keeping with the more recently recognized importance of adaptive mechanisms such as amine synthesis changes (Mandell et al., 1972) and amine receptor function changes (Bunney and Murphy, 1975) in behavioral regulation and in the mediation of psychoactive drug effects. This information has helped shift the time frame for the evaluation of biochemical effects of these drugs from hours and days to weeks—and hence closer to the time usually required for their clinical antidepressant effects to appear. These longer-term adaptive and regulatory processes delineated from studies of psychoactive drugs are now coming under scrutiny in relation to their possible contribution to the genesis of mood, behavioral, and neuroendocrine changes in depressed patients.

CONCLUDING REMARKS

There have been a number of developments over the past several years contributing to the understanding of psychoactive drug effects relevant to depression. Recent studies indicate that clinical factors may predict antidepressant drug responses, since some clinically defined subgroups of depressed patients have been demonstrated to respond differentially to various antidepressant drugs. Some biological predictors of antidepressant drug response have also been described, including genetically based differences in the metabolism of tricyclic and MAO-inhibiting antidepressants.

Investigations of the biochemical effects accompanying the long-term administration of antidepressant agents in animals and man have suggested that early attempts to understand their mechanisms of behavioral action on the basis of acute, high-dosage studies in animals may be incorrect. Similarly, some components of the early biological models of depression derived from these mechanisms no longer appear valid. Hypotheses based primarily on norepinephrine alterations in brain as representing mediating or even etiological mechanisms in depressed behavior have been replaced by more complex formulations involving interactions between catecholamines and other brain neurotransmitter systems. In addition, increased knowledge of synaptic mechanisms has permitted more detailed specification not only of some additional biochemical sites of action of antidepressant drugs but also of hypothesized sites of synaptic abnormalities that may contribute to depressed behavior.

REFERENCES

Alexanderson, B., Sjöqvist, F., and Price Evans, D. A. (1969): Steady-state plasma levels of nortriptyline in twins: Influence of genetic factors and drug therapy. *Br. Med. J.*, 4:764–768.

Asberg, M., Bertilsson, L., Tuck, D., Cronholm, B., and Sjöqvist, F. (1973): Indoleamine metabolites in the cerebrospinal fluid of depressed patients before and during treatment with nortriptyline. *Clin. Pharmacol. Ther.,* 14:277–286.

Asberg, M., Crönholm, B., Sjöqvist, F., and Tuck, D. (1971): Relationship between plasma level and therapeutic effect of nortriptyline. *Br. Med. J.,* 3:331–334.

Beckmann, H., and Goodwin, F. K. (1975): Central norepinephrine metabolism and the prediction of antidepressant response to imipramine or amitriptyline: Studies with urinary MHPG in unipolar depressed patients. *Arch. Gen. Psychiatry (in press).*

Braithwaite, R. A., Goulding, R., Theano, G., Bailey, J., and Coppen, A. (1972): Plasma concentration of amitriptyline and clinical response. *Lancet,* 1:1297–1300.

Bunney, W. E., Jr., Brodie, H. K. H., Murphy, D. L., and Goodwin, F. K. (1970): Psychopharmacological differentiation between two subgroups of depressed patients. In: *Proceedings of the American Psychological Association.*

Bunney, W. E., Jr., and Davis, J. M. (1965): Norepinephrine in depressive reactions. *Arch. Gen. Psychiatry,* 13:483–494.

Bunney, W. E., Jr., Goodwin, F. K., Murphy, D. L., House, K. M., and Gordon, E. K. (1972): The "switch process" in manic-depressive illness. II. Relationship to catecholamines, REM sleep and drugs. *Arch. Gen. Psychiatry,* 27:304–309.

Bunney, W. E., Jr., and Murphy, D. L. (1975): Strategies for the study of neurotransmitter receptor function in man. In: *Pre and Post-Synaptic Receptors,* edited by E. Usdin and W. E. Bunney, Jr. Marcel Dekker, New York (in press).

Burrows, G. D., and Davies, B. (1971): Antidepressants and barbiturates. *Br. Med. J.,* 4:113.

Burrows, G. D., Davies, B., and Scoggins, B. A. (1972): Plasma concentration of nortriptyline and clinical response in depressive illness. *Lancet,* 2:619–623.

Carlsson, A. (1970): Structural specificity for inhibition of (^{14}C)-5-hydroxytryptamine uptake by cerebral slices. *J. Pharm. Pharmacol.,* 22:729–732.

Carlsson, A., Fuxe, K., Hamberger, B., and Malmfors, T. (1969): Effect of a new series on bicyclic compounds with potential thymoleptic properties on the reserpine-resistant uptake mechanism of central and peripheral monoamine neurones in vivo and in vitro. *Br. J. Pharmacol.,* 36:18–28.

Carroll, B. J. (1971): Monoamine precursors in the treatment of depression. *Clin. Pharmacol. Ther.,* 12:743–761.

Colburn, R. W., Goodwin, F. K., Bunney, W. E., Jr., and Davis, J. M. (1967): Effect of lithium on the uptake of noradrenaline by synaptosomes. *Nature (Lond.),* 215:1395–1397.

Costa, E., and Sandler, M. (1972): Monoamine oxidases—new vistas. *Adv. Biochem. Psychopharmacol.,* 5:1–447.

Fann, W. E., Davis, J. M., Janowsky, D. S., Kaufman, J. S., Griffith, J. D., and Oates, J. A. (1972): Effect of iprindole on amine uptake in man. *Arch. Gen. Psychiatry,* 26:158–162.

Fawcett, J., Maas, J. W., and Dekirmenjian, H. (1972): Depression and MHPG excretion. *Arch. Gen. Psychiatry,* 26:246–251.

Fischer, E., Spatz, H., Saavedra, J. M., Reggiani, H., Miro, A. H., and Heller, B. (1972): Urinary elimination of phenethylamine. *Biol. Psychiatry,* 5:139–147.

Glowinski, J., and Axelrod, J. (1964): Inhibition of uptake of tritiated-noradrenaline in the intact rat brain by imipramine and structurally related compounds. *Nature (Lond.),* 204:1318–1319.

Goodwin, F. K., and Murphy, D. L. (1974): Biological factors in the affective disorders and schizophrenia. *Psychopharmacol. Agents,* 3:5–26.

Goodwin, F. K., Murphy, D. L., Brodie, H. K. H., and Bunney, W. E., Jr. (1970): L-DOPA, catecholamines and behavior: A clinical and biochemical study in depressed patients. *Biol. Psychiatry,* 2:341–366.

Goodwin, F. K., Murphy, D. L., Dunner, D. L., and Bunney, W. E., Jr. (1972): Lithium response in unipolar versus bipolar depression. *Am. J. Psychiatry,* 129:44–47.

Goodwin, F. K., Post, R. M., Dunner, D. L., and Gordon, E. K. (1973): Cerebrospinal fluid amine metabolites in affective illness: The probenecid technique. *Am. J. Psychiatry,* 130:73–79.

Gram, L. F., and Overø, K. F. (1972): Drug interaction: Inhibitory effect of neuroleptics on metabolism of tricyclic antidepressants in man. *Br. Med. J.,* 1:463–465.

Gyermek, L. (1966): The pharmacology of imipramine and related anti-depressants. *Int. Rev. Neurobiol.,* 9:95–143.

Hammer, W., and Sjöqvist, F. (1967): Plasma levels of monomethylated tricyclic anti-depressants during treatment with imipramine-like compounds. *Life Sci.,* 6:1895–1903.

Hollister, L. E. (1973): *Clinical Use of Psychotherapeutic Drugs.* Charles C Thomas, Springfield, Ill.

Hollister, L. E., Overall, J. E., Shelton, J., Pennington, V., Kimbell, I., and Johnson, M., (1967): Drug therapy of depression: Amitriptyline, perphenazine, and their combination in different syndromes. *Arch. Gen. Psychiatry,* 17:486–498.

Janowsky, D. S., El-Yousef, M. K., Davis, J. M., Hubbard, B., and Sekerke, H. J. (1972): Cholinergic reversal of manic symptoms. *Lancet,* 1:1236–1237.

Johnstone, E. C., and Marsh, W. (1973): Acetylator status and response to phenelzine in depressed patients. *Lancet,* 1:567–570.

Kannengiesser, M. H., Hunt, P., and Raynaud, J-P. (1973): An in vitro model for the study of psychotropic drugs and as a criterion of antidepressant activity. *Biochem. Pharmacol.,* 22:73–84.

Klein, D. F., and Davis, J. M. (1969): *Diagnosis and Drug Treatment of Psychiatric Disorders.* Williams & Wilkins, Baltimore.

Kragh-Sørensen, P., Eggert-Hansen, C., and Asberg, M. (1975): Plasma levels of nortriptyline in the treatment of endogenous depression. *Lancet (in press).*

Lahti, R. A., and Maickel, R. P. (1971): The tricyclic antidepressants—inhibition of norepinephrine uptake as related to potentiation of norepinephrine and clinical efficacy. *Biochem. Pharmacol.,* 20:482–486.

Lapin, I. P., and Oxenkrug, G. F. (1969): Intensification of the central serotoninergic processes as a possible determinant of the thymoleptic effect. *Lancet,* 1:132–136.

Maas, J. W., Fawcett, J. A., and Dekirmenjian, H. (1972): Catecholamine metabolism, depressive illness, and drug response. *Arch. Gen. Psychiatry,* 26:252–261.

Mandell, A. J., Segal, D. S., Kuczenski, R. T., and Knapp, S. (1972): Some macromolecular mechanisms in CNS neurotransmitter pharmacology and their physiological organizations. In: *The Chemistry of Mood, Motivation and Memory,* edited by J. McGaugh, pp. 105–148. Plenum Press, New York.

Medical Research Council (1965): Clinical trial of treatment of depressive illness. *Br. Med. J.,* 1:881–886.

Mendlewicz, J., Fieve, R. R., and Stallone, F. (1972): Genetic history as a predictor of lithium response in manic-depressive illness. *Lancet,* 1:599–600.

Moody, J. P., Tait, A. C., and Todrick, A. (1967): Plasma levels of imipramine and desmethylimipramine during therapy. *Br. J. Psychiatry,* 113:183–193.

Murphy, D. L. (1972): Amine precursors, amines and false neurotransmitters in depressed patients. *Am. J. Psychiatry,* 129:141–148.

Murphy, D. L., Baker, M., Goodwin, F. K., Miller, H., Kotin, J., and Bunney, W. E., Jr. (1974a): L-Tryptophan in affective disorders: Indoleamine changes and differential clinical effects. *Psychopharmacologia,* 34:11–20.

Murphy, D. L., Brand, E., Baker, M., van Kammen, D. P., and Gordon, E. (1974b): Phenelzine effects in hospitalized unipolar and bipolar depressed patients: Behavioral and biochemical relationships. *J. Pharmacol. (Suppl. 1),* 5:102–103.

Murphy, D. L., Brodie, H. K. H., Goodwin, F. K., and Bunney, W. E., Jr. (1971a): L-DOPA: Regular induction of hypomania in bipolar manic-depressive patients. *Nature (Lond.),* 229:135–136.

Murphy, D. L., and Costa, J. L. (1975): Utilization of cellular studies of neurotransmitter-related enzymes and transport processes in man for the investigation of biological factors in behavioral disorders. In: *Recent Biological Studies of Depressive Illness,* edited by J. Mendels. Spectrum Publications, New York (in press).

Murphy, D. L., Colburn, R. W., Davis, J. M., and Bunney, W. E., Jr. (1970): Imipramine and lithium effects on biogenic amine transport in depressed and manic-depressed patients. *Am. J. Psychiatry,* 127:339–345.

Murphy, D. L., Goodwin, F. K., Brodie, H. K. H., and Bunney, W. E., Jr. (1973): L-DOPA, dopamine, and hypomania. *Am. J. Psychiatry,* 130:79–82.

Murphy, D. L., Goodwin, F. K., and Bunney, W. E., Jr. (1971b): Clinical and pharmacological investigations of the psychobiology of the affective disorders. *Int. Pharmacopsychiatry,* 6:137–146.

Murphy, D. L., Goodwin, F. K., and Bunney, W. E., Jr. (1975): The psychobiology of mania. In: *American Handbook of Psychiatry,* Vol. 6, edited by D. Hamburg. Basic Books, New York (*in press*).

Murphy, D. L., and Kopin, I. J. (1972): The transport of biogenic amines. In: *Metabolic Transport,* edited by L. E. Hokin, pp. 503–542. Academic Press, New York.

Murphy, D. L., and Redmond, D. (1975): The catecholamines: Possible role in affect, mood and emotional behavior in man and animals. In: *Catecholamines and Behavior,* edited by A. J. Friedhoff, pp. 73–117. Plenum Press, New York.

Overall, J. E., Hollister, L. E., Johnson, M., and Pennington, V. (1966): Nosology of depression and differential response to drugs. *J.A.M.A.,* 195:946–948.

Overall, J. E., Hollister, L. E., Meyer, F., Kimbell, I., Jr., and Shelton, J. (1964): Imipramine and thioridazine in depressed and schizophrenic patients: Are there specific antidepressant drugs? *J.A.M.A.,* 189:605–608.

Pare, C. M. B., Rees, L., and Sainsbury, M. J. (1962): Differentiation of two genetically specific types of depression by the response to antidepressants. *Lancet,* 2:1340–1343.

Paykel, E. S. (1972): Depressive typologies and response to amitriptyline. *Br. J. Psychiatry,* 120:147–156.

Post, R. M., and Goodwin, F. K. (1973): Stimulated behavior states: An approach to specificity in psychobiological research. *Biol. Psychiatry,* 7:237–254.

Prange, A. J., Jr., Wilson, I. C., Lynn, C. W., Alltop, L. B., and Stikeleather, R. A. (1974): L-Tryptophan in mania. *Arch. Gen. Psychiatry,* 30:56–64.

Price Evans, D. A., Davison, K., and Pratt, R. T. C. (1964): The influence of acetylator phenotype on the effects of treating depression with phenelzine. *Clin. Pharmacol. Ther.,* 6:431–435.

Prien, R. F., Klett, C. J., and Caffey, E. M., Jr. (1974): Lithium prophylaxis in recurrent affective illness. *Am. J. Psychiatry,* 131:198–203.

Raskin, A. (1974): A guide for drug use in depressive disorders. *Am. J. Psychiatry,* 131:181–185.

Raskin, A., Schulterbrandt, J. G., Reatig, N., and McKeon, J. J. (1970): Differential response to chlorpromazine, imipramine, and placebo: A study of subgroups of hospitalized depressed patients. *Arch. Gen. Psychiatry,* 23:164–173.

Reid, W. D., Stefano, F. J. E., Kurzepa, S., and Brodie, B. B. (1969): Tricyclic antidepressants: Evidence for an intraneuronal site of action. *Science,* 164:437–439.

Rosenblatt, S., and Chanley, J. D. (1974): Measuring the pharmacological action of imipramine in the treatment of depressions. *Arch. Gen. Psychiatry,* 30:456–460.

Schanberg, S. M., Schildkraut, J. J., and Kopin, I. J. (1967): The effects of psychoactive drugs on norepinephrine-^{3}H metabolism in brain. *Biochem. Pharmacol.,* 16:393–399.

Schildkraut, J. J. (1965): The catecholamine hypothesis of affective disorders: A review of supporting evidence. *Am. J. Psychiatry,* 122:509–522.

Schildkraut, J. J. (1973): Norepinephrine metabolites as biochemical criteria for classifying depressive disorders and predicting responses to treatment: Preliminary findings. *Am. J. Psychiatry,* 130:695–699.

Schildkraut, J. J. (1974): Biogenic amines and affective disorders. *Ann. Rev. Med.,* 25:333–348.

Schildkraut, J. J. (1975): Depressions and biogenic amines. In: *American Handbook of Psychiatry,* Vol. 4, edited by D. Hamburg. Basic Books, New York (*in press*).

Schildkraut, J. J., Keeler, B. A., Grab, E. L., Kantrowich, J. (1973): MHPG excretion and clinical classification in depressive disorders. *Lancet,* 1:1251–1252.

Schildkraut, J. J., and Kety, S. S. (1967): Biogenic amines and emotion. *Science,* 156:21–30.

Tyrer, P., Candy, J., and Kelly, D. (1973): A study of the clinical effects of phenelzine and placebo in the treatment of phobic anxiety. *Psychopharmacologia,* 32:237–254.

Weiner, N., and Bjur, R. (1972): The role of intraneuronal monoamine oxidase in the regulation of norepinephrine synthesis. *Adv. Biochem. Psychopharmacol.,* 5:409–419.

West, E. D., and Dally, P. J. (1959): Effects of iproniazid in depressive syndromes. *Br. Med. J.,* 1:1491–1494.

Wharton, R. N., Perel, J. M., Dayton, P. G., and Malitz, S. (1971): A potential clinical use for the interaction of methylphenidate (Ritalin) with tricyclic antidepressants. *Am. J. Psychiatry,* 127:1619–1625.

Wilson, I. C., and Prange, A. J., Jr. (1972): Tryptophan in mania: Theory of affective disorders. *Psychopharmacologia (Suppl.),* 26:76.

Woodruff, R. W., Goodwin, D. W., and Guze, S. B. (1974): *Psychiatric Diagnosis.* Oxford University Press, New York.

Zeidenberg, P., Perel, J. M., Kanzler, M., Wharton, R. N., and Malitz, S. (1971): Clinical and metabolic studies with imipramine in man. *Am. J. Psychiatry,* 127:1321–1326.

Chapter 9

Tricyclic Antidepressants

John M. Davis

A new dimension was added to the treatment of depressive illness during the late 1950s with the development of two classes of drugs—the tricyclic antidepressants (imipramine-type drugs) and the monoamine oxidase (MAO) inhibitors. Prior to these discoveries the principal treatment approaches to depression were based predominantly on the use of psychotherapy, psychomotor stimulants, narcotics, sedatives, and electroconvulsive therapy (ECT). Over the last decade tricyclic agents, because of their therapeutic efficacy in the treatment of approximately 70% of depressed patients, have received widespread clinical application. Nonetheless, in spite of their distinct therapeutic advantages, there remain problems with their use; these difficulties underscore the importance of adopting a judicious approach to their clinical application and alert and discriminating attention to the ongoing clinical research with them.

In this connection the clinician's task is complicated by the multiple uses of the concept of depression and by the relatively undeveloped state of knowledge concerning the causes of the affective disorders in general. In time it seems probable that the pharmacological effects of antidepressant drugs may produce important clues concerning the causes of depression.

HISTORY

The discoveries of the antidepressant properties of both tricyclic agents and the MAO inhibitors were the fortuitous and unexpected consequences of tangential avenues of research. While investigating the antipsychotic activity of imipramine (which is structurally similar to the phenothiazines), the Swiss clinical researcher Kuhn (1958) found that although it was ineffective in schizophrenia it did produce considerable improvement in depressed patients. Similar serendipitous findings contributed to the development of the MAO inhibitors when iproniazid, the first of these agents, was found to produce mood elevation and euphoria (side effects) in tuberculous patients. On the basis of the preliminary clinical observations, later researchers administered this agent to depressed patients with favorable results.

Subsequent to the discovery that imipramine functions as an active antidepressant, the pharmaceutical industry proceeded with the development of numerous antidepressant agents similar to imipramine in their structural and pharmacological properties. The early development of this class of drugs, as well as the MAO inhibitors—both of which have revolutionized the treatment of depression—emphasized that not all critical pharmacological discoveries are made deductively from general theory or in the course of basic animal research and laboratory experiments. Pharmaceutical researchers have frequently found in their work with antidepressants that relationships between chemical structure and pharmacological activity which evolved from animal test systems clearly do not predict a drug's antidepressant activity in man. In the case of the antidepressant medications, as with the antipsychotic agents, it is instructive to note the crucial importance of alert clinical observations in the early development of these drugs.

PHARMACOLOGICAL ACTIVITY

Unlike the amphetamines, which are not antidepressants in the precise sense of the word, tricyclic agents are not general stimulants and euphoriants and do not appreciably influence the normal organism in a baseline state. The action of these agents seems to become pronounced in the presence of an abnormal condition. It is similar, for example, to the action of aspirin, which reduces ordinary hyperpyrexia but does not reduce the temperature of the normal organism. Hence although there is adequate evidence that the imipramine-type drugs have no substantial effect on normal persons, they have a marked antidepressant effect on depressed patients.

EVALUATION AND METHODOLOGICAL ISSUES

The comparison in controlled trials of a new antidepressant drug with other standard treatment methods (e.g., ECT, placebo, or a well-studied drug such as imipramine) is a critical aspect in assessing the efficacy of the new agent in ameliorating depression. In such comparisons the use of a placebo control group is particularly important, since many controlled studies show that 30 to 50% of depressed patients receiving only placebo improve during the investigative period. This group includes patients who improve spontaneously owing to a variety of endogenous and exogenous factors, those who respond to the nonpharmacological aspects of their treatment regimen, and those who fall into the classic category for placebo-induced improvement; i.e., the patient is taking a pill which he reasons must be helping him to get better.

Examination of uncontrolled studies of new psychoactive drugs almost always reveals a higher rate of improvement than is found in controlled studies. One may hypothesize that this is in part due to the bias of the clinical investigator, who has a strong desire to help his patients and who therefore "sees" more improvement than has actually occurred. Conversely, well-controlled double-blind studies characterized by a highly skeptical approach may serve to reduce the actual rate of improvement occurring in patients under investigation.

Identification of the type of patient who responds to a given drug and the composition of the patient population under investigation are probably the most crucial factors in drug efficacy studies. Results pooled from many controlled studies (Klerman and Cole, 1965) reveal that 46% of acutely depressed, recently hospitalized patients improved during the first few weeks of placebo treatment, whereas only 16% of chronically depressed hospitalized patients improved with placebo. Outpatients treated with placebo exhibited a 21% improvement rate. Reasons for these differences are by no means clear, but variability in the types of depression exhibited by different members of the sample is most certainly a contributing factor. For example, the hospital atmosphere may prove unpleasant to the inpatient, or he may be experiencing pressure from home, causing him to complain less and therefore be discharged sooner. Furthermore, some patients may not possess a true depressive disorder (e.g., schizophrenics, patients with chronic character disorders, paranoid patients with depression) and hence may not respond to antidepressant drugs alone. Thus the reported ineffectiveness of a drug in a controlled investigation may be a function of the proportion of "poor responders" or inappropriately diagnosed patients within the sample, rather than the ineffectiveness of the drug used.

One further research finding noteworthy for both the researcher and the clinician is the proportion, if any, of patients who are made worse by the drug. This information should always be reported in one's findings, and well-done controlled studies not only report global judgments but also describe in detail changes in the various aspects of the depressive psychopathology of the patients studied (e.g., agitation, retardation, guilt, anxiety).

Drug combinations must always be considered in clinical evaluation, since agents such as the phenothiazines may themselves provide some benefit in relieving depressive symptoms. Another drug-related problem arises when an active agent such as amphetamine or atropine is used as the comparison drug in a controlled study. These drugs may cause a patient to become better or worse, hence providing a different basis for comparison than does an inert placebo or a standard antidepressant drug.

Finally, side effects "produced" by antidepressant drugs constitute an important methodological problem. Many of the side effects commonly associated with antidepressive drugs are also fairly typical symptoms of depression itself (e.g., fatigue, dry mouth, dizziness, constipation, profuse sweating, tremor, nausea and vomiting, drowsiness, insomnia, sexual impotence). Thus some of these symptoms may have been present prior to initiation of treatment, and others may spontaneously appear during treatment but may be unrelated to the drug, being caused instead by the depressive disorder itself. Here we once again see the importance of using a control group receiving placebo. Interpretation of the possible relationship between the drug and the exhibited side effects becomes as important as the possible relationship between the drug and the observed clinical improvement. Specifically, one must demonstrate that the frequency with which any side effect appears in conjunction with administration of the drug is greater than its base rate occurrence in a comparable, untreated population.

A summary of the results of some well-controlled studies of antidepressant drugs is contained in Table 1, which provides a "box score" of the results of all the double-blind studies that have compared the antidepressants with a placebo, or imipramine with other antidepressants. Double-blind studies that used random assignment of patients to different treatment groups are included. Each study was reviewed and a decision was made as to whether it had shown the drug to be more effective than a placebo or other control medication. Global judgments were based on the entire body of evidence presented. When

TABLE 1. *Summary of the controlled double-blind studies of the tricyclic antidepressants*

Drug or other treatment	No. of studies of tricyclic drugs	
	Drug more effective than placebo	Drug equal to or less effective than placebo
Tricyclic drugs		
Imipramine (Tofranil)	26	12
Amitriptyline (Elavil)	9	2
Desipramine (Norpramin, Pertofrane)	3	2
Nortriptyline (Aventyl)	4	0
Protriptyline (Vivactil)	2	0
Opipramol (Ensidon)	4	0
Trimipramine (Surmontil)	1	0

	No. of studies of other antidepressant therapies		
	Treatment more effective than imipramine	Treatment equal to imipramine	Treatment less effective than imipramine
MAO inhibitors			
Tranylcypromine (Parnate)	0	3	0
Iproniazid (Marsilid)	0	1	1
Isocarboxazid (Marplan)	0	2	2
Nialamide (Niamid)	0	0	1
Pheniprazine (Catron)	0	1	1
Phenelzine (Nardil)	0	4	3
Pargyline (Eutonyl)	0	0	0
Etryptamine (Monase)	0	0	0
Other treatments			
Electroshock therapy	4	3	0
Chlorpromazine (Thorazine)	0	3	0
Thioridazine (Mellaril)	0	1	0
Chlorprothixene (Taractan)	0	1	0

necessary, statistics were recalculated using different methods than those used by the original author in order to arrive at the appropriate categorization.

TRICYCLIC ANTIDEPRESSANTS

The major imipramine-like antidepressants—imipramine, desipramine, amitriptyline, nortriptyline, and protriptyline—are quite similar structurally to the phenothiazines (Fig. 1). The synthesis of imipramine, from which the other tricyclic drugs are derived, entails replacing the sulfur atom in the phenothiazine molecule with a dimethyl bridge. Although this is a relatively minor structural alteration, it produces a critical difference in pharmacological

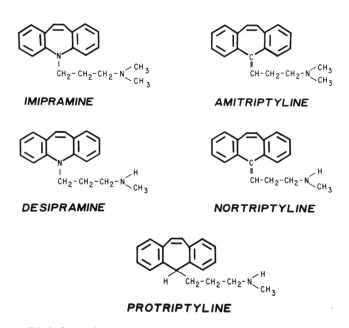

FIG. 1. Chemical structures of the major tricyclic antidepressant drugs.

activity and is illustrative of the significant pharmacological effects of highly discrete structural modifications.

The tricyclic antidepressants are readily absorbed from the gastrointestinal tract. In humans imipramine and amitriptyline are partially metabolized to their desmethyl derivatives (desipramine and nortriptyline). Knowledge of this process led to the synthesis of desipramine in the hope that it would exert its antidepressant action more rapidly than its parent compound does. Clinical studies, however, clearly demonstrate no difference in speed or action of the newer compounds. The side effects of the desmethyl derivatives are said to be less sedating than their parent compounds. Amitriptyline is reported to be more sedating than imipramine, and protriptyline less so.

CLINICAL EFFECTS

The principal tricyclic antidepressants—imipramine, amitriptyline, nortriptyline, desipramine, protriptyline—constitute the most effective class of antidepressants and are beneficial to approximately 70% of depressed patients. This incidence of improvement may be contrasted to the roughly 20 to 40% who are helped by placebo within the same time period. When considered from the patient's perspective, his chance of recovery within 3 to 4 weeks is doubled if he receives tricyclic medication instead of a placebo. Because of their relatively greater therapeutic effectiveness when compared with other antidepressant medications, and because they have the least risk of side effects, the tricyclic drugs are probably the drugs of choice for most depressive illness.

In general, it is the severe psychotic or endogenous depressive who responds best to tricyclic drugs, whereas the chronic characterologic depressive responds less well. The therapeutic response, when it occurs, develops after a lag period of 3 to 14 days and results in marked improvement in behavior and a striking decrease in depression. Patients who remain unresponsive after 3 weeks of treatment at adequate dosage levels will probably not respond at all and consequently should be shifted to another drug or receive ECT. Most well-controlled investigations show few tangible statistical differences between the tricyclics with regard to efficacy or speed of onset.

One hopes that more effective antidepressants will be developed in the future. Although a class of drugs that is effective in 70% of depressed patients is less than optimal, one should not forget the other side of the coin, i.e., that these medications bring about marked improvement in almost twice the number of patients who improve on placebo.

CLINICAL USE AND DOSAGE

In the treatment of depression with drugs, dosage is a particularly important variable. Prior to medication it is essential first to make a careful determination of the patient's psychiatric, medical, and medication status. The patient's age, severity of depression, and medical (especially cardiovascular) status bear on the rapidity of dosage increase. For patients with pre-existing cardiovascular disease, a cautious approach and careful monitoring are required: lower initial doses with smaller and less rapid increases are used. If the patient is extremely depressed and suicidal but medically sound, prompt movement to a higher dosage (or to ECT) may be indicated.

Under ordinary circumstances the physician starts the patient on a modest dose, e.g., imipramine or amitriptyline, 25 mg t.i.d. If the dosage is well tolerated, within several days the patient is graduated to 50 mg t.i.d. After 1 week the dose may be increased to 200 mg/day or in some cases to 250 mg/day. A critical dosage exists for each individual, and the physician should bear in mind that this level must be reached for clinical response to occur. Systematic attention to side effects and therapeutic results, as well as the monitoring of postural hypotension with lying and standing blood pressures, are important in dosage adjustments.

After the patient is stabilized on a safe and clinically effective dose and has recovered from the depression, the dosage is gradually reduced by 25% to 50%. Because there is ample evidence that patients may not take their drugs, at this point it is advisable to administer the total daily medication at bedtime. This procedure proves as satisfactory as divided doses because of the long half-lives of the tricyclic drugs. This regimen is simpler for the patient to remember and permits the most pronounced side effects to occur during sleep when they are not noticed. The physician also may utilize the sedative effects of tricyclic agents such as amitriptyline to induce adequate sleep without the necessity of giving a sleeping medication. Furthermore, this procedure permits a substantial reduction in the vast amount of staff time spent in the multiple, daily administration of medications. Finally, by giving the total daily dose in a single capsule, rather than in divided doses, the cost of the daily medication may be reduced by as much as 50%.

MAINTENANCE

After remission in the patient's depression is achieved and he has been discharged from the hospital, the clinician faces the decision of when to discontinue the antidepressant medication. For many patients depression is a recurrent disorder, so the issue of whether continued treatment with tricyclic drugs will prevent relapse is an important one. In an effort to develop evidence pertinent to this question, Mindham, Howland, and Shepherd (1972) pursued a collaborative study in cooperation with 34 psychiatrists in Great Britain. The subject population was limited to depressed patients who had responded to treatment with either imipramine or amitriptyline in doses of at least 150 mg/day. The patients were assigned to one of two groups; one was placed on a placebo for 15 months, while the other was maintained on tricyclic agents at 75 to 100 mg/day. At the end of 15 months 50% of the placebo group had relapsed compared to a relapse rate of only 22% in the tricyclic maintenance group. In both groups the rate of relapse was approximately linear (Fig. 2). No data are yet available that yield adequate predictors of which patients require tricyclic medication to prevent relapse, except that those with incomplete remissions relapse more regularly (Mindham et al., 1972). The clinical implication of this finding and four other studies is that maintenance treatment is indicated in some patients for at least a year or so.

Consequently once remission is achieved, patients should be continued at full dosage for 1 month. The dosage is then reduced by approximately 50% for maintenance treatment (e.g., to 75 mg imipramine). Extended medication

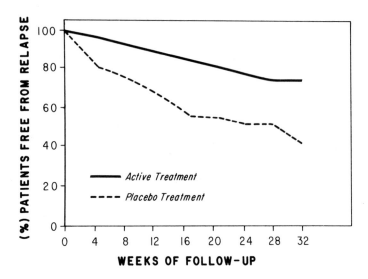

FIG. 2. Comparison of relapse rates in depressed patients receiving either a tricyclic drug or a placebo. (Adapted from Mindham et al., 1972.)

with tricyclic agents or lithium may be indicated for unipolar patients prone to frequent recurrences. Maintenance lithium is recommended for bipolar patients to prevent the recurrence of both aspects of this disorder.

BLOOD LEVELS

Approximately 70% of depressed patients are helped by tricyclic drugs. It is probable that some of the nonresponders are suffering from forms of depression unresponsive to this class of medications. However, others may not respond for two further reasons related to abnormalities in the metabolic rate of tricyclic drugs.

Under ordinary circumstances, as the tricyclic agents are administered blood levels build up until they reach a fairly constant level within about a week. There are considerable individual differences in plasma levels. It appears that some patients have a metabolic defect that results in the accumulation of unusually high plasma and brain levels. Consequently these patients may fail to improve clinically because they are receiving a toxic dose. Others appear to metabolize the tricyclic drugs with unusual rapidity; as a result they fail to develop adequate blood levels and hence have low brain levels. These patients may prove especially slow in responding to the medication and are likely to remain unresponsive to lower dosages.

Using variable treatment dosages, Asberg and her colleagues (Asberg, Cronholm, Sjoqvist, and Tuck, 1971a; Asberg, Price-Evans, and Sjoqvist, 1971b) explored the relationships between therapeutic response and plasma concentrations of nortriptyline. Among those patients who failed to respond were two subgroups with very high and very low blood levels of nortriptyline. Kragh-Sorensen, Asberg, and Eggert-Hansen (1973) replicated these studies using a constant dose of 150 mg. A number of patients were found to have relatively high plasma levels of nortriptyline, and these patients did significantly less well. After reducing their dose, five of these patients responded rapidly and were discharged from the hospital within a week—a finding which suggests that their initial unresponsiveness to the drug was due to having a plasma concentration that was too high.

Further studies of blood levels of tricyclic agents were developed by Braithwaite, Goulding, Theano, Bailey, and Coppen (1972). In an investigation of plasma amitriptyline and nortriptyline in patients receiving amitriptyline, they found that low plasma levels of these two tricyclic agents were not effective, whereas moderate levels produced a good therapeutic response. No interpretation was made, however, of possible relationships between high blood levels and poor clinical response. When these findings were reanalyzed by Gruvstad (1973), the evidence suggested a tendency for patients with elevated blood levels to have a poorer response than the group with intermediate levels. It should be noted that although these results are suggestive and have potential clinical importance, a definitive interpretation of the significance of plasma levels awaits further efforts designed to replicate and clarify these data.

Desipramine and nortriptyline, the desmethyl derivatives of both amitriptyline and imipramine, are also active antidepressants; hence this metabolic transformation probably has little effect on these drugs' therapeutic activities. This group of compounds are hydroxylated on the ring, which then undergoes conjugation. The site of the rate-limiting metabolism of the tricyclic drugs is probably the liver. The hydroxylation rate can be affected by previous drug treatment which alters liver enzymes, but is also determined by genetic factors, the mode of inheritance probably being polygenic (Asberg et al., 1971b).

There is a very high correlation between the reciprocal single-dose plasma clearance rates and the multiple-dose steady-state plasma levels (Alexanderson, 1972). Consequently it should be possible to use single-dose plasma clearance levels as a predictor of steady-state levels. If these correlations conform to a curvilinear relationship, clinicians will have an important basis for predicting plasma levels and hence avoiding levels that are too high or low to induce a therapeutic response.

Many clinicians have formed the impression that different patients respond to different doses of tricyclics. This clinical finding is consistent with available plasma level data, which indicate that there are wide individual differences in the rate at which these drugs are metabolized. Hence preliminary evidence suggests that the clinician should make an effort to find the best tricyclic dose for a particular patient, keeping in mind that nonresponse may indicate an overly high dose as well as inadequate dosage. At this point in the state of the art, adjustment of medication to achieve therapeutic blood levels must be carried out purely on the basis of clinical acumen. In the future, laboratory studies may provide us with procedures to achieve the desired result in a more precise and rapid fashion.

SIDE EFFECTS AND ADVERSE REACTIONS

The tricyclic medications produce roughly comparable side effects, although there are some slight quantitative differences worthy of note: Amitriptyline is reported to be more sedating and protriptyline less sedating than imipramine.

Autonomic Effects

Minor differences notwithstanding, all the tricyclic antidepressants can cause the autonomic effects that might be expected as a result of their anticholinergic pharmacological properties. Dry mouth, palpitations, tachycardia, loss of accommodation, postural hypotension, fainting, dizziness, vomiting, constipation, edema, and aggravation of narrow-angle glaucoma are among the more frequently appearing autonomic side effects. More rarely, urinary retention and paralytic ileus leading to serious or even fatal complications have been reported, particularly when the tricyclic drugs are combined with other anticholinergic agents. Among the more common side effects, dry mouth is the most frequent, and patients should be warned of its potential occurrence. Postural hypotension, when it occurs, is not usually a problem. For the most part, autonomic effects tend to be mild and usually grow less distressing after the initial weeks of treatment. However, should they remain troublesome they may be effectively controlled by adjusting the dosage level.

Tricyclic antidepressants possess two important properties which may play a role in producing many of the observed autonomic side effects: (1) they inhibit the reuptake of released norepinephrine, thereby potentiating noradrenergic function (norepinephrine remains at the receptor site for a longer time since its action is not terminated by the reuptake pump); and (2) they produce cholinergic blockade, thus producing an atropine-like effect. Blockage of the reuptake pump is important in explaining the drug-drug interaction between guanethidine-type drugs and tricyclic antidepressants. Guanethidine-type antihypertensive medications are also pumped into the peripheral noradrenergic neuron by the membrane pump and are thereby concentrated in the noradrenergic nerve, where they exert their hypotensive effects. When this pump is blocked, the uptake of the hypertensive agent guanethidine is also blocked, thus preventing it from getting to its neuronal site of activity. For this reason treatment with tricyclic antidepressants interferes with the therapeutic effects of guanethidine-type antihypertensive agents, through inhibition of the membrane uptake pump.

Central Nervous System Effects

Tricyclic drugs may induce a fine, persistent tremor, particularly in the upper extremities but also in the tongue. Insomnia and disturbance of motor function may also rarely occur, usually in elderly patients. The insomnia is generally transitory and responds well to nightly sedation. Other central nervous system (CNS) effects that may rarely accompany the administration of tricyclic agents are twitching, convulsions, dysarthria, paresthesia, ataxia, and peroneal palsies.

Occasionally both amitriptyline and imipramine engender episodes of confusion, mania, or schizophrenic excitement. These episodes usually occur in patients manifesting a predisposition to schizophrenia, a chronic brain syndrome, or bipolar manic-depressive psychosis, rather than in patients manifesting a neurosis. This fact suggests that a pre-existing substratum of disease must be present in order for the drug to exert its psychotomimetic properties. In general, these symptoms subside within 1 to 2 days of withdrawing the drug; should they fail to subside, they can be controlled by administering the phenothiazine derivatives.

Mild withdrawal reactions characterized by nausea, vomiting, and general malaise have been reported subsequent to abrupt termination of imipramine. These reactions should not present a clinical problem since gradual dosage reduction is the more frequent procedure; they do not appear when this method is followed.

Allergic and Hypersensitivity Effects

Skin reactions are the most frequently reported allergic reactions to the antidepressant drugs, and they often subside with reduced dosage. Jaundice sometimes occurs early in the treatment program and is of the cholestatic type, similar to that associated with chlorpromazine. Very rarely cases of agranulocytosis, leukocytosis, leukopenia, and eosinophilia have been reported.

Cardiovascular Effects

Tricyclic drugs may cause flattened T-waves, prolonged Q-T intervals, and depressed S-T segments in the electrocardiogram when administered in therapeutic doses. The causative role of antidepressant agents in these side effects remains unclear since it is exceedingly difficult to distinguish a side effect causally related to the drug from a cardiovascular incident precipitated by other factors but which occurs coincidentally with drug therapy. This determination of causality notwithstanding, caution must be exercised in treating the cardiac patient since cardiovascular incidents have occurred in patients with pre-existing heart disease (Moir, Crooks, Sawyer, Turnbull, and Weir, 1972). Hence predisposed patients should be started with lower doses and should have cardiac function monitored carefully, with very gradual dose increment.

Drug Interactions

Severe toxic reactions and extreme hyperpyrexia often leading to death may result when tricyclic antidepressants and MAO inhibitors are used in close conjunction. For this reason a patient receiving an MAO inhibitor should have this medication discontinued at least 1 week prior to commencing tricyclic therapy.

OVERDOSAGE

Since a severe overdosage of tricyclic antidepressants may result in extremely serious life-threatening consequences, it is important that physicians be capable of differentially diagnosing this class of poisoning. The clinical picture is characterized by temporary agitation, delirium, convulsions, hyperreflexive tendons, bowel and bladder paralysis, disturbance of temperature regulation, and mydriasis, with the patient subsequently progressing to coma accompanied by shock and respiratory depression. Cardiac rhythm may be disturbed, resulting in tachycardia, arterial fibrillation, ventricular flutter, and atrioventricular or intraventricular block. Coma generally does not last more than 24 hr.

Treatment should begin with gastric aspiration and lavage, and the diagnosis is confirmed by analyzing the gastric lavage material. Intramuscular anticonvulsants such as diazepam are used to control seizures, the respiration is supported and coma care is applied.

Management of cardiac function is critical during coma, as death can result from cardiac arrhythmia. If the patient survives this period, vigorous resuscitative measures, cardioversion, continuous cardiac monitoring, and chemotherapy to manage arrhythmias should be applied in an intensive care unit. Physostigmine (0.25 to 4 mg i.v. or i.m.) is useful to counteract anticholinergic toxicity and tachycardia, and propranolol is helpful in preventing arrhythmias. The patient must be kept under constant medical supervision for several days to permit immediate attention to any delayed cardiac difficulties that may arise.

Ingestion of several grams (20 to 40 of the 50-mg tablets) can be fatal. Consequently care must be exercised to prevent suicidal depressed patients from gaining access to large numbers of antidepressant tablets.

ANXIETY-DEPRESSION SYNDROME

The nonpsychotic, mixed anxiety-depression syndrome is a common complaint among psychiatric patients. Doxepin, a tricyclic antidepressant drug with both antidepressant and antianxiety properties has been found to be equal in efficacy to diazepam (Valium) and chlordiazepoxide (Librium), and to be superior to placebo. In one study doxepin was slightly superior to diazepam, but this may have been due to the facts that (1) many patients with depression were included in the population studied, and (2) a low dose of diazepam was used. This syndrome has also been treated with conventional tricyclic antidepressants, and doxepin has been approximately equal in therapeutic efficacy to the former drugs.

A combination of amitriptyline and perphenazine has also been used to treat the mixed anxiety-depression syndrome. The rationale for this treatment is presumably that the phenothiazine would be effective in patients who manifest a psychotic process in their illness, whereas the tricyclic agent would be specific for the depressive component of the disorder. Ideally it would be desirable to be specific in diagnosis, so that a specific syndrome would be treated with a single agent, rather than adopting a blanket approach with a broad-spectrum drug or a combination of drugs. The reality of psychiatric practice, however, is that many patients manifest both anxiety and depression, and it is exceedingly difficult to determine which is the primary symptom. Six controlled studies have shown doxepin to be approximately equal to the amitriptyline-perphenazine combination in treating this disorder, and it may be advisable to use one drug rather than a combination.

Rickels and co-workers performed three related studies designed to acquire more specific information regarding the choice of drugs, using psychopharmacology clinic patients, general practice patients, and private psychiatric patients (Rickels, Hutchinson, Weise, Csanalosi, Chung, and Case, 1972). The clinic patients responded slightly more favorably to doxepin than to the amitriptyline-perphenazine combination, whereas the general practice patients responded about equally to doxepin and the combination. The combination appeared to be slightly superior to doxepin in the private psychiatric patients, who tended to be middle class and to suffer from more depression; the phenothiazine-tricyclic combination produced greater improvement in depression and anger-hostility in these patients than did doxepin. Conversely, doxepin proved to be more acceptable in the lower socioeconomic group patients, who exhibited relatively little depression. Other studies have also shown doxepin to be superior to placebo and to be about equal in efficacy to tricyclic antidepressants and phenothiazine-tricyclic combinations. Thus there is clear evidence of doxepin's usefulness in treating outpatient anxiety and depression, the typical dose being 100 to 150 mg/day. However, it has not received extensive testing in psychotic inpatients exhibiting endogenous depression or the depressive phase of a manic-depressive psychosis. Hence more evidence is needed to define the role of the drug in these disorders (i.e., elucidation of its purely antidepressant qualities). Nevertheless there is no doubt of its efficacy in treating the anxiety-depression mixture. Pharmacologically doxepin bears a close structural resemblance to the tricyclic antidepressants and inhibits the membrane uptake pump for the biogenic amines. Consequently it interferes with the antihypertensive actions of guanethidine.

It should be noted that there are at least two ways in which a drug combination may be more advantageous than a single drug in treating depression. The first of these is the synergistic effect in which the combination helps the patient achieve a degree of improvement greater than that seen with either of the drugs singly. The second type of effect is one in which, for example, 90% of population A responds to drug 1 and only 10% to drug 2. The reverse may be true of population B. Hence if the combined population (A + B) is treated with either drug alone, only 50% of the population is helped; whereas if the combination of drugs 1 and 2 is used, 100% of this combined population is helped.

It should be noted that the phenothiazines themselves possess antidepressant properties, particularly in connection with anxious or hostile depressions. The perphenazine-amitriptyline combination appears to be particularly promising with patients manifesting a hostile type of depression. In several studies based on outpatient populations exhibiting mixed anxiety and depression, the amitriptyline-perphenazine combination was superior to chlordiazepoxide and placebo.

However, in the absence of studies that clearly establish which drugs or combinations of drugs to use with which patients, it is reasonable to use antipsychotic drugs alone or in combination with amitriptyline in treating the anxiety-depression syndrome when it appears in patients who also exhibit signs of schizophrenia, endogenous depression, psychotic (delusional) depression, or manic-depressive illness. The presence of psychosis in any form, either schizophrenic symptoms or depressive delusions, is a clear and important indication for use of neuroleptics. However, when this syndrome shades into a nonpsychotic anxiety, which is amenable to treatment on an outpatient basis, doxepin or perphenazine-amitriptyline appears to be effective.

CHOICE OF TREATMENT

Perhaps the major therapeutic question in the treatment of depression is whether drugs or ECT is the more effective treatment modality. In four of seven studies comparing imipramine with electroshock, ECT was found to be more effective, and in the remaining three studies it was equally effective (Clinical Psychiatry Committee, 1965; Wilson, Vernon, Guin, and Sandifer, 1963). These findings suggest that ECT is the preferred mode of treatment. However, other factors merit consideration as well: ECT acts faster than imipramine, a factor of considerable importance in a suicidal patient. Unfortunately ECT produces temporary memory loss, postshock confusion, and perhaps subtle but permanent CNS changes. Therefore many psychiatrists prefer not to use it as a routine measure. It should be noted that even when ECT is used, maintenance tricyclic medication is necessary to prevent recurrence of depression subsequent to the ECT-produced remission. Research studies by Kay, Fahy, and Garside (1970) found that maintenance amitriptyline patients relapsed at a rate of 15%, whereas those maintained on diazepam had a 38% relapse rate. Seager and Bird (1962) found the imipramine maintenance relapse rate to be 17%, and that of placebo 69%.

The recurrence rate of depression subsequent to ECT is high: 18 to 46% after 6 months. Nevertheless, whatever the disadvantages of ECT, it is significant that 50% of those patients who do not respond to imipramine, amitriptyline, or phenelzine do respond to ECT. Clearly it is important to develop methods of pretreatment identification of patients who will not be helped by pharmacotherapy but who will respond to ECT so that they may be started on the treatment of choice as soon as possible.

Studies have found the MAO inhibitors phenelzine and isocarboxazid to be less effective than ECT. However, a tranylcypromine-trifluoperazine combination has been reported to result in relatively rapid antidepressant action, and there is some evidence that this combination can be uniquely effective in a small proportion of patients (Schiele, Vestre, and Skin, 1961). However, methods must be developed which enable us to identify these patients.

It is necessary to underscore the value of pretreatment determination of differential response to various types of treatment. In this regard some observations have already been made that may provide clues to potential response. For example, Pare, Rees, and Sainsbury (1962) suggested that a patient with a genetic relative who responded well to either an imipramine-type drug or an MAO inhibitor responds more favorably to that type of drug than to another. It has also been suggested that hysteria with secondary depression responds best to MAO inhibitors. However, until there is sufficient cross validation of these results such hypotheses must be considered tentative, for when one considers these data in relation to a large number of clinical dimensions it becomes obvious that in some cases good responders are separated from poor responders only by chance. Thus one must look hopefully toward future research to resolve the question of drug specificity for a given patient subtype.

Given this absence of clear-cut difference among drugs, it is wiser for a clinician to be intimately familiar with the assets and liabilities of a small number of drugs than to possess merely a cursory familiarity and experience with a large number. In addition, the physician should be aware of the fact that, in general, imipramine-type (tricyclic) drugs are probably slightly more effective and slightly safer than MAO inhibitors, but that the phenothiazine derivatives and the MAO inhibitors may also be of value in selected cases of depression. While bearing these guidelines in mind, one should continue to examine the literature on new antidepressants to determine whether these newer agents are demonstrably more efficacious than the older drugs, or if more clear-cut differential indications for the use of older drugs in specific types of depressed patients have been developed.

Antidepressant drugs are generally quite safe. Dangerous side effects do occur, but their incidence is quite rare. However, the potency of antidepressant agents and the fact that side effects do occur requires that these drugs be prescribed only when there are definite indications for their use. Thus although there is no need for weekly routine laboratory tests under normal circumstances, appropriate medical investigations should be made before administering the drug, especially if there is evidence of possible physical disease.

Adjunctive psychotherapy may greatly enhance the patient's response to antidepressant drugs in terms of ultimate social adjustment and can greatly facilitate the patient's adaptation to the outside world. Furthermore, some apparently depressed patients possessing an underlying neurosis or a personality disorder may respond dramatically to psychotherapy and display no response at all to existing drugs.

The stakes are high in serious depressions—especially the ones which, if untreated, often last 6 months or more before remission. It has been estimated that approximately 15% of those patients with recurrent depressive disease eventually commit suicide. Acute depression is the cause of much pain, and chronic depression leads to marked disability and unhappiness for both the patient and his family. Since most cases of true depression are readily treatable, therapy should be vigorously and quickly applied.

SPECIFIC TRICYCLIC ANTIDEPRESSANTS

Imipramine

Combined statistics from studies of imipramine (Tofranil, Presamine) effectiveness demonstrate that, as in studies of other tricyclic drugs, approximately 70% of depressed patients respond with significant improvement. Table 1 displays the number of double-blind studies in which the therapeutic effectiveness of imipramine and other medications was compared to placebo. As these findings indicate, most of the studies demonstrated the therapeutic efficacy of imipramine. Furthermore, a significant proportion of those studies which failed to show a positive effect suffered from important methodological difficulties, including insufficient dosage, inadequate rating scales, small patient populations, or populations that encompassed high percentages of diverse clinical characteristics (e.g., elderly patients, schizoaffective patients, and patients with compensation neuroses).

Of the 38 controlled studies in this survey which compared imipramine and placebo, 26 enumerated the percentages of patients improved by drug or placebo. Combining the data from these latter studies shows that 39% of patients on placebo and 70% of those on imipramine improved; in no studies from this group did placebo produce greater improvement than imipramine. The average difference between the rates of improvement produced by placebo and imipramine was 31%, leaving only a negligible statistical probability that chance could account for these results.

Relatively few studies have claimed to isolate variables associated with good drug response. However, findings by Kiloh, Ball, and Garside (1962), who performed a discriminant function analysis in patients treated with imipramine, suggest that predictors of a favorable response to imipramine are predominantly those associated with the more severe endogenous depressions, i.e., those depressions involving incapacitating feelings of worthlessness and overwhelming guilt, severe agitation or retardation, and such symptoms as weight loss and early morning awakening. Conversely, there appears to be a tendency for patients with neurotic and characterological depressions (whose premorbid personalities show hysterical, hypochondriacal, and self-pitying traits) to respond less favorably to imipramine. Paranoid patients also often tend to respond poorly to imipramine (Whittenborn, Plant, Burgess, and Maurer, 1962). Hordern, Burt, and Holt (1965) found a poor response on the part of delusional patients. It seems reasonable to consider a neuroleptic combination or ECT in some of these cases.

Imipramine appears to be specific for a class of patients who suffer from severe panic attacks associated with phobic anxiety syndrome (Klein, 1964). It has a dramatic effect in preventing the massive panics that phobic patients may associate with certain situations: traveling alone in open spaces, on bridges, or in tunnels. The childhood version of this syndrome, school phobia, is also responsive to imipramine. However, the minor tranquilizers are more specific for the strictly anticipatory features of the anxiety associated with the phobic stimulus, which are less responsive to imipramine.

It is quite clear from the available research that depression is not a unitary phenomenon and that there are several populations of drug responders. It is unfortunate from a clinical standpoint, however, that efforts to identify drug-susceptible populations of depressed patients, as opposed to populations whose response is minimal, have not been sufficiently exhaustive. Nor have many of the major studies been cross validated. It is evident that the matching of clinical subtypes of depression to effective medication by a specific drug must await further research. The effective dose of imipramine is 150 to 300 mg/day.

Amitriptyline

Most studies comparing amitriptyline (Elavil) with imipramine have found that the two drugs are approximately equal in therapeutic efficacy. No studies have demonstrated amitriptyline to be less effective than imipramine. Although a number of double-blind studies have shown amitriptyline to be superior to imipramine, this finding may be an artifact of dosage. It appears that amitriptyline may be slightly more potent on a milligram per milligram basis and consequently more effective at lower dosage levels. In two double-blind studies Hordern et al. (1965) found amitriptyline to be slightly superior at the end of 1 week when both medications were administered at a dosage of 200 mg/day. However, when Sandifer, Wilson, and Gambill (1965) administered the two drugs in different dose ratios—maximum dose: amitriptyline 150 mg/day and imipramine 240 mg/day—the drugs were roughly similar in therapeutic efficacy.

Desipramine and Nortriptyline

Desipramine (Pertofrane, Norpramin) and nortriptyline (Aventyl) are the demethylated derivatives of imipramine and amitriptyline, respectively, and resemble their parent compounds in many pharmacological respects. On the basis of drug-placebo and drug-imipramine comparisons, it appears that these drugs are approximately comparable to imipramine in their effectiveness. In controlled studies nortriptyline was an effective antidepressant. Desipramine was equally effective as imipramine in six studies and less effective in one. In a study of depressed Veterans Administration patients—a population which might be expected to contain a proportionately higher number of schizoaffective psychoses and compensation neuroses with depression—desipramine showed no superiority over placebo.

Desipramine was initially claimed to have a shorter lag period than its parent compound on the basis of animal studies and uncontrolled trials with depressed patients. However, recent findings based on controlled comparisons of these two tricyclic drugs have clearly disconfirmed initial claims that desipramine is faster in action than imipramine.

Protriptyline

Among the various tricyclic agents, protriptyline (Vivactil) is the least sedative. Consequently it may be particularly useful in outpatient depression when sedation is undesirable. Protriptyline is more potent than imipramine on a milligram per milligram basis; its effective dose is 15 to 40 mg/day divided into three or four doses.

Doxepin

Doxepin (Sinequan) has been suggested to have properties in common with both imipramine and diazepam, an antianxiety agent. There is clear evidence of doxepin's usefulness in the treatment of mixed anxiety-depression (nonpsychotic) syndrome, a frequent disorder among outpatients. The typical dose of doxepin for mixed outpatient anxiety-depression is 150 to 300 mg/day. Slightly lower doses (100 to 200 mg) are indicated for anxiety. The effect of doxepin on endogenous depression has not been adequately assessed.

TREATMENT SUMMARY

Generic name	Trade name	Daily dosage range (mg)
Imipramine	Tofranil, Presamine	150–300
Desipramine	Pertofrane, Norpramin	150–250
Amitriptyline	Elavil	150–300
Nortriptyline	Aventyl	50–150
Protriptyline	Vivactyl	10–60
Doxepin	Sinequan	150–300

REFERENCES

Alexanderson, B. (1972): Pharmacokinetics of nortriptyline in man after single and multiple oral doses. *Eur. J. Clin. Pharmacol.,* 4:82–91.

Asberg, M., Cronholm, B., Sjoqvist, F., and Tuck, D. (1971a): Relationship between plasma levels and therapeutic effect of nortriptyline. *Br. Med. J.,* 3:331–334.

Asberg, M., Price-Evans, D., and Sjoqvist, F. (1971b): Genetic control of nortriptyline kinetics in man: A study of relatives of propositi with high plasma concentrations. *J. Med. Genet.,* 8:129–135.

Braithwaite, R. A., Goulding, R., Theano, G., Bailey, J., and Coppen, H. (1972): Plasma concentration of amitriptyline and clinical response. *Lancet,* 1:1297–1300.

Clinical Psychiatry Committee of the British Medical Rsearch Council (1965): Clinical trial of the treatment of depressive illness. *Br. Med. J.,* 1:881–886.

Gruvstad, M. (1973): Plasma levels of antidepressants and clinical response. *Lancet,* 1:95–96.

Hordern, A., Burt, C. G., and Holt, N. F. (1965): *Depressive States.* Charles C Thomas, Springfield, Ill.

Kay, D. W. K., Fahy, T., and Garside, R. F. (1970): A seven month double blind trial of amitriptyline and diazepam in ECT-treated depressed patients. *Br. J. Psychiatry,* 117:667–671.

Kiloh, L. G., Ball, J. R. B., and Garside, R. F. (1962): Prognostic factors in treatment of depressive states with imipramine. *Br. Med. J.,* 1:1225–1227.

Klein, D. F. (1964): Delineation of two-drug responsive anxiety syndromes. *Psychopharmacologia,* 5:397–408.

Klerman, G. L., and Cole, J. O. (1965): Clinical pharmacology of imipramine and related antidepressant compounds. *Pharmacol. Rev.,* 17:101–141.

Kragh-Sorenson, P., Asberg, M., and Eggert-Hansen, C. (1973): Plasma nortriptyline levels in endogenous depression. *Lancet,* 1:113–115.

Kuhn, R. (1958): The treatment of depressive states with G 22355 (imipramine hydrochloride). *Am. J. Psychiatry,* 115:459–464.

Mindham, R. H. S., Howland, C., and Shepherd, M. (1972): Continuation therapy with tricyclic antidepressants in depressive illness. *Lancet,* 2:854–855.

Moir, D. C., Crooks, J., Sawyer, P., Turnbull, M. J., and Weir, R. D. (1972): Cardiotoxicity of tricyclic antidepressants. *Br. J. Pharmacol.,* 44:371–372.

Pare, C. M. B., Rees, L., and Sainsbury, M. J. (1962): Differentiation of two genetically specific types of depression by the response to antidepressants. *Lancet,* 2:1340–1343.

Rickels, K., Hutchinson, J. C., Weise, C. C., Csanalosi, I., Chung, H. R., and Case, W. G. (1972): Doxepin and amitriptyline-perphenazine in mixed anxious-depressed neurotic outpatients: A collaborative controlled study. *Psychopharmacologia,* 23: 305–318.

Sandifer, M. G., Wilson, I. C., and Gambill, J. M. (1965): The influence of case selection and dosage in antidepressant drug trial. *Br. J. Psychiatry,* 111:142–148.

Schiele, B. C., Vestre, N. D., and Stein, K. E. (1961): A comparison of thioridazine, trifluoperazine, chlorpromazine, and placebo: A double blind controlled study on the treatment of chronic, hospitalized, schizophrenic patients. *J. Clin. Exp. Psychopathol.*, 22:151–162.

Seager, C. P., and Bird, R. L. (1962): Imipramine with electrical treatment in depression controlled trial. *J. Ment. Sci.,* 108:704–707.

Wilson, I. C., Vernon, J. T., Guin, T., and Sandifer, M. G., Jr. (1963): A controlled study of treatments of depression. *J. Neuropsychiatry,* 4:331–337.

Wittenborn, J. R., Plante, M., Burgess, F., and Maurer, H. A. (1962): Comparison of imipramine, electroconvulsive therapy and placebo in the treatment of depression. *J. Nerv. Ment. Dis.,* 135:131–137.

Chapter 10

Monoamine Oxidase Inhibitors

Lance L. Simpson and Bruce Cabot

More often than not, serendipity has been a major force in psychopharmacology. The introduction of monoamine oxidase inhibitors (MAOI) as antidepressant drugs is certainly an example of a chance observation that was later converted into a useful therapeutic strategy. During the early 1950s a series of drugs—which were later found to be MAOIs—were being used in the treatment of tuberculosis. It was noted that some patients under treatment with these drugs experienced an elevation in mood. Accordingly, the MAOIs were tested for possible efficaciousness in the treatment of depression. The original reports were favorable, and so MAOIs were introduced into clinical psychiatry.

Although the initial enthusiasm for MAOIs was high, their value has been subsequently reassessed. At present MAOIs are not commonly used in medical practice. Most physicians restrict the use of these agents to those patients who have a demonstrated refractoriness to other antidepressants, particularly the tricyclic drugs.

There are two major factors that have contributed to the demise of MAOIs. The first of these is their ability to interact adversely with a number of drugs, including the dietary amino acid tyramine; their interaction with tyramine can produce a hypertensive crisis. This adverse reaction is potentially so grave that it has discouraged most physicians from prescribing MAOIs. A second factor is that, as the literature on clinical studies comparing MAOIs and tricyclics has grown, it has become apparent that the latter agents should be regarded as the drugs of choice for treating most types of depressive illness. Thus the MAOIs currently enjoy only limited use in psychiatry.

BASIC PHARMACOLOGY

Monoamine oxidase (MAO) is the name given to the enzyme that catalyzes the oxidative deamination of monoamines. It is distributed somewhat ubiquitously throughout the body, but there are high concentrations in blood, liver, and nervous tissue. The function of MAO in blood, liver, and other nonnervous tissue is to inactivate circulating monoamines. Since these compounds (e.g., norepinephrine, dopamine, serotonin) have many pharmacological actions, it is essential that the body have some mechanism for keeping them at low levels in the circulation. MAO is that mechanism.

In neurons that utilize monoamines as synaptic transmitters, the role of MAO is somewhat more complex. Monoamines synthesized within the nerve terminal undergo one of two fates: They are either stored in synaptic vesicles for release during synaptic transmission, or they are deaminated by MAO. Hence MAO serves as a regulatory enzyme to ensure that cytoplasmic levels of monoamines do not exceed those necessary for synaptic transmission. The enzyme serves a similar function at a later step during transmission. When a monoamine is released by a nerve, it diffuses across the synapse to interact with a postsynaptic receptor. Thereafter the monoamine can either diffuse away from the synapse, or it can diffuse back toward the presynaptic cell. In the latter case the presynaptic neuron has an active pump mechanism for transporting monoamines back into the cells from which they were released. In fact, the neuronal pump is the major mechanism for terminating the synaptic effects of monoamines. When these substances are pumped into the nerve ending, they undergo the same fate as newly synthesized monoamines; i.e., they are either stored for later use, or they are enzymatically deaminated. Once again, MAO serves to regulate the cytoplasmic levels of monoamines.

When MAO is inhibited, the intraneuronal levels of monoamines increase (Spector, Hirsch, and Brodie, 1963). This increase has long been assumed to be the mechanism that accounts for the antidepressant effects of MAOIs. In large part this assumption stems directly from the catecholamine hypothesis of mood (Schildkraut, 1965). In its simplest form the hypothesis suggests that depression may be due to a functional deficit of neurotransmitter monoamines. Administration of an MAOI would cause neuronal levels of monoamines to rise, and thus the functional deficit would be overcome. This might lead to alleviation of a depressed mood.

The proposed mechanism of the antidepressant action of MAOIs has many attractive features, not the least of which is its relative simplicity. Unfortunately there are a number of arguments against the idea, four of which are particularly noteworthy.

1. *Reserpine model:* Much of the early work on laboratory models of depression employed the drug reserpine (Brodie, Pletscher, and Shore, 1956). When this agent is administered to laboratory animals, it causes a state of profound psychomotor retardation that is often labeled "depression." To some extent MAOIs can antagonize reserpine-induced depression. Since reserpine acts to deplete neuronal stores of monoamines, it was reasoned that MAOIs could reverse the depression by counteracting monoamine depletion. Regardless of the merit in this reasoning, it is now believed that the reserpinized animal is a poor model for human depression (Mendels and Frazer, 1974). Therefore the ability of MAOIs to counteract the cellular effects of reserpine in animals may provide little insight into the therapeutic effects of MAOIs in human patients.

2. *Catecholamine hypothesis of mood:* One of the prevailing hypotheses to explain the underlying cause of depression is that there is a functional deficit of monoamines, particularly of catecholamines. However, as detailed elsewhere in this volume, there are no compelling data to support the catecholamine hypothesis. In the absence of a demonstrated catecholamine deficit, there is no obvious reason to expect MAO inhibition to be therapeutic in depression.

3. *Transmitter release:* Although the catecholamine hypothesis of mood has no clear experimental support, the hypothesis has had tremendous heuristic value. It has stimulated a wide-ranging and intense effort to understand the pharmacology and physiology of synaptic transmission. As part of this research effort, a great deal has been learned about the uptake, storage, and release of neurotransmitter monoamines (Patil, Miller, and Trendelenburg, 1974). Among other things, we learned that these amines are stored and subsequently released from a small intraneuronal pool, and that this pool is only a fraction of the total monoamine present in nerves. Although evidence to date is rather sparse, it is thought that the pool of monoamine available for synaptic transmission is *not* the pool that increases after MAO inhibition. In fact, no one has demonstrated that MAO inhibition can effectively increase nerve stimulation-induced release of monoamines.

4. *Hypertension:* Perhaps the most problematic issue in understanding why MAO inhibition should relieve depression arises from the fact that some MAOIs (e.g., pargyline) are antihypertensive drugs. The explanations proposed to account for the antihypertensive actions of MAOIs seem to be totally contrary to the explanations for their antidepressant actions. The contradictions become apparent when one examines two hypotheses that have been advanced to explain why MAO inhibition should lower blood pressure. According to one explanation (Kopin, Fischer, and Musacchio, 1965), chronic MAO inhibition leads to intraneuronal accumulation of a false transmitter. (A false transmitter is a substance that is synthesized, stored, and released by a nerve ending but which is usually much less potent than the endogenous transmitter.) Accumulation and subsequent release of a false transmitter impairs synaptic transmission. More precisely, release of a false transmitter from peripheral sympathetic neurons could lead to diminished vascular tone and a resultant fall in blood pressure. It is generally agreed that chronic MAO inhibition alters the metabolism of sympathetic neurons such that a false transmitter (octopamine) does appear. On the other hand, there is disagreement as to whether a sufficient amount of octopamine accumulates to impair sympathetic transmission (Antonaccio and Smith, 1969).

Another putative explanation for why MAO inhibition lowers blood pressure relates to intraneuronal kinetics. The neuron has many regulatory mechanisms for governing the rate of monoamine synthesis. One of these mechanisms is known as "feedback inhibition." When the intraneuronal level of a monoamine surpasses a certain threshold, the monoamine can block its own synthesizing enzymes. Following MAOI administration the levels of cytoplasmic mono-amines increase so much that they begin to produce feedback inhibition of their own synthesis (Neff and Costa, 1968; Ngai, Neff, and Costa, 1968; Berkowitz, Tarver, and Spector, 1974). One result of this could be diminished release of monoamines. Needless to say, this proposed explanation for why MAO inhibition should lower blood pressure is diametrically opposed to earlier explanations of why MAO inhibition should relieve depression.

The literature on MAO inhibition is currently at an impasse. No one has advanced an acceptable explanation for why MAOIs should be both anti-depressants and antihypertensives. In the absence of sound explanations, at least a score of speculations have emerged. These range from the conservative (MAOIs relieve depression and hypertension at different dosages) to the extreme (MAO inhibition is an ancillary action of the drugs which is not central to their antidepressant and/or antihypertensive properties).

There are no data available which would permit us to choose among the various speculations. However, there is a line of investigation that may hold promise for eventually understanding the various actions of MAOIs. Historically, MAO was regarded as a single enzyme. Research during the past few years has revealed that there are actually a host of isoenzymes that can deaminate monoamines (Youdim, Collins, and Sandler, 1969). Interestingly, these isoenzymes have different substrate specificities and are vulnerable to different inhibitors (Johnston, 1968; Costa and Sandler, 1972). As fate would have it, all of the clinically useful MAOIs are broad-spectrum inhibitors; i.e., they tend to inhibit all of the isoenzymes. There are experimental inhibitors that are much more specific than the therapeutic inhibitors now available. It may be that study of these specific inhibitors will ultimately help us to understand what mechanisms account for the various therapeutic actions of MAOIs.

CLINICAL PHARMACOLOGY

The first MAO inhibitor to be used in psychiatric patients was iproniazid. This agent is a derivative of isoniazid and, like isoniazid, has antituberculosis activity. Since it also has mood-elevating properties, it was tested in depressed patients. Early reports on the efficacy of iproniazid were favorable, and the drug enjoyed a brief reign in psychopharmacology (Crane, 1957; Loomer, Saunders, and Kline, 1957).

During its brief tenure as an antidepressant drug, iproniazid was implicated in a number of adverse reactions, the most troublesome of which was hepato-toxicity. The seriousness of the medical complications associated with iproniazid use led to its discontinuance as a therapeutic agent. Prior to this, it had been determined that iproniazid was an MAOI (Zeller, Barsky, Fouts, Kirch-heimer, and Van Orden, 1952). Therefore efforts were launched to synthesize MAOIs that would not produce hepatotoxicity or other untoward effects. This research resulted in the introduction of two broad groups of MAOIs.

One group, known as the hydrazines, is composed of substances structurally related to iproniazid. Examples of this group are phenelzine, nialamide, and isocarboxazid (Fig. 1). A second group, known as the nonhydrazines, are heterogeneous in structure and not related to iproniazid. The only antidepressant of this group currently marketed is tranylcypromine. As Fig. 2 illustrates, tranylcypromine was derived from a slight modification of amphetamine; i.e., an isopropyl side chain was converted to a cyclopropyl sidechain.

There are a number of features common to all the clinically useful MAOIs. They are all reasonably lipophilic and hence are well absorbed from the gut and can penetrate the blood-brain barrier with ease. They are all broad-spectrum MAOIs and to varying degrees can inhibit MAO in all body tissues. As would be expected, the drugs differ in their potency as inhibitors, which

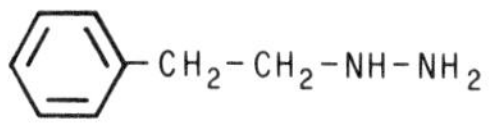

$$\text{\raisebox{0pt}{⟨benzene ring⟩}} - CH_2 - CH_2 - NH - NH_2$$

PHENELZINE

$$\underset{\text{⟨pyridine ring⟩}}{\overset{\displaystyle O}{\overset{\|}{C}}} - NH - NH - CH_2 - CH_2 - \overset{\displaystyle O}{\overset{\|}{C}} - NH - CH_2 \;\text{⟨benzene ring⟩}$$

$$\text{⟨benzene ring⟩} - CH_2 - NH - NH - \overset{\displaystyle O}{\overset{\|}{C}} - \overset{}{C} - CH \quad \substack{\| \; \| \\ N \; C - CH_3 \\ \diagdown \diagup \\ O}$$

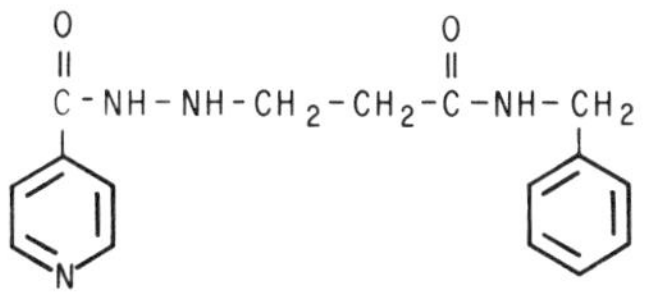

NIALAMIDE 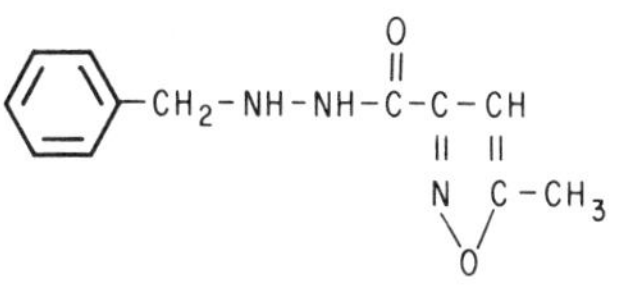   **ISOCARBOXAZID**

FIG. 1. Chemical structure of hydrazine-type MAOIs.

presumably contributes to the fact that equiefficacious doses are not equimolar. The drugs also differ in terms of their molecular action. The main difference is that hydrazine derivatives produce irreversible inhibition of MAO, whereas the nonhydrazine derivatives are reversible (albeit slowly).

There is an important clinical implication to some MAOIs being irreversible. When a patient has received a drug of this type, MAO activity does not recover as a function of the inhibitor being eliminated from the body. Indeed, even with total elimination of circulating inhibitor, there can still be appreciable loss of enzyme activity. Following the administration of an irreversible inhibitor, MAO activity recovers as a function of the synthesis of new MAO. The rate of synthesis of new MAO is slow compared to the rate of metabolism and/or elimination of an irreversible inhibitor. Therefore even though blood levels of inhibitor may be absolutely zero, the body may not have had time to resynthesize enzyme to replace that which was lost. Failure on the part of a physician to take this matter into account can have serious consequences for the patient.

There is no doubt that in man, just as in laboratory animals, MAOIs have pronounced effects on monoamine metabolism. One of the first studies to illustrate this point was published by Sjoerdsma, Oates, and Gillespie (1960). These investigators administered various inhibitors to hypertensive patients and subsequently monitored the rates of urinary excretion of monoamine metabolites. Their techniques were indirect, but their data did suggest that at equiefficacious doses the various MAOIs produced equivalent amounts of enzyme inhibition. Their study represented one of the original attempts to demonstrate a relationship between therapeutic action and enzyme inhibition.

For obvious reasons the number of studies that provide direct evidence of enzyme inhibition in human brain are quite limited. Those which have appeared (Ganrot, Rosengren, and Gottfries, 1962; MacLean, Nicholson, Pare, and Stacey, 1965; Pare, 1971) tend to support several conclusions, as follows:

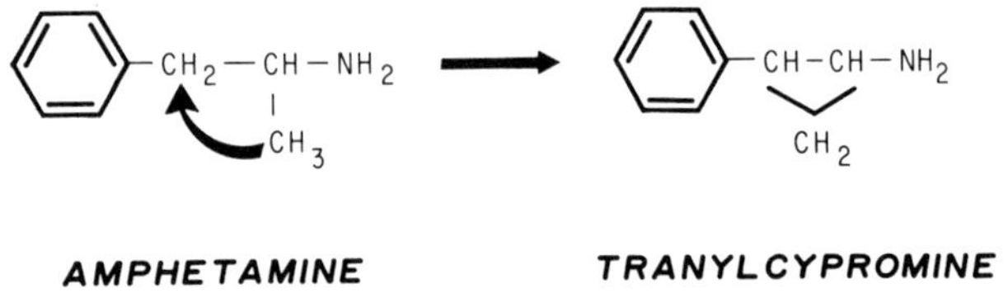

AMPHETAMINE   **TRANYLCYPROMINE**

FIG. 2. Chemical structure of a nonhydrazine MAOI, tranylcypromine, which is a derivative of amphetamine.

(1) All clinically useful MAOIs produce significant loss of brain MAO activity. (2) Equiefficacious doses of MAOIs produce equivalent amounts of total enzyme inhibition. (3) Patients under treatment with MAOIs have elevated levels of brain monoamines. (4) The time course of increase in brain monoamines roughly parallels the time course of onset of MAOI antidepressant activity.

On the surface these findings seem to be quite promising. Nevertheless, the small number of studies involved means that the work remains to be confirmed. Moreover, the brain tissue that was assayed (autopsy specimens from terminal patients) was not obtained from depressed patients. Furthermore, there was no evidence that the MAOIs had exerted any effect on behavior. It remains to be determined whether relief from depression is closely or causally linked to MAO inhibition in brain.

Experiments that resolve some of the drawbacks in earlier work have been published by Youdim and his associates (Youdim, Collins, Sandler, Bevan Jones, Pare, and Nicholson, 1972). Their work differs from previous reports in that autopsy material was obtained from depressed patients. Moreover, they studied the effects of inhibitors on the activity of several isoenzymes rather than on total MAO activity. Their findings indicate that various MAOIs differ in their ability to inhibit various forms of MAO. There were too few patients in the study to establish a link between enzyme inhibition and therapeutic response, however. As the authors point out, more work will be necessary to establish how MAO inhibition can lead to relief of depression.

The majority of studies dealing with MAOIs have focused on the manner in which such inhibitors alter the metabolism of monoamines. It should be pointed out that there is an important line of investigation dealing with alterations in the metabolism of inhibitors themselves. In this regard, hydrazine-type MAOIs (e.g., phenelzine) are partially metabolized by acetylation. It has been demonstrated that there is polymorphism of acetylator status among humans, and that random samples of a human population would yield approximately equal pools of "fast" and "slow" acetylators.

Two prospective studies have sought to relate acetylator status and therapeutic response to phenelzine. In the earlier study (Price Evans, Davison, and Pratt, 1965), patients were treated for both endogenous and neurotic depression. The dosage of phenelzine was 15 mg t.i.d. In the later study (Johnstone and Marsh, 1973), there was a concentration of neurotic depressives. Phenelzine was initiated at 15 mg t.i.d., but at 1 week the dosage was doubled. The results of the two studies were similar in that slow acetylators tended to be more susceptible to serious adverse side effects. The tendency was more significant in the earlier study. The two reports differed in their conclusions about acetylator status and therapeutic response. Price Evans et al. (1965) found that the improvement rate did not correlate with acetylator status. By contrast, Johnstone and Marsh (1973) concluded that slow acetylators were more likely than fast acetylators to respond favorably to phenelzine. Whether the opposing conclusions relate to drug dosage or patient characteristics remains undetermined. The matter is sufficiently important to warrant further study.

PSYCHIATRIC INDICATIONS

MAOI are indicated in the treatment of some types of depression, and they may be useful in the treatment of phobias. Treatment of depression is central to the present discussion.

Depression

There seems to be an inevitable sequence of events that accompanies the introduction of any drug or group of drugs as therapeutic agents. According to this sequence, initial reports tend to be highly favorable, sometimes to the extent that discovery of a panacea is suggested. These favorable reports are followed by more somber accounts, and these in turn are followed by damaging reports. Only after the entire sequence has been enacted does there emerge a well-reasoned effort to establish the precise role a new drug should play in therapeutics. The literature on MAOIs is a classic illustration of the sequence

An example of an early favorable report is that of Agin (1963). In this study MAOI treatment produced responses in 82% of all depressed patients; psychotic depressives had a 70% response rate. These improvement data are quite impressive; sadly enough, they are also quite unreproducible. The cumulative literature, and especially the literature based on well-controlled, double-blind studies, reveals that MAOIs are not notably effective in psychotic (or endogenous) depressions. Furthermore, their precise value in neurotic depressions is a matter of some debate.

For the purpose of simplifying the literature, we designate the year 1965 as being pivotal in the evaluation of MAOIs. Prior to that year many reports of varying quality had appeared concerning efficacy of the inhibitors. The role of these drugs in clinical psychiatry was unsettled. In 1965 two articles were published that have often been cited and that in general marked the end of vigorous research on antidepressant MAOIs. In one of these articles electroconvulsive therapy, imipramine, phenelzine, and placebo were evaluated in a large study of a mixed population of depressed patients (Clinical Psychiatry Committee, 1965). Germane to the present discussion was the finding that phenelzine was not very effective as an antidepressant. During the same year Atkinson and Ditman (1965) published a thorough review on tranylcypromine. The authors concluded that "the drug alone was beneficial in reactive and psychoneurotic depressions, while it tended not to influence agitated, psychotic, or endogenous depression." They further concluded that MAOI therapy, in the main, should be restricted to patients who are unresponsive to tricyclic antidepressants.

The near termination of MAOI research that occurred after 1965 left many unanswered questions and unresolved points. In an extensive review on psychotherapeutic drug efficacy, Klein and Davis (1969) point out the incompleteness of the literature. Within this context, they propose several tentative conclusions, two of which are generally shared by psychopharmacologists. First, phenelzine and tranylcypromine have a useful although limited value in certain depressions; the value of isocarboxazid and nialamide is less certain. Second, because of the greater incidence of hypertensive crises associated with tranylcypromine, phenelzine may be the favored drug among MAOIs. These conclusions have been sustained in a more recent review of antidepressant drug efficacy (Morris and Beck, 1974).

The main thrust of current research has been to identify a subpopulation of depressed patients likely to respond to MAO inhibition. In this vein there are several groups of investigators who believe that MAOIs may be useful in neurotic depression and in patients with "atypical depression." This belief derives from early work, mainly British, that proposed the inhibitors as being notably effective in reactive depressions characterized by somatization of symptoms (West and Dally, 1959; Dally and Rohde, 1961; Sargant, 1961, 1962). The inclination of some British workers to view MAO inhibitors favorably has continued (Mackinnon, 1973).

The number of American investigators actively involved in evaluating MAOIs is small. However, one group has recently published findings that attracted much attention. Robinson, Nies, Ravaris, and Lamborn (1973b) conducted a prospective, controlled, double-blind study involving patients with symptoms of atypical depression. The investigators selected 16 indices of depression that they predicted would respond to inhibitor (phenelzine) therapy. Of these, 15 responded better to phenelzine than to placebo. Irritability, hypochondriasis-agitation, and psychomotor activity responded especially well to phenelzine. In a related study (Robinson, Nies, Ravaris, Ives, and Lamborn, 1973a) the same investigators examined blood platelet MAO activity. They found that patients with 80% or greater MAO inhibition were very likely to be responsive to phenelzine therapy.

Other groups have similarly noted that phenelzine may be useful in depression, but they have been unable to identify a specific subpopulation as being peculiarly responsive to the drug (Raskin, 1974a,b). It may be that differences in the outcome of MAO studies relate to the criteria used to select depressed patients for study.

Because of the number of conflicts and controversies in the literature, the MAOIs have not emerged as drugs of choice in the treatment of any type of depressive illness. Furthermore, in studies seeking to compare MAOIs with tricyclic drugs, the latter have usually been rated superior; occasionally MAOIs have been rated equivalent to tricyclics, but they have never been deemed superior (Klerman and Cole, 1965; Klein and Davis, 1969; Morris and Beck, 1974). It could be that MAOIs are singularly effective in a subpopulation of depressed patients, but there is no consensus on how to identify these patients. When such a consensus is forthcoming, the MAOIs will occupy a more significant position in psychopharmacology.

Phobic Neurosis

The treatment of neurosis is described in an earlier section of this book. We confine ourselves here to mentioning three studies that relate phenelzine treatment to phobic states. Two of these studies were prospective in nature, and one was retrospective.

In 1970 Kelly and his associates reported a retrospective study involving 246 phobic patients (Kelly, Guirguis, Frommer, Mitchell-Heggs, and Sargant, 1970). A variety of MAOIs were used in the study, and the general conclusion was that these drugs were effective in diminishing the number of panic attacks. Two prospective studies followed shortly thereafter. Tyrer, Candy, and Kelly (1973) confirmed that phenelzine was useful in phobic anxiety; i.e., it reduced the number of panic attacks. Solyom, Heseltine, McClure, Solyom, Ledwidge, and Steinberg (1973) found that both phenelzine and brief psychotherapy were effective in phobic neurosis. The combination of drug plus psychotherapy produced the most rapid therapeutic response. It is likely that these positive reports will encourage additional work on drug treatment of phobias.

ADVERSE SIDE EFFECTS

Iproniazid and other MAOIs that have been withdrawn from the market were implicated in serious adverse reactions. By contrast, the MAOIs currently available seldom produce adverse reactions serious enough to limit their use in patients. Evidence for this conclusion is provided by a recent study on adverse effects of phenelzine (Raskind, 1972). This prospective, double-blind study was part of a multihospital survey of all untoward effects to phenelzine, diazepam, and placebo in a population of newly admitted, depressed patients. Of the 110 patients who received phenelzine, only three had to discontinue the drug. Close examination of the data reveals that even this ratio (three of 110) may be an inflated estimate of phenelzine-induced severe reactions. One of the three patients taken off phenelzine complained of headaches, but this symptom was present both before phenelzine treatment and after its discontinuance. Another patient had several reactions, none of which was medically serious; the patient was taken off the drug because of the intensity of her complaints. The third patient, whose reaction was serious, had several problems, including possible liver damage. The problems disappeared shortly after phenelzine treatment was stopped.

There are a number of minor side effects that may be associated with MAOI therapy. These include hypotension (usually orthostatic but occasionally resting), insomnia, restlessness or agitation, dry mouth, constipation, impotence, and dizziness (perhaps secondary to orthostatic hypotension). The reactions can be troubling and uncomfortable to the patient, but the benefit of relieving depression normally outweighs the discomfort of side effects. Candor about the nature and intensity of adverse reactions plus good patient-physician rapport tend to enhance the patient's acceptance of drug-induced side effects.

The MAOIs are known to be involved in several adverse drug interactions. Indeed, the interaction between MAOIs and sympathomimetic amines is one of the classic drug-drug interactions in medicine and pharmacology. This interaction can involve amines which are dietary in origin—e.g., tyramine (Bethune, Burrell, Culpan, and Ogg, 1964; Blackwell, Marley, Price, and Taylor, 1967)—as well as amines in proprietary and prescription drugs, e.g., ephedrine (Cuthbert, Greenberg, and Morley, 1969). The result of the interaction can be a hypertensive crisis.

There seem to be at least two mechanisms that may account for a pronounced increase in blood pressure (Stockley, 1973). MAOIs act at several sites to inhibit the metabolism of sympathomimetic amines, so the biological half-life of these substances is prolonged. In addition, MAO inhibition leads to increased stores of norepinephrine in nerve endings, particularly those which innervate the vasculature. Exogenous sympathomimetic amines can displace norepinephrine from the nerve ending onto vascular receptors. By prolonging the biological activity of sympathomimetic amines and by increasing the pool of norepinephrine available for displacement, the MAOIs promote hypertensive episodes.

Given the mechanisms proposed above, it is easily understood why hypertensive crises can occur even when blood levels of irreversible MAOIs are zero. The enzymes that degrade exogenous sympathomimetic amines and endogenous norepinephrine remain inhibited, and full activity is not restored until the body synthesizes new enzyme. Until this new enzyme appears, the patient remains vulnerable to interactions with exogenous sympathomimetic amines. Accordingly, a patient's diet and drug intake must be closely monitored not only while he is on MAOI therapy but also for several days after MAOI therapy stops. The lag period after cessation of drug therapy permits the patient the needed time to replace lost enzyme.

MAOIs can inhibit liver enzymes other than MAO. Therefore drugs which are normally metabolized or detoxified by the liver may interact adversely with MAOIs. Important examples of such drugs are barbiturates (Laroche and Brodie, 1960) and narcotic analgesics and related agents (Eade and Renton, 1970). Prior administration of an MAOI inhibits the metabolism of these drugs. As would be expected, this prolongs and enhances the activity of drugs whose hepatic metabolism is retarded.

CONCLUSIONS

The idea of defining a role for MAOIs in psychiatry is unsettling. Simple observation reveals that most psychiatrists use MAOIs in depressed patients who have not responded to tricyclic agents. A smaller number of psychiatrists regard MAOIs as drugs of choice in atypical depression. The empirical basis for either of these strategies is something less than awesome.

There is reasonable agreement that at least two MAOIs, phenelzine and tranylcypromine, have antidepressant properties. A difficulty arises in trying to specify the extent to which these antidepressant properties can or should be utilized in clinical psychiatry. It may be that this difficulty will be resolved in the course of research on MAOIs that inhibit specific MAO activity rather than total activity. In fact, research of this nature could be very exciting; it might generate drugs of greater antidepressant efficacy and lesser potential for adverse interactions. These possibilities prompt us to conclude that, although MAOI's are currently drugs of narrow therapeutic utility, there is good reason to reintensify both basic and clinical pharmacological research on specific inhibitors. Such future research may enhance the role of MAOIs as therapeutic agents.

TREATMENT SUMMARY

Generic name	Trade name	Daily dosage range (mg)
Phenelzine	Nardil	45–75
Nialamide	Niamid	150–225
Isocarboxazid	Marplan	10–30
Tranylcypromine	Parnate	20–40

REFERENCES

Agin, H. V. (1963): Phenelzine in the treatment of depression. *Am. J. Psychiatry,* 119:1173–1174.

Antonaccio, M. J., and Smith, C. B. (1969): Effects of chronic pretreatment with pargyline upon responses of the atrial pacemaker and of left atrial strips of guinea pigs to tyramine, mephentermine, d-amphetamine and adrenergic nerve stimulation. *J. Pharmacol. Exp. Ther.,* 170:97–107.

Atkinson, R. M., and Ditman, K. S. (1965): Tranylcypromine: A review. *Clin. Pharmacol. Ther.,* 6:631–655.

Berkowitz, B. A., Tarver, J. J., and Spector, S. (1974): Control of norepinephrine synthesis in blood vessels and the effects of monoamine oxidase inhibition. *J. Pharmacol. Exp. Ther.,* 190:21–29.

Bethune, H. C., Burrell, R. H., Culpan, R. H., and Ogg, G. J. (1964): Vascular crises associated with monoamine-oxidase inhibitors. *Am. J. Psychiatry,* 121:245–248.

Blackwell, B., Marley, E., Price, J., and Taylor, D. (1967): Hypertensive interactions tween monoamine oxidase inhibitors and foodstuffs. *Br. J. Psychiatry,* 113:349–365.

Brodie, B. B., Pletscher, A., and Shore, P. A. (1956): Possible role of serotonin in brain function and in reserpine action. *J. Pharmacol.,* 116:9.

Clinical Psychiatry Committee (1965): Clinical trial of the treatment of depressive illness. *Br. Med. J.,* 1:881–886.

Costa, E., and Sandler M. (editors) (1972): *Advances in Biochemical Psychopharmacology, Vol. 5: Monoamine Oxidases—New Vistas.* Raven Press, New York.

Crane, G. E. (1957): Iproniazid phosphate (Marsilid), a therapeutic agent for mental disorders and debilitating diseases. *Psychiatr. Res. Rep.,* 8:142–152.

Cuthbert, M. F., Greenberg, M. P., and Morley, S. W. (1969): Cough and cold remedies: A potential danger to patients on monoamine oxidase inhibitors. *Br. Med. J.,* 1:404–406.

Dally, P. J., and Rohde, P., (1961): Comparison of antidepressive drugs in depressive illnesses. *Lancet,* 1:18–20.

Eade, N. R., and Renton, K. W. (1970): The effect of phenelzine and tranylcypromine on the degradation of meperidine. *J. Pharmacol. Exp. Ther.,* 173:31–36.

Ganrot, P. O., Rosengren, E., and Gottfries, C. G. (1962): Effect of iproniazid on monoamines and monoamine oxidase in human brain. *Experientia,* 18:260–261.

Johnston, J. P. (1968): Some observations upon a new inhibitor of monoamine oxidase in brain tissue. *Biochem. Pharmacol.,* 17:1285–1297.

Johnstone, E. C., and Marsh, W. (1973): Acetylator status and response to phenelzine in depressed patients. *Lancet,* 1:567–570.

Kelly, D., Guirguis, W., Frommer, E., Mitchell-Heggs, N., and Sargant, W. (1970): Treatment of phobic states with antidepressants. *Br. J. Psychiatry,* 116:387–398.

Klein, D. F., and Davis, J. M. (1969): *Diagnosis and Drug Treatment of Psychiatric Disorders.* Williams & Wilkins, Baltimore.

Klerman, G. L., and Cole, J. O. (1965): Clinical pharmacology of imipramine and related antidepressant compounds. *Pharmacol. Rev.,* 17:101–141.

Kopin, I. J., Fischer, J. E., Musacchio, J. M., Horst, W. D., and Weise, V. K. (1965):

"False neurochemical transmitters" and the mechanism of sympathetic blockade by monoamine oxidase inhibitors. *J. Pharmacol. Exp. Ther.,* 147:186–193.

Laroche, M. J., and Brodie, B. B. (1960): The lack of relationship between the inhibition of monoamine oxidase and the potentiation of hexobarbital hypnosis. *J. Pharmacol. Exp. Ther.,* 130:134–137.

Loomer, H. P., Saunders, J. C., and Kline, N. S. (1957): A clinical and pharmacodynamic evaluation of iproniazid as a psychic energizer. *Psychiatr. Res. Rep.,* 8:129–141.

Mackinnon, A. U. (1973): Psychiatry viewed from general practice. *Practitioner,* 210: 135–143.

MacLean, R., Nicholson, W. J., Pare, C. M. B., and Stacey, R. S. (1965): Effect of monoamine-oxidase inhibitors on the concentrations of 5-hydroxytryptamine in the human brain. *Lancet,* 2:205–208.

Mendels, J., and Frazer, A. (1974): Brain biogenic amine depletion and mood. *Arch. Gen. Psychiatry,* 30:447–451.

Morris, J. B., and Beck, A. T. (1974): The efficacy of antidepressant drugs. *Arch. Gen. Psychiatry,* 30:667–674.

Neff, N. H., and Costa, E. (1968): Application of steady state kinetics to the study of catecholamine turnover after monoamine oxidase inhibition or reserpine administration. *J. Pharmacol. Exp. Ther.,* 160:40–47.

Ngai, S. H., Neff, H. H., and Costa, E. (1968): Effect of pargyline treatment on the rate of conversion of tyrosine ^{14}C to norepinephrine ^{14}C. *Life Sci.,* 7:847–855.

Pare, C. M. B. (1971): Monoamine oxidase inhibitors and brain monoamines in clinical conditions. *Biochem. J.,* 121:36P–37P.

Patil, P. N., Miller, D. D., and Trendelenburg, U. (1974): Molecular geometry and adrenergic drug activity. *Pharmacol. Rev.,* 26:323–392.

Price Evans, D. A., Davison, K., and Pratt, R. T. C. (1965): The influence of acetylator phenotype on the effects of treating depression with phenelzine. *Clin. Pharmacol. Ther.,* 6:430–435.

Raskin, A. (1972): Adverse reactions to phenelzine: Results of a nine-hospital depression study. *J. Clin. Pharmacol.,* 12:22–25.

Raskin, A. (1974*a*): A guide for drug use in depressive disorders. *Am. J. Psychiatry,* 131:181–185.

Raskin, A. (1974*b*): Depression subtypes and response to phenelzine, diazepam, and a placebo: Results of a nine hospital collaborative study. *Arch. Gen. Psychiatry,* 30:66–75.

Robinson, D. S., Nies, A., Ravaris, C. L., Ives, J. O., and Lamborn, K. R. (1973*a*): Treatment response to MAO inhibitors: relation to depressive typology and blood platelet MAO inhibition. In: *Classification and Prediction of Outcome of Depression,* edited by J. Angst. Schattauer Verlag, New York.

Robinson, D. S., Nies, A., Ravaris, L., and Lamborn, K. R. (1973*b*): The monoamine oxidase inhibitor, phenelzine, in the treatment of depressive-anxiety states. *Arch. Gen. Psychiatry,* 29:407–413.

Sargant, W. (1961): Drugs in the treatment of depression. *Br. Med. J.,* 1:225–227.

Sargant, W. (1962): The treatment of anxiety states and atypical depressions by the monoamine oxidase inhibitor drugs. *J. Neuropsychiatry (Suppl.),* 3:96–103.

Schildkraut, J. J. (1965): The catecholamine hypothesis of affective disorders: A review of supporting evidence. *Am. J. Psychiatry,* 122:509–522.

Sjoerdsma, A., Oates, J. A., and Gillespie, L. (1960): Quantitation of monoamine oxidase inhibition produced with various drugs in man. *Proc. Soc. Exp. Biol. Med.,* 103: 485–487.

Solyom, L., Heseltine, G. F. D., McClure, D. J., Solyom, C., Ledwidge, B., and Steinberg, G. (1973): Behavior therapy versus drug therapy in the treatment of phobic neurosis. *Can. Psychiatr. Assoc. J,* 18:25–32.

Spector, S., Hirsch, C. W., and Brodie, B. B. (1963): Association of behavioral effects of pargyline, a non-hydrazine MAO inhibitor with increase in brain norepinephrine. *Int. J. Neuropharmacol.,* 2:81–93.

Stockley, I. H. (1973): Monoamine oxidase inhibitors. I. Interactions with sympathomimetic amines. *Pharm. J.,* 210:590–594.

Tyrer, P., Candy, J., and Kelly, D. (1973): Phenelzine in phobic anxiety: A controlled trial. *Psychol. Med.*, 3:120–124.

West, E. M., and Dally, P. J. (1959): Effects of iproniazid in depressive syndromes. *Br. Med. J.*, 1:1491–1494.

Youdim, M. B. H., Collins, G. G. S., and Sandler, M. (1969): Multiple forms of rat brain monoamine oxidase. *Nature (Lond.)*, 223:626–628.

Youdin, M. B. H., Collins, G. G. S., Sandler, M., Bevan Jones, A. B., Pare, C. M. B., and Nicholson, W. J. (1972): Human brain monoamine oxidase: Multiple forms and selective inhibitors. *Nature (Lond.)*, 236:225–228.

Zeller, E. A., Barsky, J., Fouts, J. R., Kirshheimer, W. F., and Van Orden, L. S. (1952): Influence of isonicotinic acid hydrazine (INH) and 1-isonicotinyl-2-isopropyl hydrazine (IIH) on bacterial and mammalian enzymes. *Experientia*, 8:349–350.

Chapter 11

Amphetamines and Related Stimulants

Lance L. Simpson

Amphetamine has been and continues to be one of the most intensively studied drugs in medical pharmacology. Its actions have been investigated on essentially every organ system of every common laboratory animal and on most organ systems in man. The intensity of research on amphetamine derives from the fact that at various times during the past four decades the drug has been used clinically in the treatment (or intended treatment) of illnesses as diverse as narcolepsy, obesity, and depression. More recently amphetamine has been proposed as a useful drug for helping to understand the pathophysiology of schizophrenia; and as an overlay to these medical applications, amphetamine has a long history of abuse and misuse.

Because of—and sometimes in spite of—the many contexts in which amphetamine has been used, a great deal has been learned about the basic pharmacology and the clinical pharmacology of the drug. In this chapter the basic pharmacology of amphetamine is reviewed briefly, followed by a discussion of the clinical pharmacology of amphetamine, particularly as it relates to the treatment of psychiatric depression.

BASIC PHARMACOLOGY

There is a wide array of drugs that have in common an ability to produce behavioral stimulation. Among this array, the four drugs of major interest are amphetamine (both the dextro and levo isomers), methylamphetamine, methylphenidate, and cocaine (Fig. 1). All of these drugs are known to act on catecholamine nerves, and all probably share some common mechanism(s) of action. Since amphetamine has been more thoroughly investiagted than the other stimulants, it can serve as a prototype for the group.

When amphetamine is administered orally to laboratory animals, it is rapidly absorbed and widely distributed. The extent of plasma protein binding varies from species to species, but it never exceeds 45% of the total drug in plasma (Baggot, Davis, and Neff, 1972). Whether administered orally or parenterally, the drug easily passes the blood-brain barrier and accumulates in the central nervous system (Maickel, Cox, Miller, Segal, and Russell, 1969; Baggot et al., 1972). There appears to be a reasonable degree of correlation between brain levels of amphetamine and behavioral responses evoked by the drug (Maickel et al., 1969; Fuller, Molloy, Roush, and Hauser, 1972; Taylor and Sulser, 1973).

The rate and extent of amphetamine metabolism varies tremendously among species. In the rat the plasma half-life of amphetamine is about 1 hr (Sulser, Owens, and Dingell, 1966; Miller, Freeman, Dingell, and Sulser, 1970). In some other species the plasma half-life is much longer; for example, Baggot and Davis (1972) reported that amphetamine has a biological half-life of 4.5 hr in dogs. In addition to having variable rates of metabolism, different species also have various metabolic routes. To date two major pathways for metabolic

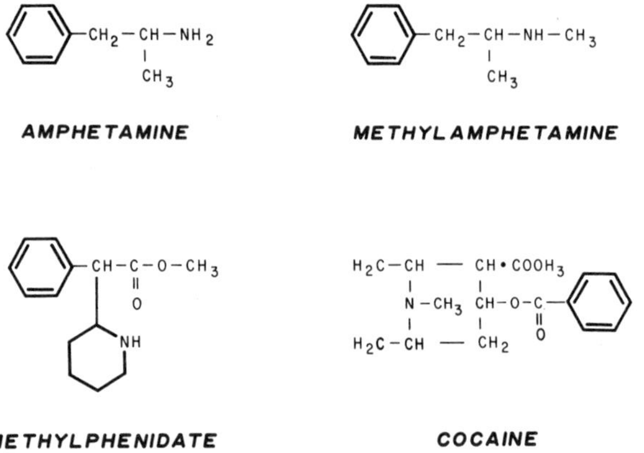

FIG. 1. Chemical structures of the major stimulant drugs.

degradation of amphetamine have been described: deamination and hydroxylation (Dring, Smith, and Williams, 1970). The guinea pig is an example of a creature that relies primarily on deamination; approximately two-thirds of an orally administered dose of amphetamine is excreted in a deaminated form. The rat, on the other hand, uses hydroxylation; it excretes approximately two-thirds of an orally administered dose of amphetamine in the hydroxylated form. Both creatures excrete approximately 10% to 20% of the administered amphetamine in an unchanged form.

It has been suggested that the hydroxylated metabolites of amphetamine may have important pharmacological actions. Therefore the metabolites themselves have been the subject of some research. Hydroxylation of amphetamine proceeds in a two-step sequence (Fig. 2). Para-hydroxylation, which is the initial step, occurs in the liver; the kinetics of this reaction have been studied in detail (Jonsson, 1974). The second step is β-hydroxylation, a reaction that can occur in several organs, including the brain (Freeman and Sulser, 1974). The latter reaction is of special importance to psychopharmacologists. Amphetamine is β-hydroxylated by the enzyme dopamine β-oxidase. This is the same enzyme that converts dopamine to norepinephrine. Because of this, there has been continuing interest in the possibility that hydroxylated metabolites of amphetamine might enter and impair the function of noradrenergic nerves. The potential significance of this possibility is discussed below.

Amphetamine itself exerts several effects on the nervous system; most of these effects relate to synaptic transmission. Although amphetamine can affect acetylcholine-mediated transmission (Ho and Gershon, 1972; Vasko, Domino, and Domino, 1974) and serotonin-mediated transmission (Leonard, 1972; Knapp, Mandell and Geyer, 1974), its major actions are probably related

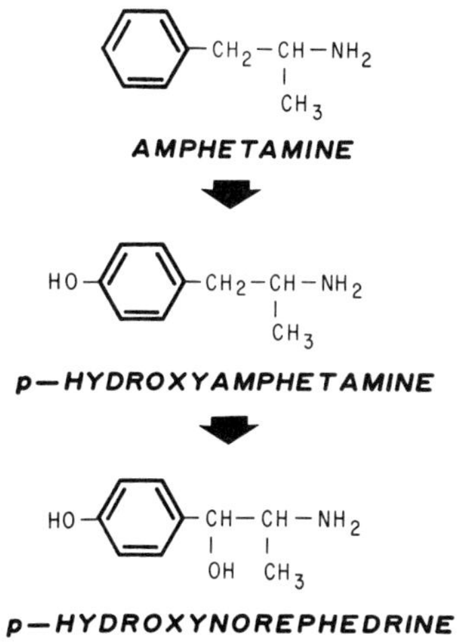

$CH_2-CH-NH_2$
CH_3

AMPHETAMINE

$HO-$ $CH_2-CH-NH_2$
CH_3

p—HYDROXYAMPHETAMINE

$HO-$ $CH-CH-NH_2$
OH CH_3

p—HYDROXYNOREPHEDRINE

FIG. 2. Metabolic pathway for hydroxylation of amphetamine. Amphetamine is converted to p-hydroxyamphetamine by liver hydroxylating enzymes. p-Hydroxyamphetamine is converted to p-hydroxynorephedrine by the enzyme dopamine β-oxidase, an enzyme found in noradrenergic nerves.

to catecholamine-mediated transmission. In all likelihood amphetamine exerts effects on both of the major brain catecholamines, i.e., norepinephrine and dopamine.

Much of the current research on amphetamine stems from the classic experiments of Burn and Rand (1958). These workers described amphetamine as being an indirectly acting sympathomimetic agent. This term was meant to imply that amphetamine can enter catecholamine nerve endings and evoke the release of endogenous catecholamines. Hence amphetamine works indirectly to activate or potentiate catecholamine transmission. During the years since the early studies of Burn and Rand, it has been determined that amphetamine has yet another important action. Like all of the behavioral stimulants (methylamphetamine, methylphenidate, cocaine) and most of the tricyclic antidepressants (imipramine, amitriptyline, etc.), amphetamine can block the neuronal uptake of catecholamines. Nerve endings are known to have a pump mechanism by which they capture catecholamines that have been released into the synaptic space. Pumping catecholamines back into the nerves from which they were released is an important mechanism for terminating synaptic activity. By blocking this pump, amphetamine and other stimulants potentiate catecholamine transmission.

Studies on the ability of amphetamine to evoke catecholamine release and block its uptake have now reached a relatively high level of sophistication. For example, it is possible to install perfusion cannulas in the lateral ventricles of animals, and in so doing monitor the release of norepinephrine and dopamine. Using this technique several investigators demonstrated that amphetamine causes a sharp increase in the release of newly synthesized catecholamines (Chiueh and Moore, 1974; Philippu, Glowinski, and Besson, 1974). Another technique, microiontophoresis, has permitted the injection of minute quantities of amphetamine onto single cells in the brain; this work has confirmed the belief that amphetamine acts centrally on catecholamine nerve cells (Bunney, Aghajanian, and Roth, 1973).

There is little question that amphetamine potentiates catecholamines in the brain. Therefore recent research has sought to localize those regions of the brain in which amphetamine acts to initiate certain behaviors, e.g., psychomotor stimulation. There is an emerging body of neuroanatomical and neuropharmacological data suggesting that the striatum is an important site of amphetamine action (Creese and Iversen, 1973, 1975; Neill, Boggan, and Grossman, 1974). These data are very encouraging because the striatum is a region of the brain that is particularly rich in catecholamines.

CLINICAL PHARMACOLOGY

As might be expected, our knowledge of the clinical pharmacology of amphetamine does not equal our knowledge of its animal pharmacology. Nevertheless, there is a modest amount of information on the human pharmacology of the drug.

Following oral administration, amphetamine is rapidly absorbed from the gut and begins to be distributed throughout the body within approximately 30 min. In common with lower animals, man shows significant (16%) plasma protein binding of amphetamine (Baggot et al., 1972). The binding appears to be associated with plasma albumin. The biological half-life of amphetamine in man has been reported to be approximately 12 hr (Rowland, 1969), but more work is necessary to confirm this estimate.

One of the more detailed studies on amphetamine metabolism in man was reported by Dring et al. (1970). These investigators determined the fate of ^{14}C-amphetamine after its administration to human volunteers. They reported that 60% to 65% of the total ^{14}C was excreted in urine within 24 hr. Of this total, approximately half was unchanged drug and half deaminated metabolite. Only a small fraction of the administered amphetamine appeared in the urine as a hydroxylated metabolite. Approximately 30% more of the total ^{14}C was excreted over the next 2 to 3 days. Therefore of the total administered dose, approximately 90% was excreted in urine over a 3- to 4-day period. These findings are in general agreement with other reports on amphetamine metabolism in man (Beckett and Rowland, 1965; Vree and van Rossum, 1970).

Once it has been distributed to the nervous system, amphetamine presumably exerts the same actions in man as in laboratory animals. At a systemic or a behavioral level, there is evidence to support this assumption. Amphetamine exerts both sympathomimetic and psychomotor stimulant effects in man (Cameron, Specht, and Wendt, 1965; Martin, Sloan, Sapira, and Jasinski, 1971). On the other hand, it is difficult to establish a similarity between man and other animals in terms of the cellular pharmacology of amphetamine. Nevertheless there is one line of research which suggests that amphetamine acts in man by potentiating catecholamine transmission. Approximately a decade ago it was demonstrated that the stimulant properties of amphetamine in laboratory animals could be diminished or abolished by pretreating the animals with drugs that block catecholamine synthesis (Weissman, Koe, and Tenen, 1966). This observation has been reproduced many times, and it serves to support the belief that amphetamine acts indirectly via catecholamine neurons. If this mechanism of action is applied to man, then one would predict that blockade of catecholamine synthesis should obtund the euphoriant effect of amphetamine. This possibility was actually tested by Jonsson, Anggard, and Gunne (1971). These investigators pretreated a small group of amphetamine users with α-methyltyrosine, an effective inhibitor of catecholamine synthesis. As expected, the subsequent administration of amphetamine failed to elicit or elicited only a mild euphoriant effect. This finding suggests that in man, as in laboratory animals, there is a link between amphetamine-induced behavioral stimulation and catecholamine transmission.

PSYCHIATRIC INDICATIONS

Stimulants are commonly used in two quite distinct populations of patients: those who suffer from depression and those who suffer from minimal brain dysfunction (MBD; hyperkinesia). The latter disorder and its treatment with amphetamine-like drugs is discussed elsewhere in this volume. The present discussion focuses on the treatment of depression.

In any discussion of the drug treatment of affective disorders, it is essential to clarify terminology. More precisely, one must differentiate the terms "stimulant" and "antidepressant." These terms differ in many respects, but there are three areas of central importance to understanding the treatment of depression. First, stimulants have a primary effect on psychomotor activity, whereas antidepressants have no direct effect on it. Second, stimulants have the potential to alter mood in all patients, but antidepressants alter mood only in patients whose depression is manifest. Third, stimulants and antidepressants have different temporal characteristics. Stimulants have a rapid onset of action, but this action can be sustained for a period of only a few days or weeks; antidepressants have a slow onset of action, but the action may be sustained indefinitely.

Ideally, a therapeutic choice between stimulants and antidepressants should be made on the basis of patient symptoms and diagnosis, and thereafter a particular stimulant drug selected on a rational pharmacological basis. Unfortunately these desirable therapeutic aims are difficult to achieve. Given the data currently available, one can make only general statements about the bases on which to choose between stimulants and antidepressants. Furthermore, choosing the appropriate stimulant from among those available nearly defies rationale.

For depressive disease, diagnosis plays a moderately important role in influencing the selection of a particular drug therapy. Although there are shortcomings to the *Diagnostic and Statistical Manual* (*DSM-II*), especially as it relates to affective disorders, the *DSM-II* is nonetheless the classification scheme currently used in psychiatry. According to *DSM-II*, depressive illness can occur in a variety of forms, as indicated in Table 1. Of the three major

TABLE 1. *Major categories of depression*

A. Psychoses
    1. Major affective disorders
        a. Involutional melancholia
        b. Unipolar depression
        c. Bipolar depression (manic-depressive illness)
    2. Psychotic depressive reaction
B. Neuroses
    1. Depressive neurosis
C. Personality disorders
    1. Cyclothymic personality

A summary of the major depressive illnesses as categorized by the *Diagnostic and Statistical Manual* (*DSM-II*).

groupings (psychoses, neuroses, and personality disorders), the psychoses are the ones in which a physician would be least inclined to use a stimulant. For unipolar and bipolar depressions, as well as for psychotic depressive reactions, the drugs of choice are the tricyclic antidepressants. Should these agents fail, a trial with monoamine oxidase (MAO) inhibitors would be in order. For involutional melancholia the primary therapy is not pharmacological in nature; electroconvulsive therapy appears to be of greater value. Although stimulants have been used in the past for depressions of psychotic intensity, such use met with little or no gain. Besides, this early use of stimulants predated the introduction and widespread acceptance of antidepressants (see Leake, 1958 for a review of the early literature).

At the other end of the spectrum is the cyclothymic personality disorder. By definition, a personality disorder is neither severe nor deteriorative. As such, it should require little if any physical treatment. Should drug therapy become necessary, Klein and Davis (1969) proposed instituting the same drug regimen that would be used in manic-depressive illness.

Lying between the depressive psychoses and the depressive personality disorders, but certainly not a pathological continuum between them, are the depressive neuroses. It is in patients with depressive neuroses that one might consider the use of stimulants. In particular, a stimulant might be prescribed for those patients with a mild depressive episode. It should be noted that tricyclic antidepressants are usually the favored drugs even in depressive neuroses. However, a short trial with a stimulant drug may be appropriate if a patient shows fatigue or lassitude, has a clear subjective sense of depression, is not suffering notable agitation, and appears to need little assistance to recover normal mood.

As mentioned earlier, there are four major drugs in the stimulant class: amphetamine, methylamphetamine, methylphenidate, and cocaine. Of these four, the first to be used in the treatment of depression was cocaine. Freud introduced cocaine as a remedy for his own depressive moods, as well as for those suffered by other members of his family. During the years since Freud's work, little attention has been focused on cocaine as a psychotherapeutic agent, and it currently has no accepted indications in psychiatry. Because of the scarcity of well-controlled clinical trials with cocaine, Post, Kotin, and Goodwin (1974) recently evaluated the drug in 16 patients hospitalized with "endogenous" depression. When cocaine was administered orally, it did not have a consistently therapeutic effect; when administered by intravenous infusion, it occasionally produced an elevation in mood, but this favorable response was often marred by the simultaneous appearance of dysphoria. The authors concluded that cocaine should not be recommended for the treatment of depression.

Of the remaining stimulants, there is little comparative data on which to base decisions about which agent to use. Even for amphetamine, which has been more thoroughly studied than methylamphetamine and methylphenidate, there is a striking paucity of well-controlled clinical studies. In one of the few studies seeking to compare subjective responses to stimulants, Martin et al. (1971) reported that amphetamine, methylamphetamine, and methylphenidate produced equivalent mood changes. No clear criteria emerged from their study by which to select one stimulant over the others. Indeed until evidence to the contrary is forthcoming, amphetamine, methylamphetamine, and methylphenidate can be regarded as stimulants of equivalent efficacy.

In addition to their use as therapeutic agents in depression, stimulants may also have an adjunctive role in influencing therapy to antidepressant drugs. Two of these adjunctive roles merit comment. According to Wharton and coworkers, methylphenidate can potentiate the clinical effects of tricyclic antidepressant drugs (Wharton, Perel, Dayton, and Malitz, 1971). The potentiation may result from the fact that methylphenidate can act in the liver to retard the metabolism of tricyclic drugs. As a result, addition of methylphenidate to a constant regimen of a tricyclic antidepressant results in elevated plasma levels of the latter drug. Presumably the change in plasma levels of tricyclic drug could have therapeutic consequences. The interaction between methylphenidate and tricyclic antidepressants is not a common feature of all stimulants. Accordingly, amphetamine has little effect on metabolizing enzymes in the liver, and it does not potentiate antidepressants.

A second adjunctive role for stimulants is as a predictor of subsequent responses to tricyclic drugs (Fawcett and Siomopoulos, 1971; Fawcett, Maas, and Dekirmenjian, 1972). The cumulative literature on tricyclic antidepressants indicates that approximately two-thirds of all depressed patients have some measure of favorable response, and one-third do not. Since antidepressant drugs may require a lengthy time for onset of action, it would be useful to have a quick predicative technique for distinguishing potential responders from potential nonresponders. According to Fawcett and his associates, challenge with amphetamine might be such a technique. These authors have reported that depressed patients who respond favorably to a short trial on amphetamine are very likely to respond to subsequent treatment with a tricyclic drug. By contrast, those patients who have little or no elevation in mood during amphetamine therapy tend not to respond to later therapy with tricyclic drugs. These findings, if generally confirmed, might have some implications in terms of clinical psychiatry; but perhaps more importantly, the finding may have relevance to research into the biochemical basis of depressive disease.

ADVERSE SIDE EFFECTS

Amphetamine and other stimulants can produce a number of adverse side effects. Some of the more serious of these effects are discussed below. However, as a prelude to this discussion, it is important to establish a sense of perspective about the frequency of adverse reactions. At the doses at which these agents are used clinically, side effects tend to be relatively infrequent.

Systemic Reactions

The use of stimulants may be accompanied by a variety of mild systemic reactions, including such phenomena as perspiration, dry mouth, gastrointestinal disorders, transient anorexia, and difficulties in ejaculation and urination. Only infrequently is there a systemic effect of sufficient magnitude to warrant discontinuation of drug therapy.

The adverse systemic effect that seems to concern physicians most is hypertension. Based on the fact that amphetamine is an indirectly acting sympathomimetic agent, one would expect the drug to be a reasonably potent pressor agent. Indeed, the stimulants are capable of producing transient elevations in blood pressure (Martin et al., 1971). However, this effect tends to be of minor importance because pressor responses are usually short in duration and minimal in amplitude. In fact, orally administered amphetamine at thera-peutically useful doses has little cardiovascular activity.

It may seem paradoxical that amphetamine can act via catecholamines to produce striking behavioral effects and at the same time fail to elicit striking cardiovascular effects. The explanation of this paradox probably involves two factors. First, both norepinephrine and dopamine in the brain appear to be involved in psychomotor activity, but only norepinephrine in the periphery is involved in cardiovascular activity. Therefore the central effects of ampheta-mine are surely far more complex than the peripheral effects. A second factor is that there are well-developed reflex mechanisms for regulating blood pres-sure but no such mechanisms for reflexly regulating behavior. When blood pressure reflexes are surgically abolished in laboratory animals, the pressor effects of amphetamine are profoundly enhanced (Simpson, 1975a,b).

Although therapeutic doses of amphetamine and other stimulants typically do not produce alarming cardiovascular sequelae, large doses (e.g., those used by drug abusers) can have serious or fatal consequences. In a number of cases stimulant drug abuse has been associated with intracranial hemorrhage (Zalis and Parmley, 1963; Goodman and Becker, 1970; Weiss, Raskind, Morganstern, Pytlyk, and Baiz, 1970). Presumably these misadventures were secondary to hypertensive episodes caused by excessive amounts of stimulant.

Interestingly, there are some patients who become *hypo*tensive rather than *hyper*tensive after prolonged amphetamine use. The explanation for this phenomenon is not entirely clear, but according to one school of thought hypotension and shock could be due to the accumulation of *p*-hydroxynore-phedrine (Cavanaugh, Griffith, and Oates, 1970). This compound, which is a hydroxylated metabolite of amphetamine, can impair sympathetic transmis-sion. Thus hypotension might be secondary to *p*-hydroxynorephedrine-induced failure of transmission between sympathetic nerves and vascular smooth muscle. This putative explanation for hypotension deserves further explora-tion. In the meantime, it is gratifying to report that depressed patients seldom develop significant hypotension.

Behavioral Reactions

In a small percentage of patients, stimulants may produce agitation, dys-phoria, and insomnia. The latter of these effects is a common patient com-plaint. Of greater medical concern are two behavioral effects that are the center of great research interest: psychological dependence and drug-induced psychosis.

Repeated administration of stimulants leads to the development of toler-ance (Kosman and Unna, 1968). With most but not all drugs, the develop-ment of tolerance is accompanied by dependence, which can be either physical or psychological in nature. It appears that psychological dependence may de-velop with stimulants, but that physical dependence is unlikely. Needless to say, a dependence liability narrows the utility of stimulant drugs in depressed patients.

Perhaps the most stunning adverse effect one sees with stimulant drugs is precipitation of an acute paranoid-schizophrenic syndrome. This psychosis-like syndrome was described in detail by Bell (1965) and Ellinwood (1967). The phenomenon is ordinarily encountered among chronic abusers of stimulants, but it can be iatrogenic (McDonald, 1964; Ney, 1967). It is important to note that schizophrenic patients, whether their psychosis is latent or manifest, are especially vulnerable to the reaction (Janowsky, El-Yousef, Davis, and Sekerke, 1973; West, 1974).

When one encounters a dysphoric or paranoic reaction to a stimulant drug, there is a graded system of therapeutic approach. If the condition is mild, reassurance in a stimulus-damped environment may be adequate. If the reaction is truly a behavioral crisis, use of an antianxiety agent such diazepam can be helpful (Solursh and Clement, 1968). If the reaction is severe, phenothiazines (Espelin and Done, 1969) or butyrophenones (Angrist, Lee, and Gershon, 1974) can be used to obtund the behavioral reaction. The use of an antianxiety or an antipsychotic agent does not obviate the need for reassurance or stimulus damping.

Drug Interactions

Although there are several drug interactions that involve stimulant drugs, only one consistently assumes alarming proportions. The combination of an MAO inhibitor and an indirectly acting sympathomimetic agent (e.g., amphetamine) can produce a rapid and life-threatening hypertensive crisis (Bethune, Burrell, Culpan, and Ogg, 1964; Blackwell, Marley, Price, and Taylor, 1967). The MAO inhibitors, by blocking the enzymatic degradation of catecholamines, permit accumulation of an abnormally large pool of norepinephrine, which is susceptible to the releasing action of amphetamine. As a result, the combination of the MAO inhibitor plus amphetamine leads to extraordinary release of norepinephrine from sympathetic nerves, in turn leading to vasoconstriction and a hypertensive crisis. The release of norepinephrine is apparently so intense that the baroceptor mechanism cannot reflexly control blood pressure. The combination of an MAO inhibitor and an indirectly acting sympathomimetic agent can produce all of the untoward effects normally associated with a sustained hypertensive episode. If a patient should present in the midst of such a crisis, the use of α-adrenergic blocking agents (phentolamine, phenoxybenzamine) is in order.

Contraindications

There are relatively few contraindications to the use of stimulants. Those that do exist are predictable based on the adverse side effects. More precisely, one should be wary of using stimulants in patients with cardiovascular or cerebrovascular disorders, those with schizophrenia, or those receiving anti-depressant drugs, particularly of the MAO inhibitor type.

An additional contraindication is pheochromocytoma. Because this form of tumor leads to excessive synthesis of endogenous catecholamines, such patients are especially vulnerable to indirectly acting sympathomimetic amines. The administration of such drugs can lead to a hypertensive crisis.

CONCLUDING REMARKS

There are few drugs better known to the lay public and to the medical profession than the stimulants. These drugs have been available for several decades and have been used in an extraordinary breadth of medical contexts. Because of this widespread use, there has been a remarkably intense effort to describe their precise mechanism of action. Ironically, as our understanding of the basic pharmacology of the stimulants has increased, our need for the drugs as therapeutic agents has decreased. In part, this irony is due to the development of newer and more efficacious drugs for the treatment of depression.

Although it is difficult to predict the future role of stimulants as psycho-therapeutic agents, it is possible to identify a factor which will play a dominant role in deciding that future. In the past, stimulants were used somewhat indiscriminately in depressive illness. At present, effort is being spent in determining with some exactness the patients most likely to benefit from the drugs. To the extent that it is possible to identify a population of patients who respond favorably to stimulants but who derive little benefit from other drugs, the therapeutic future of stimulants will be ensured.

TREATMENT SUMMARY

Generic name	Trade name	Daily dosage range (mg)
D-Amphetamine	Dexedrine	5–30
D,L-Amphetamine	Benzedrine	5–30
Methylamphetamine	Desoxyn (and others)	5–15
Methylphenidate	Ritalin	20–60

REFERENCES

Angrist, B., Lee, H. K., and Gershon, S. (1974): The antagonism of amphetamine-induced symptomatology by a neuroleptic. *Am. J. Psychiatry*, 131:817–819.

Baggot, J. D., and Davis, L. E. (1972): Pharmacokinetic study of amphetamine elimination in dogs and swine. *Biochem. Pharmacol.*, 21:1967–1976.

Baggot, J. D., Davis, L. E., and Neff, C. A. (1972): Extent of plasma protein binding of amphetamine in different species. *Biochem. Pharmacol.*, 21:1813–1816.

Beckett, A. H., and Rowland, M. (1965): Urinary excretion kinetics of amphetamine in man. *J. Pharm. Pharmacol.,* 17:628–639.
Bell, D. S. (1965): Comparison of amphetamine psychosis and schizophrenia. *Br. J. Psychiatry,* 111:701–707.
Bethune, H. C., Burrell, R. H., Culpan, R. H., and Ogg, G. J. (1964): Vascular crises associated with monoamine-oxidase inhibitors. *Am. J. Psychiatry,* 121:245–248.
Blackwell, B., Marley, E., Price, J., and Taylor, D. (1967): Hypertensive interactions between monoamine oxidase inhibitors and foodstuffs. *Br. J. Psychiatry,* 113:349–365.
Bunney, B. S., Aghajanian, G. K., and Roth, R. H. (1973): Comparison of effects of L-dopa, amphetamine and apomorphine on firing rate of rat dopaminergic neurones. *Nature (Lond.),* 245:123–125.
Burn, J. H., and Rand, M. J. (1958): The action of sympathomimetic amines in animals treated with reserpine. *J. Physiol. (Lond.),* 144:314–336.
Cameron, J. S., Specht, P. G., and Wendt, G. R. (1965): Effects of amphetamines on moods, emotions, and motivations. *J. Psychol.,* 61:93–121.
Cavanaugh, J. H., Griffith, J. D., and Oates, J. A. (1970): The effect of acute and chronic amphetamine administration on the adrenergic neuron in man. In: *Amphetamine and Related Compounds,* edited by E. Costa and S. Garattini, pp. 551–556. Raven Press, New York.
Chiueh, C. C., and Moore, K. E. (1974): In vivo release of endogenously synthesized catecholamines from the cat brain evoked by electrical stimluation and by d-amphetamine. *J. Neurochem.,* 23:159–168.
Creese, I., and Iversen, S. D. (1973): Blockage of amphetamine induced motor stimulation and stereotypy in the adult rat following neonatal treatment with 6-hydroxydopamine. *Brain Res.,* 55:369–382.
Creese, I., and Iversen, S. D. (1975): The pharmacological and anatomical substrates of the amphetamine response in the rat. *Brain Res.,* 83:419–436.
Dring, L. G., Smith, R. L., and Williams, R. T. (1970): The metabolic fate of amphetamine in man and other species. *Biochem. J.,* 116:425–435.
Ellinwood, E. H. (1967): Amphetamine psychosis: I. Description of the individuals and process. *J. Nerv. Ment. Dis.,* 144:273–283.
Espelin, D. E., and Done, A. K. (1969): Amphetamine poisoning: Effectiveness of chlorpromazine. *N. Engl. J. Med.,* 278:1361–1365.
Fawcett, J., Maas, J. W., and Dekirmenjian, H. (1972): Depression and MHPG excretion: Response to dextroamphetamine and tricyclic antidepressants. *Arch. Gen. Psychiatry,* 26:246–251.
Fawcett, J., and Siomopoulos, V. (1971): Dextroamphetamine response as a possible predictor of improvement with tricyclic therapy in depression. *Arch. Gen. Psychiatry,* 25:247–255.
Freeman, J. J., and Sulser, F. (1974): Formation of p-hydroxynorephedrine in brain following intraventricular administration of p-hydroxyamphetamine. *Neuropharmacology,* 13:1187–1190.
Fuller, R. W., Molloy, B. B., Roush, B. W., and Hauser, K. M. (1972): Disposition and behavioral effects of amphetamine and β,β-difluoroamphetamine in mice. *Biochem. Pharmacol.,* 21:1299–1307.
Goodman, S. J., and Becker, D. P. (1970): Intracranial hemorrhage associated with amphetamine abuse. *J.A.M.A.,* 212:480.
Ho, A. K. S., and Gershon, S. (1972): Drug-induced alterations in the activity of rat brain cholinergic enzymes. I. In vitro and in vivo effect of amphetamine. *Eur. J. Pharmacol.,* 18:195–200.
Janowsky, D. S., El-Yousef, M. K., Davis, J. M., and Sekerke, H. J. (1973): Provocation of schizophrenic symptoms by intravenous administration of methylphenidate. *Arch. Gen. Psychiatry,* 28:185–191.
Jonsson, J. A. (1974): Hydroxylation of amphetamine to parahydroxyamphetamine by rat liver microsomes. *Biochem. Pharmacol.,* 23:3191–3197.
Jonsson, L-E., Anggard, E., and Gunne, L-M. (1971): Blockade of intravenous amphetamine euphoria in man. *Clin. Pharmacol. Ther.,* 12:889–896.
Klein, D. F., and Davis, J. M. (1969): *Diagnosis and Drug Treatment of Psychiatric Disorders.* Williams & Wilkins, Baltimore.

Knapp, S., Mandell, A. J., and Geyer, M. A. (1974): Effects of amphetamines on regional tryptophan hydroxylase activity and synaptosomal conversion of tryptophan to 5-hydroxytryptamine in rat brain. *J. Pharmacol. Exp. Ther.,* 189:676–689.

Kosman, M. E., and Unna, K. R. (1968): Effects of chronic administration of the amphetamines and other stimulants on behavior. *Clin. Pharmacol. Ther.,* 9:240–254.

Leake, C. D. (1958): *The Amphetamines.* Charles C Thomas, Springfield, Ill.

Leonard, B. E. (1972): Effect of four amphetamines on brain biogenic amines and their metabolites. *Biochem. Pharmacol.,* 21:1289–1297.

Maickel, R. P., Cox, R. H, Jr., Miller, F. P., Segal, D. S., and Russell, R. W. (1969): Correlation of brain levels of drugs with behavioral effects. *J. Pharmacol. Exp. Ther.,* 165:216–224.

Martin, W. R., Sloan, J. W., Sapira, J. D., and Jasinski, D. R. (1971): Physiologic, subjective, and behavioral effects of amphetamine, methamphetamine, ephedrine, phenmetrazine, and methylphenidate in man. *Clin. Pharmacol. Ther.,* 12:245–258.

McDonald, R. L. (1964): Iatrogenic amphetamine psychosis. *Am. J. Psychiatry,* 120:1200–1201.

Miller, K. W., Freeman, J. J., Dingell, J. V., and Sulser, F. (1970): On the mechanism of amphetamine potentiation by iprindole. *Experientia,* 26:863–864.

Neill, D. B., Boggan, W. O., and Grossman, S. P. (1974): Behavioral effects of amphetamine in rats with lesions in the corpus striatum. *J. Comp. Physiol. Psychol.,* 86:1019–1030.

Ney, P. G. (1967): Psychosis in a child, associated with amphetamine administration. *Can. Med. Assoc. J.,* 97:1026–1029.

Philippu, A., Glowinski, H., and Besson, M. J. (1974): In vivo release of newly synthesized catecholamines from the hypothalamus by amphetamine. *Naunyn Schmiedebergs Arch. Pharmacol.,* 282:1–8.

Post, R. M., Kotin, J., and Goodwin, F. K. (1974): The effects of cocaine on depressed patients. *Am. J. Psychiatry,* 131:511–517.

Rowland, M. (1969): Amphetamine blood and urine levels in man. *J. Pharm. Sci.,* 58:508–509.

Simpson, L. L. (1975a): The effect of behavioral stimulant doses of amphetamine on blood pressure. *Arch. Gen. Psychiatry (in press).*

Simpson, L. L. (1975b): Blood pressure and heart rate responses evoked by d- and l-amphetamine in the pithed rat preparation. *J. Pharmacol. Exp. Ther.,* 193:149–159.

Solursh, L. P., and Clement, W. R. (1968): Use of diazepam in hallucinogenic drug crises. *J.A.M.A.,* 205:644–645.

Sulser, F., Owens, M. L., and Dingell, J. V. (1966): On the mechanism of amphetamine potentiation by desipramine (DMI). *Life Sci.,* 5:2005–2010.

Taylor, W. A., and Sulser, F. (1973): Effects of amphetamine and its hydroxylated metabolites on central noradrenergic mechanisms. *J. Pharmacol. Exp. Ther.,* 185:620–632.

Vasko, M. R., Domino, L. E., and Domino, E. F. (1974): Differential effects of d-amphetamine on brain acetylcholine in young, adult and geriatric rats. *Eur. J. Pharmacol.,* 27:145–147.

Vree, T. B., and van Rossum, J. M. (1970): Kinetics of metabolism and excretion of amphetamines in man. In: *Amphetamines and Related Compounds,* edited by E. Costa and S. Garattini, pp. 165–190. Raven Press, New York.

Weiss, S. R., Raskind, R., Morganstern, N. L., Pytlyk, P. J., and Baiz, T. C. (1970): Intracerebral and subarachnoid hemorrhage following use of methamphetamine ("speed"). *Int. Surg.,* 53:123–127.

Weissman, A., Koe, B. K., and Tenen, S. S. (1966): Anti-amphetamine effects following inhibition of tyrosine hydroxylase. *J. Pharmacol. Exp. Ther.,* 151:339–352.

West, A. P. (1974): Interaction of low-dose amphetamine use with schizophrenia in outpatients: Three case reports. *Am. J. Psychiatry,* 131:321–323.

Wharton, R. N., Perel, J. M., Dayton, P. G., and Malitz, S. (1971): A potential clinical use for methylphenidate with tricyclic antidepressants. *Am. J. Psychiatry,* 127:1619–1625.

Zalis, E. G., and Parmley, L. F. (1963): Fatal amphetamine poisoning. *Arch. Intern. Med.,* 112:822–826.

Chapter 12

Neuropsychopharmacology of Mania

Baron Shopsin, Samuel Gershon, and Gerard Selzer

We are here concerned with exploring possible relationships between some biological and pharmacological findings and the clinical entity of mania.[1] It might appear that in dealing with mania we are clinically on fairly reasonable ground, perhaps on firmer ground than with other psychiatric disorders. However, in carefully examining some of the published data in the field, we find it overwhelmingly obvious that this assumption of diagnostic clarity is illusive. Therefore before we examine the biological and pharmacological findings, we must comment on some of the problems of diagnosis and also give some consideration to other behavioral variables that may confound the data. In addition, we must note that methodological problems are perhaps greater in the study of mania than in other disorders. These problems arise from special difficulties in differential diagnosis and in the lack of rating devices specifically related to the disease.

The initial issue in any research study, particularly one in which we are looking for specific biological changes, is the specificity and homogeneity of the clinical study sample. A semantic confusion also exists: Gross psychomotor overactivity may suggest use of the term mania to describe the patient. To attest to the arbitrariness of diagnosis, Noyes (1954) reports that some centers claim nearly 30% of admissions are due to manic-depressive psychosis; others report only 5%. The diagnosis of mania by our research unit at Bellevue Psychiatric Hospital accounts for approximately one in 1,999 admissions (0.1%). One standard source gives the incidence as very low, i.e., three to four per 100,000 of the general population (Redlich and Freedman, 1966). Other authors give quite different figures. It is clear that diagnostic features and fashions thereof could account for differences in manic-depressive disease that would outweigh differences due to almost any other variable.

Bratfos and Haug (1968) note that manic-depressive disease is the admission diagnosis for 5% of patients in their institution. They report also that 3% have subsequently taken a schizophrenic or schizoaffective course. Other investigators give an incidence of subsequent schizophrenic diagnosis ranging from 3% to 14% for patients originally diagnosed as manic-depressive (Rennie, 1942; Lundquist, 1945; Poort, 1945; Kinkelin, 1954; Astrup, Fossum,

---

[1] There are many different biological determinants that have been studied in relation to mania, including neurotransmitters, enzymes, hormones, and electrolytes. In keeping with the scope of this text, the present chapter focuses of neurotransmitter amines.

and Holmboe, 1959). However, Book (1953) conducted an extensive, careful survey and found an incidence of 82% for whom diagnoses changed from manic-depressive disease to schizophrenia. In a similar situation Asano (1967) gives 81.5% as the proportion of cases classified as "atypical" manic-depressive disease. These "atypical" cases showed clouding of consciousness and pathological features resembling schizophrenic symptoms.

The rarity of manic-depressive disease and the even greater rarity of cases presenting in the manic phase increase the problems in studies on this disorder. In Bratfos and Haug's (1968) study of 215 manic-depressives, only 20% either presented with or had a history of a manic episode. The incidence of a manic phase in Asano's (1967) study of 162 cases was 14.2%. This raises the question of whether there is a unipolar manic subgroup. The existence of such an entity is difficult to determine because of the limitation of follow-up and of the possibility of a depressive episode occurring at a subsequent time. Bratfos and Haug (1968) give an incidence of this entity (unipolar mania) as 2% of their sample; recently Abrams, Taylor, and Gaztanagu (1974) reported an incidence of 28%. Again, diagnostic criteria are an issue. A diagnosis of mania was applied on the criteria of hyperactivity, rapid pressured speech, and a euphoric, expansive, or irritable mood. Cases are included with auditory hallucinations (36% to 50%), persecutory delusions (50% to 57%), confusion (19% to 43%), visual hallucinations (14% to 28%), olfactory hallucinations (14%), catatonia (7% to 17%), and first-rank symptoms (21%).

Thus the heterogeneity of patient populations poses a problem in selecting and defining the patient groups suitable for specific biochemical studies. Despite the fact that this problem has led to differences across various studies in either treatment outcome or biochemical data, the problem has not yet been adequately resolved. Thus we are faced with one of the most perplexing problems in differential diagnosis in clinical psychiatry: the ill-defined interface between the manic phase of manic-depressive illness and schizophrenia of the schizoaffective type. Others, like ourselves, believe that "pure" mania should be the only criterion used when making a diagnosis of manic phase, manic-depressive illness; still others hold that a diagnosis of schizoaffective illness is never applicable. The latter group would place any patient showing affective overlay in the manic-depressive rubric and would accept the existence of profound thought disorder. At the moment these differences in diagnostic approach remain unsettled and so serve to cloud any effort to search out and explore a particular biological variable that might be unique to mania. This difficulty must be borne in mind while reading the following review of biological studies.

BIOGENIC AMINES IN MANIA

The current biological theories of mania, like those of depression, are united in postulating a role for brain monoamines in these disorders. The catecholamines of importance include dopamine (DA) and norepinephrine (NE); serotonin (5-hydroxytryptamine, 5-HT) is the putative indoleamine involved. The catecholamine and indoleamine theories of affective illness, simply stated, suggest that there is a functional deficit of brain neurotransmitter amines at specific central synapses in depression and, conversely, a functional excess of these amines in mania. The indoleamine hypothesis has been modified in recent years to suggest a deficit of indoleamines in both mania and depression, with a greater functional deficit of serotonin in depression.

These biological theories of mania have led to the idea that catecholamine or indoleamine metabolites in urine and/or cerebrospinal fluid (CSF) might vary with mood state. Therefore a number of investigators have sought to correlate mania with changes in monoamine excretion. The preponderance of these studies have focused on NE and its metabolites.

Urine

There have been a number of studies on urinary excretion of NE and two of its major metabolites, normetanephrine (NM) and 3-methoxy-4-hydroxy-phenylglycol (MHPG). Early studies reported increases in urinary excretion of NE during the manic phase of manic-depressive disorder. For example, Bergsman (1959) reported elevated excretion of NE in a series of manic patients. Shinfuku, Michio, and Masao (1961) reported increases in urinary excretion of NE during mania in a single patient with regular manic-depressive mood changes. Greenspan, Schildkraut, Gordon, Levy, and Durell (1969) found that excretion of NE and NM was greater during hypomania than during normothymic periods or periods of retarded depression. Bunney, Goodwin, Murphy, House, and Gordon (1972) reported that NE and DA were elevated before and during the manic episode. In particular, NE was significantly increased the day before the shift from depression to mania. Considering changes in catecholamine excretion, Bunney et al. (1972) commented that the days just before the manic episode may represent an initial phase of mania.

Although these studies suggest a consistent trend, the fact is that work on urinary NE has been highly contradictory. There are several reports that fail to correlate NE excretion with mania. (For extended critiques on clinicobiochemical studies, the reader should consult the reviews by Shopsin, Wilk, Gershon, Roffman, and Goldstein, 1973b; and Shopsin, Wilk, Sathananthan, Gershon, and Davis, 1974.) Furthermore, urinary NE is derived mainly from peripheral structures, and so centrally derived NE is greatly diluted. In response to these facts, many investigators have turned to the study of MHPG.

The concentration of MHPG was not elevated during a longitudinal study, including the manic phase, of three patients with manic-depressive illness (Bunney et al., 1972). However, there was a trend toward increased MHPG excretion preceding the onset of mania. In another longitudinal study Bond, Jenner, and Sampson (1972) also suggested that an increase in urinary

MHPG excretion preceded the "switch" into mania; furthermore, the excretion of this metabolite during mania was higher than baseline levels before mania. Jones, Maas, Dekirmenjian, and Fawcett (1973) reported on MHPG and NM in daily urine specimens from a patient with manic-depressive cycles. The quantities of these catecholamine metabolites excreted in urine were decreased during periods of depression as compared with periods of mania. The authors showed that the changes in MHPG and perhaps NM preceded the affective and behavioral state.

We have not found a significant correlation between mood state and MHPG excretion. In longitudinal studies of patients with manic-depressive illness, we did not find that MHPG excretion correlated with mania; in addition, it was not clear that the switch into the manic phase was associated with elevated MHPG excretion (Shopsin et al., 1973b).

An alternative approach to relating mood to MHPG excretion has been to study excretion of the metabolite in patients receiving amphetamine. Once again, the results have not been consistent. According to Schildkraut, Watson, Draskoczy, and Hartman (1971), urinary MHPG was elevated when amphetamine was taken, and it declined precipitously after the drug was withdrawn. MHPG excretion appeared to correlate with patients' moods, which were hypomanic while receiving amphetamine and depressed after discontinuance of the drug. These findings contrast with those of the present authors (Angrist, Shopsin, Gershon, and Wilk, 1972). We have found no consistent directional change in urinary MHPG excretion during amphetamine administration to healthy subjects.

The most serious criticism of studies which measure urinary MHPG in psychiatric patients is the fact that such measurements reflect total body change, of which the central nervous system (CNS) contribution is likely minimal. Therefore the percentage of urinary MHPG derived from brain may be quite small. If this were indeed the case, then changes in urinary MHPG would largely reflect changes in peripheral sympathetic activity, and small changes in central NE metabolism would be obscured. Consequently human studies utilizing urinary MHPG as a measure of central events should be viewed with reservation.

Cerebrospinal Fluid

Studies of amines and their metabolites in CSF probably represent the most direct available means of evaluating amine metabolism in the human subject (Moir, Ashcroft, Crawford, Eccleston, and Guldberg, 1970). Based on the interpretation of available data, the measurement of CSF MHPG in man likely yields the most direct information on the relationship between catecholamines and affective disorders. With several modifications of the gas-liquid chromatographic technique developed for measuring MHPG in urine, our group has analyzed CSF MHPG levels in carefully selected patient groups before and after drug therapy (Wilk, Shopsin, Gershon, and Suhl, 1972*a*; Wilk, Shopsin, Gershon, Davis, and Stuhl, 1972*b*). Our studies collectively indicate that the vast majority of psychiatric patients investigated to date, regardless of diagnosis, show CSF MHPG levels falling within the range of values seen in normal control subjects. All depressed patients—whether endogenous or reactive, bipolar or unipolar, and irrespective of the degree of psychomotor agitation or retardation—show normal MHPG levels in CSF.

We have previously shown that some manic and schizophrenic patients have CSF MHPG levels elevated beyond the range of our normal controls; for the manic and schizophrenic groups taken as a whole, statistical significance was attained for each group, with greatest significance in the manics ($p < 0.01$). There was no statistically significant difference between the manic and schizophrenic groups. We have now studied more patients; currently there are 15 manic individuals, 10 endogenous depressives, two reactive depressives, and 26 schizophrenics who have been studied with regard to CSF MHPG values. The greater number has eliminated any significance between the manic or schizophrenic populations when compared to controls. Again, the additional endogenously depressed patients show normal values of CSF MHPG, and for the depressed population as a whole there is no statistical difference compared to the mean of the control group.

Coppen (1970) recently found that MHPG in the CSF of his endogenously depressed and manic individuals is within the normal range. Post, Kotin, Goodwin, and Gordon (1973) found low CSF MHPG levels in some depressed individuals, but they suggest that motor activity is probably responsible for this result. They recorded normal values of CSF MHPG in manic patients.

It is noteworthy that clinical change in some of our bipolar manic-depressives is clearly associated with a marked shift in MHPG levels corresponding to the direction of mood swing (Shopsin. Wilk, Gershon, Green, and Davis, 1971). Although this cannot be duplicated in all bipolar subjects, the finding would be consistent with previous data suggesting that catecholamines may be involved only in the "switch process" rather than the steady state, i.e., that only the onset and cessation of the manic state may be associated with abnormal catecholamine metabolism (Goodwin, Murphy, Brodie, and Bunney, 1970).

The interpretation of data on CSF MHPG is itself not free from criticism and must be approached with caution. Some of the limiting factors in the interpretation of these data are as follows: (1) the origin of CSF MHPG has not been firmly established, and at least a small fraction of it may be peripheral in origin. (2) There are difficulties in determining the relative contributions of the brain as opposed to the spinal cord in producing total CSF MHPG. (3) MHPG may not be the principal brain metabolite of NE. The latter point is currently somewhat controversial. There is a possibility that other metabolites—e.g., vanillylmandelic acid (VMA)—could be the major product of brain NE. However, the levels of CSF VMA are so low that measuring it would be an extremely difficult if not questionable approach to studying central catecholamine metabolism (Shopsin et al., 1974).

Relatively few studies have engaged in attempts to assess the dopamine metabolite homovanillic acid (HVA) in the CSF of psychiatric patients. Normal values in both mania and depression have been recorded (Ashcroft, Blackburn, Eccleston, Glen, Hartley, Kinlock, Lonergan, Murray, and Pullar, 1973; Sathananthan, Wilk, Angrist, Shopsin, and Gershon, 1975).

In contrast to the paucity of studies on dopamine metabolites, there are a wealth of studies on central metabolism of 5-HT. The major metabolite of 5-HT is 5-hydroxyindoleacetic acid (5-HIAA). There are many published reports on CSF 5-HIAA in psychiatric patients. Unfortunately the data are not consistent. As yet, there has emerged no clear trend of investigation to show that mood changes are associated with characteristic changes in CSF 5-HIAA levels.

Critical Assessment of Biogenic Amine Data

In reviewing the vast literature dealing with the role of amines in affective disorders, we are struck by the staggering array of investigations reporting various experimental approaches to different biological determinants. In our overview of published findings, we find that in attempting to extract material from the available literature the story and the label do not readily fit; support or confirmation of hypotheses linking either catecholamines or indoleamines to the pathogenesis of affective disorders does not readily emerge.

Differences in methodology and experimental design make direct data comparison difficult from one study to another. In this regard the problem of diagnostic discrepancies; the patient's age, sex, diet, and physical activity; the influence of pharmaceutical agents; the diurnal variation in endogenous amine release; and the discrepant findings in different as well as the same biological determinants explored contribute to the difficulties in assessing human studies.

Studies exploring the role of amines and/or their metabolites in affective states have employed urine or CSF as the two principal media with which to formulate experimental approaches to the problem. If one examines the available literature dealing with MHPG, HVA, or 5-HIAA in the CSF of psychiatric patients, it is apparent that data cannot be duplicated by different investigators, or sometimes even by the same investigator at different times. Even when changes in biogenic amines of psychiatric patients are recorded, the data cannot be consistently correlated with behavioral and affective changes in the clinical state. Furthermore, and of even greater significance, similar findings have been found in psychiatric populations having diagnoses other than affective illness, as well as in individuals showing a wide variety of neurological diseases with no demonstrable psychiatric impairment. Hence it remains to be established that either the absolute level or the rate of metabolism of any biogenic amine is a major factor in affective disease.

PSYCHOPHARMACOLOGY OF MANIA

The monoamine hypothesis of affective illness largely germinated from retrospective observations concerning the biochemical activity of certain psychoactive drugs used in the treatment of mental patients. For example, reserpine produces a marked degree of behavioral control as well as a calming effect in manic patients; it is also capable of producing depression. Since reserpine is known to deplete the brain of monoamines, it was logical to propose that the amines must be related to affect. A difficulty in pursuing the hypothesis has arisen on many counts, one of which has been an inability to pinpoint definitively the particular amine(s) responsible for the clinical changes observed in reserpine-treated patients. Therefore a number of other research strategies have evolved to help determine the particular amine that underlies affect or changes in affect. These strategies can be grouped into four broad categories:

1. Administration of drugs that selectively block the synthesis of monoamines

2. Administration of precursors that may lead to increased brain levels of monoamines

3. Use of selective blocking agents to diminish or abolish the postsynaptic activity of monoamines

4. Use of drugs that alter the metabolism of monoamines

It would be gratifying to report that all of these strategies have been rationally applied to the study of all brain amines. Unfortunately that is not the case. Each method has been used to a different extent with different monoamines. Some of the more important studies are described below. (Interested readers may also consult the 1974 review by Mendels and Frazer.)

Blockade of Synthesis

Two inhibitors have been used in the study of mania: parachlorophenylalanine (PCPA) and α-methylparatyrosine (α-MPT). The former agent is a specific inhibitor of tryptophan hydroxylase, the rate-limiting enzyme in the synthesis of 5-HT. No specific antimanic effects were observed with PCPA in a study in which this drug was used in doses of up to 4 g/day in a limited number of manic individuals (Post et al., 1973). α-MPT is a potent and specific inhibitor of DA and NE synthesis, centrally as well as peripherally. The effects of α-MPT have been evaluated in patients hospitalized for mania (Brodie, Murphy, Goodwin, and Bunney, 1970; Bunney, Brodie, Murphy, and Goodwin, 1971). Although the compound was found to have some antimanic properties, it was not as effective as lithium in the small series of patients studied. Other investigators have found that α-MPT lacks antimanic properties (Shopsin and Gershon, *unpublished findings*).

Precursor Loading

Wilson and Prange (1972) reported a double-blind study of tryptophan versus chlorpromazine (CPZ) in 10 manic patients; they found that tryptophan has antimanic properties, and that it was superior to CPZ in most respects, although statistical significance was apparently absent. These investigators have since, in a double-blind placebo-controlled crossover study, treated (1) five manic patients with CPZ, then with tryptophan, and (2) five patients with tryptophan first and then CPZ. The results of this more recent study indicate that tryptophan was slightly superior to CPZ in all respects. "Partial" antimanic effects of tryptophan have also been cited by Murphy, Baker, Goodwin, Miller, Kotin, and Bunney (1974).

We have not been able to duplicate the findings of Wilson and Prange (1972). In several outpatient manic-depressives, tryptophan treatment resulted in exacerbation of mania and subsequent hospitalization. In two patients exacerbation of the manic state was more pronounced than ever before in the patient's history; severe disorganization and delusional material (out of context with the manic picture) developed in one. A similar case was recorded by Murphy et al. (1974).

Postsynaptic Blocking Agents

Preliminary studies by Dewhurst (1968), Haskovec (1969), and Haskovec and Soucek (1968; 1969) indicated a marked, rapid-acting, antimanic effect for methysergide, an antiserotonin agent. This compound is obviously of tremendous tactical and theoretical interest, since several observations suggest that 5-HT metabolism may be disturbed in affective illness, as well as in the manic phenomena accompanying it. This suggested to Dewhurst that the specificity of response to methysergide could serve as a diagnostic test in cases of undiagnosed excitement, since results would be evident within 48 hr. However, controlled cross-validation studies are lacking; in fact, Coppen, Prange, Whybrow, Noguera, and Pacz (1969) indicated that this compound exhibited no apparent therapeutic action in their patients with moderate to severe mania, and that since it compared poorly with placebo effects it may even be detrimental. McCabe, Reich, and Winokur (1970) also reported on an open trial of methysergide in acute mania. Of the 12 patients in the study, only one responded during the 4- to 5-day trial. Several patients who did not respond were given a considerably longer trial than the usual 4 days, but they showed no change.

Itil, Polvan, and Holden (1971) reported efficacy for a relatively new antiserotonin compound, called cinnanserin (2′,3′-dimethylaminopropylthiocinnamanilide hydrochloride), in the treatment of manic patients. These authors indicate that the drug seems to have a very potent and dramatic effect on manic patients, with a particularly noteworthy speed of effectiveness. This finding is in agreement with a report by Kane (1970), who also observed a rapid improvement in manic patients under cinnanserin treatment. In the study by Itil et al. (1971), cinnanserin was given to manic patients in a fixed dose of 800 mg, reached after a 2- to 5-week treatment period; this was accompanied by a 4-week placebo period before and after treatment. Treatment efficacy was measured by standard rating techniques. The most common physical side effects were hyperkinesia, stimulated behavior, and insomnia.

In another study by Itil, Polvan, Dincmen, and Sungarbey (1975), another antiserotonin and antihistamine compound was found effective in bipolar patients with manic episodes. The compound, homochlorocyclazine, was given in a single-blind fashion to 10 manic patients for a period of 2 to 33 days in mean daily dosages of 120 to 300 mg. The results are highly preliminary and difficult to interpret at this point, but the investigators have indicated promising results.

In light of the negative studies following the early enthusiastic claims for methysergide in mania, it would be wise to await the results of further investigations currently underway before ascribing a definite role for cinnanserin and other antiserotonin/anhihistamine compounds in the treatment of mania.

Another compound newly tested in the treatment of manic illness is propranolol, a β-adrenergic blocking agent. Reporting on the rapid, distinct improvement with this drug in certain types of psychotic patients including manics, Atsmon, Blum, Wijsenbeck, Maoz, Steiner, and Ziegelman (1971) indicated that an outstanding impression of treatment was the "complete return to normal within hours, recovery taking place from 12 to 48 hours after initial treatment." Nearly all patients received an initial propranolol dose of 600 to 800 mg/day. The dosage was increased in some cases, in one instance reaching 5,800 mg. There was a clear-cut parallelism between the onset of amelioration of symptoms and lowering of pulse rate, followed by a lowering of blood pressure after 12 to 24 hr. The specific outcome in manic patients cannot be extracted from the overall result of treatment in all psychotics. The results of Atsmon et al. (1971) have not been duplicated by others in the United States (Orzack, Gardos, and Branconnier, 1973).

Altered Metabolism

Physostigmine is a reversible, centrally active acetylcholinesterase inhibitor. Administration of physostigmine slows the metabolism of acetylcholine. This drug has been given intravenously, under experimental conditions, to manic patients and has been reported to antagonize or neutralize mania as well as euphoric symptoms related to other illnesses (Janowsky, El-Yousef, Davis, and Sekerke, 1972). In addition, it was reported by these same authors to

cause depression and has been shown to have effects opposite to those occurring in situations in which adrenergic activation occurs (e.g., amphetamine-
induced euphoria and psychomotor stimulation). For this reason it was proposed that central cholinergic factors may play a role in the etiology of
affective disorders and specifically in the balance between central cholinergic
and adrenergic neurotransmitter activity in specific brain areas that regulate
affect, with depression being a disease of cholinergic dominance and mania
being one of adrenergic dominance. However, other studies now completed
seriously question the specificity of physostigmine in qualitatively altering
the manic state (Carroll, Frazer, Schless, and Mendels, 1973; Janowsky, El-
Yousef, Davis, and Sekerke, 1973)

The antimanic effects of physostigmine have been questioned. Both Carroll
et al. (1973) and Shopsin, Janowsky, Davis, and Gershon (1973a; a collaborative study with the original authors of the hypothesis) found that apathy
and anergia were apparent in manic patients treated with physostigmine but
that delusional quality of manic psychopathology was not basically altered.
No patient became depressed as had been previously described. Shopsin et al.
(1973a) focused on "rebound" phenomena, or postphysostigmine changes,
as a clinical index with which to characterize chemically the initial state of
amine imbalance responsible for a given affective illness. Their data, if substantiated, could be consistent with an adrenergic-dopaminergic-cholinergic
balance hypothesis of affective disorders and could provide a link in understanding the interface, or crossover, between organic and schizoaffective
illnesses.

Critical Assessment of Psychopharmacology Data

Despite persistent investigational preoccupation with brain amines over the
past decade, clinical studies have not revealed unequivocal, consistent, or
unique physiological abnormalities in mania or depression that substantiate
the pharmacologically derived monoamine theories. However, the general
monoamine theories have been remarkably productive, leading to an impressive body of experimental and clinical data that have provided new insights into brain neurotransmitter activity and affective disorders only dimly
suspected a decade ago.

METABOLIC STUDIES IN MANIA

Enzymes and Electrolytes

Because of the prevailing belief that monoamines are somehow related to
affective disorders, there have been a significant number of studies on the
enzymes involved in monoamine synthesis and degradation. Thus enzymes
such as dopamine-β-oxidase, monoamine oxidase, and catechol-O-methyl-

transferase have all been studied in relation to mania. Although the level of research interest has been high, no one has yet demonstrated a compelling link between monoaminergic enzymes and mania.

Another line of inquiry has dealt with electrolytes and hormones (renin, aldosterone, etc.) that influence electrolyte metabolism. This line of investigation arises from the fact that lithium, like sodium and potassium, is a monovalent cation that can be widely distributed in biological tissues and fluids. To date there have been many studies on sodium and potassium (levels, distribution, elimination) in patients with affective disorders. Here again, though, results have not been clear-cut. Nevertheless, the majority of studies tend to indicate that manic patients do not have any significant alterations in sodium or potassium metabolism. An extensive analysis of electrolyte studies in mania will appear shortly (Shopsin, Gershon, and Selzer, *in preparation*).

Lithium

One interesting exception to the trend of "no metabolic derangement" in mania relates to lithium, a drug used to treat mania. There is some evidence to suggest that manic patients may handle the lithium ion somewhat differently from normal subjects.

Various workers measuring urinary lithium levels report that manic patients retain more orally administered lithium than do nonmanic patients. This difference, detected as early as 4 hr after a test dose of lithium carbonate, may increase with time. Other workers dispute this and attribute apparent differences in retention to inadequate intestinal absorption, brevity of collection time, loss of urine, or sodium or water imbalance (or both). Moreover, some of the studies included patients receiving somatic treatment in addition to lithium during both the depressive and manic phases of illness. Because of the importance of these studies in delineating a possible uniqueness of manic patients with regard to specific physiological parameters, we review some of the relevant data.

Trautner, Morris, Noack, and Gershon (1955) first recorded that acutely manic patients retain more lithium ion than do normal controls or other psychiatric patients, and that on recovery manics excrete the excess lithium ion in the urine. There was no dietary control in this study, and the manic and nonmanic patients were given different lithium doses. Hullin, Swincoe, and McDonald (1968) studied 13 patients with manic psychoses in a dietary controlled study, in which intake of sodium and potassium as well as overall composition of the diet were held constant. They found in such a lithium-balance study that a significantly greater amount of lithium is retained by manic patients than by controls. Most of the controls remained in lithium balance from the sixth day of treatment on; i.e., the daily urinary output of lithium was approximately equal to the intake. The manic patients tended to remain in positive lithium balance for longer periods. Despite a cumulative retention of lithium in 12 of the 14 manics, plasma lithium concentrations did not exceed 1.4 mEq/liter.

In two reports from the National Institute of Mental Health (Greenspan, Goodwin, Bunney, and Durrell, 1968a; Greenspan, Green, and Durrell, 1968b), lithium balance studies were reported for eight patients, seven of whom had a history of bipolar manic-depressive illness. The eighth patient had a history of recurrent depressions and acute intermittent porphyria. Three patients were acutely manic when lithium administration was begun, and one of these patients was treated in two distinctly separate manic episodes. Three patients were depressed when lithium treatment was begun, and three were normothymic (during a clinical period in which normal mood and behavior were observed). One of the normothymic patients had been studied previously during an acute manic episode. It was observed that manic patients had a larger total positive lithium balance than either depressed or normothymic patients. For the four manic episodes, the total lithium retained ranged from 86 to 152 mEq. The total lithium retained by the normothymic and depressed patients varied between 32 and 50 mEq. Whereas no period of appreciable negative lithium balance was noted in the depressed or normothymic patients, a period ranging from 6 to 13 days of appreciable negative lithium balance was noted when the manic patients recovered from the manic symptoms (the period of negative lithium balance is defined as that period in which daily excretion of lithium ions exceeds the daily ingestion of lithium ions by more than 5%). The cumulative total negative lithium balance measured for the four patients to whom lithium was administered during a manic episode varied from 21 to 136 mEq. Very slight negative lithium balance (probably within experimental error) was noted for the normothymic and depressed patients, but in no case did it exceed a cumulative total of 11 mEq.

"Normalized apparent lithium space" was determined for each patient at the time of maximal lithium retention. To compute this value, the "apparent lithium space" was calculated by dividing the total amount of lithium retained by the plasma lithium concentration. The total body water was estimated by referring to Moore's nomogram relating body weight to total body water in normals. The normalized apparent lithium space was then calculated by dividing the apparent lithium space by the estimated total body water. If, as is frequently assumed, the lithium ion is distributed uniformly throughout the body water, the normalized apparent lithium space should approximate 1.0. For the normothymic patients the normalized apparent lithium space was 1.1 to 1.5, for the depressed patients 1.4 to 1.5, and for the manic patients 1.7 to 3.7.

Other groups of investigators have extended these studies, focusing on the initial period of lithium administration. Epstein, Grant, Herjanic, and Winokur (1965) studied lithium excretion for 24 hr following a single lithium dose but observed no differences between acutely manic patients and controls.

Serry (1969) used an oral loading dose of 1,200 mg lithium carbonate and measured the excretion of this ion for 4 hr. Patients were defined as "retainers" or "excreters" depending on whether they excreted less than 12 mg or more than 18 mg lithium ion during the 4-hr period, respectively. Of the 159 hospitalized psychiatric patients, 47% were labeled as retainers and 40% as excreters. The manic patients as a group showed a higher percentage of retainers; those who did not appear to respond to lithium treatment were in the excreter group. Stokes, Mendels, Secunda, and Dyson (1972) attempted to replicate these studies but found that only 6% of their patients were retainers by the definition established by Serry (1969). They were also unable to relate the retention to diagnosis or to use retention as a predictor of whether the patient would respond to lithium treatment. Their results cannot be considered entirely comparable, since the distribution of retainers and excreters was so different from that of Serry's.

In a study by Almay and Taylor (1973), consecutive hospital admissions were carefully diagnosed for use as matched groups of either acute manic patients or normal controls. Each subject ingested 900 mg lithium carbonate with water at 8:00 A.M., emptied his bladder, and began a 36-hr total urine collection. Blood was collected hourly for 12 hr after lithium ingestion, then every 6 hr for four additional samples. The total urine volume excreted every 6 hr was measured for lithium ion content. There was no dietary control. The data showed that manic patients retain significantly more orally administered lithium than do normal controls, and that this difference is apparent at the end of each measured time interval (up to 36 hr), beginning 6 hr after the test dose. The difference between groups was most apparent when total 36-hr urine lithium ion excretion levels were compared. The mean serum lithium concentrations were not significantly different between groups at any time during the 36-hr test.

The study by Almay and Taylor (1973) thus tended to confirm previous data that manic patients retain significantly more orally administered lithium ion than normals. However, they showed that this difference is detectable by comparing urine but not serum concentrations, and this retention difference increases over time. Their findings are also consistent with the suggestion that manic patients distribute lithium in their bodies differently than do normals, and so measuring the serum concentration does not reflect the differences in lithium retention between manic and nonmanic patients.

Shopsin, Gershon, and Pinckney (1969) studied lithium levels in human mixed saliva and found that manic patients comprised two groups with respect to lithium secretion into this medium. One group of manic patients reached peak lithium levels within 7 days (mean) following oral lithium administration and then showed a marked decrease over a period of days to weeks thereafter (mean, 16 days). Moreover, there was evidence to suggest a correspondence between time of clinical response and elevated lithium concentrations in such individuals. The fall in lithium levels noted thereafter may correspond to the massive lithium diuresis reported in patients after their mania breaks. The second group of manic patients demonstrated a different pattern of lithium distribution, showing a continued rise in levels that graphically assumed a monotonic pattern. This group may correspond to those not showing the characteristic lithium diuresis following clinical improvement.

Critical Assessment of Lithium Data

The box score for lithium retention/excretion studies in mania shows an approximately equal number of positive and negative reports. Data comparison is rendered difficult because of the difference in methodology and study design among the different investigations. Some of the studies (both pro and con) do not control for diet or for the ingestion of other drugs. The lithium doses vary from one study to another; in one study the dose was different in the manic patients from that in nonmanic psychiatric patients or controls. The studies differ with regard to duration of lithium treatment and urinary excretion, ranging from hours to weeks. Certainly those studies not controlled for diet, especially with regard to sodium and water intake, remain highly questionable and include the early work of Trautner et al. (1955) and the recent evaluations by Almay and Taylor (1973).

With these reservations in mind, we are inclined to conclude that lithium is probably handled in a unique manner in mania, in that differences in excretion do appear when manic patients are compared with control subjects, or in manic-depressive patients during different phases of their cyclic illness. Manic patients tend to retain more lithium during manic episodes and may even undergo a period of negative lithium balance on recovery from the manic symptoms.

CONCLUSIONS

It becomes quite evident that the intense investigational curiosity into the affective disorders, specifically with regard to manic-depressive illness, has primarily focused on depression, the unipolar or bipolar types. Relatively speaking, there have been conspicuously few studies specifically related to the manic aspects of this severe mood disorder. Electrolyte studies, neuroendocrine studies; studies into different enzyme systems, and those dealing with amines/amine metabolites exploring possible etiopathogenic mechanisms underlying the affective disorders have also focused mainly on the depressive aspects of the manic-depressive disorder.

In reviewing the available material, one is often faced with the problem of evaluating conflicting results. The study of amines in urine or CSF highlights this problem; the researcher is often confronted by six reports with one result and six with opposite conclusions. Whatever the area explored, differences in methodology and experimental design often complicate the issues;

disparate data are often a function of different diagnostic interpretations (heterogeneous populations), the absence of adequate control groups, methods of assessment, intricacies of techniques, ingestion of drugs during baseline periods in psychiatric patients, and factors such as age, sex, hospitalization, diet, physical activity, and time of testing. It would not be unfair to note that, at the present state of the art, there is no specific biochemical finding with which to make, predictably and consistently, an objective diagnosis of mania.

In spite of the fact that no biochemical determinant of mania has been identified, this should not occasion pessimism about clinicobiochemical research. Even though a cellular explanation for affective disease has not been found, the published work has had sizable impact. One major result is that during the course of efforts to unravel pathological changes, we have learned a great deal about the normal physiology of the brain and the relationship of that physiology to normal behavior. An additional gain is that clinical investigators, as a whole, have experienced a rapid increase in the level of sophistication with which they approach problems relating to neuro- and psychopharmacology. It is almost certain that the increasing level of sophistication in clinical research will ultimately lead to a biochemical explanation of mania and other affective disorders.

REFERENCES

Abrams, R., Taylor, M. A., and Gaztanagu, P. (1974): Manic depressive illness and paranoid schizophrenia. *Arch. Gen. Psychiatry,* 31:640–643.

Almay, G. L., and Taylor, M. A. (1973): Lithium retention in mania. *Arch. Gen. Psychiatry,* 29:232–234.

Angrist, B., Shopsin, B., Gershon, S., and Wilk, S. (1972): Metabolites of monoamines in urine and cerebrospinal fluid, after large dose amphetamine administration. *Psychopharmacologia,* 26:1–9.

Asano, N. (1967): Clinico-genetic study of manic-depressive psychosis. In: *Clinical Genetics in Psychiatry,* edited by H. Mitsuda. Igaku Shoin, Tokyo.

Ashcroft, G. W., Blackburn, I. M., Eccleston, D., Glen, A. I. M., Hartley, W., Kinlock, N. E., Lonergan, M., Murray, L. G., and Pullar I. A. (1973): Changes on recovery in the concentration of tryptophan and the biogenic amine metabolites in the CSF of patients with affective illness. *Psychol. Med.,* 3:319–325.

Astrup, C., Fossum, A., and Holmboe, R. (1959): A follow-up of 270 patients with acute affective psychosis. *Acta Psychiatr. Scand. [Suppl. 135],* 34:1–65.

Atsmon, A., Blum, E., Wijsenbeck, H., Maoz, B., Steiner, M., and Ziegelman, G. (1971): The short-term effects of adrenergic-blocking agents in a small group of psychotic patients. *Psychiatr. Neurol. Neurochir.,* 74:251–285.

Bergsman, A. (1959): The urinary excretion of adrenalin and noradrenalin in some mental diseases. *Acta Psychiatr. Neurol. Scand.,* 133:1–17.

Bond, P. A., Jenner, F. A., and Sampson, G. A. (1972): Daily variation of the urine content of M.H.P.G. in two manic-depressive patients. *Psychol. Med.,* 2:81–85.

Book, J. A. (1953): A genetic and neuropsychiatric investigation of a northern Swedish population. *Acta Genet.,* 4:345–414.

Bratfos, O., and Haug, J. O. (1968): The course of manic-depressive psychoses. *Acta Psychiatr. Scand.,* 44:90–112.

Brodie, H. K. R., Murphy, D. I., Goodwin, F. K., and Bunney, W. E., Jr. (1970): Catecholamines and mania: The effect of alpha-methyl-para-tyrosine on manic behavior and catecholamine metabolism. *Clin. Pharmacol. Ther.,* 12:219–224.

Bunney, W. E., Jr., Brodie, H., Murphy, D. L., and Goodwin, F. K. (1971): Studies of α-methylparatyrosine, L-dopa and L-tryptophan in depression and mania. *Am. J. Psychiatry,* 127:872–881.

Bunney, W. E., Jr., Goodwin, F., Murphy, D., House, K., and Gordon, E. K. (1972): The "switch" process in manic-depressive illness. *Arch. Gen. Psychiatry,* 27:304–309.

Carroll, B. J., Frazer, A., Schless, A., and Mendels, J. (1973): Cholinergic reversal of manic symptoms. *Lancet,* 1:427–428.

Coppen, A., Prange, A., Jr., Whybrow, P. C., Noguera, R., and Pacz, J. M. (1969): Methysergide in mania. *Lancet,* 2:338–340.

Coppen, A. J. (1970): The chemical pathology of the affective disorders. In: *The Scientific Basis of Medicine Annual Review,* pp. 179–210. Athlon Press, London.

Dewhurst, W. G. (1968): Methysergide in mania. *Nature (Lond.),* 219:506–507.

Epstein, R., Grant, L., Herjanic, M. and Winokur, G. (1965): Urinary excretion of lithium in mania. *J.A.M.A.,* 192:409.

Goodwin, F. K., Murphy, D. L., Brodie, H. K., and Bunney, W. E., Jr. (1970): L-Dopa, catecholamines and behavior: A clinical and biochemical study in depressed patients. *Biol. Psychiatry,* 2:341–366.

Greenspan, K., Goodwin, F. K., Bunney, W. E., Jr., and Durell, J. (1968a): Lithium in retention and distribution patterns in acute mania and normothymia. *Arch. Gen. Psychiatry,* 19:664–673.

Greenspan, K., Green, R., and Durell, J. (1968b): Retention and distribution patterns of lithium: A pharmacological tool in studying the pathophysiology of manic depressive psychosis. *Am. J. Psychiatry,* 125:512–519.

Greenspan, K., Schildkraut, J. J., Gordon, E. K., Levy, B., and Durell, J. (1969): Catecholamine metabolism in affective disorders. II. Norepinephrine, normetanephrine, epinephrine, metanephrine and UMA excretion in hypomanic patients. *Arch. Gen. Psychiatry,* 21:710–716.

Haskovec, L. (1969): Methysergide in mania. *Lancet,* 2:902.

Haskovec, L., and Soucek, I. (1968): Trial of methysergide in mania. *Nature (Lond.),* 219:507–508.

Haskovec, L., and Soucek, I. (1969): The action of methysergide in manic states. *Psychopharmacologia,* 15:415–424.

Hullin, R. P., Swincoe, J. C., and McDonald, R. (1968): Metabolic balance studies on the effect of lithium salts in manic depressive psychosis. *Br. J. Psychiatry,* 114:1561–1573.

Itil, T. M., Polvan, N., and Holden, J. M. C. (1971): Clinical and EEG effects of cinnanserin in schizophrenic and manic patients. *Dis. Nerv. Syst.,* 32:193–200.

Itil, T. M., Polvan, N., Dincmen, K., and Sungarbey (1975): Clinical effects of SA-97 (homochlorcyclazine) in manic patients (*in press*).

Janowsky, D., El-Yousef, M. K., Davis, J. M., and Sekerke, H. J. (1972): A cholinergic-adrenergic hypothesis of mania and depression. *Lancet,* 2:632–635.

Janowsky, D. S., El-Yousef, M. K. Davis, J. M., and Serkerke, H. J. (1973): Parasympathetic suppression of manic symptoms by physostigmine. *Arch. Gen. Psychiatry,* 28:542–547.

Jones, F. D., Maas, J. W., Dekirmenjian, H., and Fawcett, J. A. (1973): Urinary catecholamine metabolites during behavioral changes in a patient with manic-depressive cycles. *Science,* 179:300–302.

Kane, F. J. (1970): Treatment of mania with cinnanserin, an antiserotonin agent. *Am. J. Psychiatry,* 126:1020–1023.

Kinkelin, M. (1954): Verlouf und prognose des manisch-dcpressive irreseins. *Schweiz. Arch. Neurol. Psychiatr.,* 73:100–146.

Lundquist, G. (1945): Prognosis and course in manic-depressive psychosis. *Acta. Psychiatr. Scand. [Suppl.],* 35.

McCabe, M. S., Reich, T., and Winokur, G. (1970): Methysergide as a treatment for mania. *Am. J. Psychiatry,* 127:354–356.

Mendels, J., and Fraser, A. (1974): Biogenic amine depletion and mood. *Arch. Gen. Psychiatry,* 30:447–451.

Moir, A. T. B., Ashcroft, G. W., Crawford, T. B., Eccleston, D., and Guldberg, H.

(1970): Cerebral metabolites in CSF as a biochemical approach to the brain. *Brain,* 93:357–358.

Murphy, D. L., Baker, M., Goodwin, F. K., Miller, H., Kotin, J., and Bunney, W. E., Jr. (1974): L-Tryptophan in affective disorders: Indoleamine changes and differential chemical effects. *Psychopharmacologia,* 34:11–20.

Noyes, A. D. (1954): *Modern Clinical Psychiatry,* Ed. 4. Saunders, Philadelphia.

Orzack, M. H., Gardos, G., and Branconnier, R. (1973): CNS effects of propranolol in man. *Psychopharmacologia,* 29:299–306.

Poort, R. (1945): Catamnestic investigations on manic-depressive psychosis with special reference to the prognosis. *Acta. Psychiatr. Scand.,* 20:59–74.

Post, R. M., Kotin, J., Jr., Goodwin, F. K., and Gordon, E. K. (1973): Psychomotor activity and CSF amine metabolites in affective illness. *Am. J. Psychiatry,* 130:67–72.

Redlich, F. S., and Freedman, D. (1966): *The Theory and Practice of Psychiatry.* Basic Books, New York.

Rennie, T. A. C. (1942): Prognosis in manic-depressive psychosis. *Am. J. Psychiatry,* 98:801–814.

Sathananthan, G., Wilk, S., Angrist, B., Shopsin, B., and Gershon, S. (1975): An exploration of the dopamine hypothesis in psychosis (CSF-HVA). *Am. J. Psychiatry* (in press).

Schildkraut, J. J., Watson, R., Draskoczy, P. R., and Hartman, E. (1971): Amphetamine withdrawal: Depression and M.H.P.G. excretion. *Lancet,* 2:485–486.

Serry, M. (1969): Lithium retention and response. *Lancet,* 1:267–268.

Shinfuku, N., Michio, O., and Masao, K. (1961): Catecholamine excretion in manic depressive psychosis. *Yonago Acta. Med.,* 5:109–114.

Shopsin, B., Gershon, S., and Pinckney, L. (1969): The secretion of lithium in human mixed saliva: Effects of ingested lithium on electrolyte distribution in saliva and serum. *Int. Pharmacopsychiatry,* 2:148–169.

Shopsin, B., Janowsky, D., Davis, J., and Gershon, S. (1973a): Rebound phenomena in manic patients following physostigmine: Towards an understanding of the aminergic mechanisms underlying affective disorders. Presented at the ACNP Meeting, Las Vegas, Nevada.

Shopsin, B., Wilk, S., Gershon, S., Green, J., and Davis, K. (1971): Catecholamines and affective disorders: Levels of M.H.P.G. in CSF. *Pharmacologist,* 39:398.

Shopsin, B., Wilk, S., Gershon, S., Roffman, M., Goldstein, M. (1973b): Collaborative pharmacologic studies exploring catecholamine metabolism in psychiatric disorders. In: *Frontiers in Catecholamine Research,* edited by E. Usdin and S. Snyder. Pergamon Press, New York.

Shopsin, B., Wilk S., Sathananthan, G., Gershon, S., and Davis, K. (1974): Catecholamines and affective disorders revised: A critical assessment. *J. Nerv. Ment. Dis.,* 158:369–383.

Stokes, J. W., Mendels, J., Secunda, S. K., and Dyson, W. L. (1972): Lithium excretion and therapeutic response. *J. Nerv. Ment. Dis.,* 154:43–49.

Trautner, E. M., Morris, R., Noack, Ch., and Gershon, S. (1955): The excretion and retention of ingested lithium and its effect on the ionic balance in man. *Med. J. Aust.,* 2:280–291.

Wilk, S., Shopsin, B., Gershon, S., and Suhl, M. (1972a): CSF levels of M.H.P.G. in affective disorders. *Nature (Lond.),* 235:440–441.

Wilk, S., Shopsin, B., and Gershon, S. (1972b): CSF M.H.P.G.: An assessment of norepinephrine metabolism in affective disorders. *Psychopharmacologia,* 26:64. (suppl.)

Wilson, I. C., and Prange, A. J., Jr. (1972): Tryptophan in mania: Theory of affective disorders. *Psychopharmacologia,* 26:76. (suppl.)

Chapter 13

Therapeutic Uses of Lithium and Rubidium

Ronald R. Fieve

During the past 25 years, the practice of psychiatry has been revolutionized by the introduction of psychoactive drugs, and none has been so potentially revolutionary as lithium. It has been firmly established that lithium is a specific and effective antimanic agent, capable of controlling and preventing recurrence of episodes of mania. In addition there is a growing body of evidence which indicates that lithium may also control and prevent recurrent episodes of depression in both bipolar and unipolar illness. Although definitely not the panacea some supporters claim, lithium has become established as the first prophylactic drug in psychiatric history.

The emergence of lithium in psychiatric therapy is of course fraught with implications. For one thing, it lends support to the theory that major affective disorders may be organically based, i.e., the result of some chemical imbalance or genetically inherited biochemical defect. Secondly, it suggests that the entire method of treating mental disorders will undergo a radical change. Many of the hitherto employed therapies, including psychoanalysis and electroshock treatment, may eventually prove obsolete. Furthermore, as therapy becomes more effective and simpler with illness-specific drugs, the burden of psychiatric care may shift to the family practitioner, since stabilization and maintenance can easily be handled through routine laboratory testing and regular office visits.

The extraordinary promise offered by lithium has added impetus to the investigation of other potentially useful psychotropic agents. Work with rubidium, an element of the same chemical family which appears to exert neurochemical and behavioral effects "opposite" to those of lithium, is in the initial stages. In addition to these explorations, other trace metal ions await investigation.

An overview of the current findings on lithium is given here. Special attention is focused on prophylactic studies, since these have aroused considerable interest and discussion. Finally, an effort is made to define the present status of research with rubidium.

HISTORY OF LITHIUM

Lithium, the lightest of the alkali metals (which also include sodium, potassium, rubidium, and cesium), was discovered in 1817 by Johan August

Arfvedson working in the laboratory of the Swedish physician and chemist Baron Jons Jakob Berzelius. A silvery white substance, lithium does not occur freely in nature but does occur as a salt. Its distribution is almost universal; it is 20 to 70 times more prevalent than zinc in the earth's crust and more abundant than lead. Traces of lithium can be detected in many chemical compounds, in more than 150 minerals, and in sea and fresh water. It has been found in the tissues of various animals and plants, including tobacco, sugar cane, and seaweed. Its presence has also been noted in the sun's spectrum.

The use of lithium in medicine has been documented as early as the second century AD, when Seranus of Ephesus prescribed mineral waters to treat particular physical and mental complaints. Caelius Aurelianus, a fifth century physician, even recommended specific alkaline springs, many of which contained lithium, as exercising some beneficial effects.

Around 1850, investigators (Lipowitz in 1841 and Garrod in 1859) discovered that urate deposits could be dissolved by lithium salts combined with uric acid in a test tube. As a result, lithium was used to treat uremia, renal calculi, gout, rheumatism, and various other ills. European and American spas during the nineteenth and early twentieth centuries attracted patrons by advertising the lithium content (often inflated) of the mineral springs. A new industry centered around bottling the curative waters and selling them to the public. Although newer and more effective therapies for these disorders have been developed, the spas of Europe, the Soviet Union, Japan, South America, the United States, and West Germany continue to enjoy wide patronage. Enthusiasts believe that the springs are helpful in treating chronic disorders including renal, intestinal, and hepatic conditions; arthritis; rheumatism; anemia; chlorosis; gynecological complaints; heart conditions; and "nervous" disorders, e.g., neurasthenia, neuralgia, and nervous breakdowns.

During the early twentieth century lithium bromide was used as a sedative and anticonvulsant following reports of its hypnotic (Culbreth, 1917) and antiepileptic (Squire, 1908) properties. Lithium again attracted wide attention and a notorious reputation during the late 1940s when its chloride salt was introduced as a salt substitute for cardiac and hypertensive patients. Its use was quickly discontinued when reports linked it to numerous instances of severe poisoning and several deaths.

Ironically, at the same time lithium chloride was withdrawn from the market as a salt substitute, the first report of its efficacy in treating episodes of mania appeared. In 1949 in Australia Cade was examining the urine of manic patients in an attempt to identify some substance that could be responsible for triggering manic outbursts. In the course of his experiments, he noted that guinea pigs given injections of lithium urate became lethargic for several hours. Cade then tested lithium against mania in 10 human patients, all of whom responded to the drug.

His published report provoked little response, however. It was not until the mid-1960s that the psychiatric profession realized the full import of Cade's work. Between 1949 and 1964 relatively little work with lithium was undertaken. Klein and Davis (1969) attribute the "unfortunate lag between discovery and application" to several factors: (1) poor communication in the field; (2) lack of a pharmacological orientation among psychiatrists; (3) the acknowledged toxic potential of lithium; and (4) disinterest on the part of pharmaceutical companies in investigating and promoting a drug that was not commercially profitable. Cade (1970) himself suggested that the primary investigation "made by an unknown psychiatrist, working alone in a small chronic hospital with no research training, primitive techniques and negligible equipment was hardly likely to be compellingly persuasive, especially in the United States." Events appear to have borne out this assessment.

THERAPEUTIC ACTION IN MANIA

The therapeutic value of lithium in combating mania or hypomania is now firmly established. To date well over 70 reports have appeared in the literature, almost all attesting to the efficacy of lithium. Improvement rates range from 60% to 100%. However, Shull and Sapira (1970) noted that these rates for the most part reflect the results of open trials. The lack of control groups and standardized diagnostic categories makes it impossible to gauge accurately the contribution of lithium. Nevertheless, the results of these open studies, along with the findings of the regrettably few controlled single- and double-blind studies, amply demonstrate the therapeutic action of lithium. Most investigators agree that an estimate of 70 to 80% effectiveness is reasonable. This estimate takes into account possible spontaneous remissions.

Although Cade's discovery in 1949 pointed the way, it remained for other investigators to document his claims. Schou, Juel-Neilsen, Stromgren, and Voldby published the first double-blind study in 1954. Of 38 manic patients, 14 (37%) definitely improved with lithium, 18 (47%) showed possible improvement, and six (16%) had no response. Maggs (1963), in a placebo-controlled, double-blind study, assigned 18 manic patients to two groups: one treated with placebo-rest-lithium, the other with lithium-rest-placebo. Lithium was superior to placebo during the second week of treatment in both groups. Fieve, Platman, and Plutchik (1968a), in a double-blind study of 35 manic patients, showed good results in 80%, debatable response in 6%, and no improvement in 14%. A fourth double-blind study of two patients (Bunney, Goodwin, Davis, and Fawcett, 1968) involved replacing lithium with placebo at specified times. Both patients reached normal states with lithium, but they became manic again within 24 hr of lithium withdrawal. Goodwin, Murphy, and Bunney (1969), in an extension of this study with 12 manic patients, rated nine as improved with lithium and three as worse. A double-blind study of 34 manic-depressive patients (Stokes, Stoll, Shamoian, and Patton, 1971) also demonstrated lithium superior to placebo.

Studies comparing lithium with the phenothiazines or haloperidol are less conclusive. The difficulties inherent in conducting crossover double-blind drug trials in mania have limited the number of published findings. In a single-blind study Wharton and Fieve (1966) found lithium superior to chlorpromazine in a selected thorazine-refractory manic group. In a double-blind study by Johnson, Gershon, and Hekimian (1968), 27 acute manic patients showed better response to lithium (78% improvement) than to chlorpromazine (36%). In a double-blind study Platman (1970) found lithium slightly superior to chlorpromazine during a 3-week period. Spring (1971), however, had dissimilar results; in a group of 12 manics receiving chlorpromazine (five patients) or lithium (seven patients) for 3 weeks, six of the seven lithium-treated patients returned to normal states, as did three of the five chlorpromazine-treated patients. Spring concluded that neither drug was significantly better. Fieve (1970) criticized this study for its too-small sample. Prien, Caffey, and Klett (1972), in an 18-hospital study involving 255 newly admitted manic patients on either lithium or chlorpromazine, found chlorpromazine definitely superior to lithium in treating the highly disturbed, actively manic patient. However, among mildly active patients lithium appeared to be the better treatment, by a small margin.

A number of investigators have noted a qualitative difference in response to chlorpromazine and lithium. Schou, Fieve, Gershon, and others have pointed out that, although both drugs dampen overactivity, chlorpromazine in the dose required to calm moderate and severe mania also produces a sluggish, drowsy, and subjectively "drugged" feeling. Lithium has fewer side effects.

Controlled double-blind comparative studies of lithium with haloperidol or with electroshock have not as yet been reported.

THERAPEUTIC ACTION IN DEPRESSION

While by no means as conclusive as the evidence in mania, there is a growing body of data which indicate that lithium may also be helpful in controlling certain subtypes of depression. Cade (1949) was the first to evaluate lithium action in depression, observing that it had no beneficial effect. Unfortunately his observations involved only a small number of depressed patients. The results of other researchers have refuted his findings.

In 1957 Vojtechovsky reported that eight of 14 depressed patients responded favorably to lithium following failure with electroconvulsive therapy (ECT). Andreani, Caselli, and Martelli (1958) reported that 10 of 24 depressives improved on lithium. However, both studies were open and lacked controls. In another open clinical trial, Dyson and Mendels (1968) treated 31 patients with lithium, noting success with the depressed phase in 19 cases of manic depression. They reported no improvement in nine cases of neurotic depression and in three of involutional psychotic depression.

Fieve et al. (1968a), in a double-blind study, compared the antidepressant effect of lithium and imipramine in 29 depressed bipolar patients. They concluded that lithium had only a "mild antidepressant effect" compared to imipramine. Goodwin et al. (1969), in a controlled double-blind study of 30 manic depressives (which included 13 bipolar depressed and five unipolar depressed), noted a positive correlation between depressive scores and lithium treatment in 10 bipolar depressed and two unipolar depressed patients. There was a negative correlation between depressive scores and placebo treatment. Mendels, Secunda, and Dyson (1972) reported that, in a double-blind crossover study with lithium carbonate and desimipramine, lithium was as effective an antidepressant as desimipramine in "selected depressed" patients. Stokes et al. (1971), in a double-blind trial, noted a slightly better improvement rate with lithium than with placebo in 18 depressed manic-depressive patients. In an uncontrolled long-term follow-up study of 40 patients treated for "recurrent affective disorders" in private practice, Warick (1970) reported that 29 patients treated for acute manic attacks had no recurring episodes and milder depressions than were experienced before taking lithium. However, four patients needed additional antidepressant medication to reach a normal state.

It is evident that the picture is far from clear concerning any therapeutic effect of lithium against depression. Investigators believe, however, that the recent classification of depression into bipolar or unipolar subtypes may help in evaluating the action of lithium. The above double-blind studies—by Fieve et al. (1968a), Goodwin et al. (1969), Mendels et al. (1972), and Stokes et al. (1971)—indicate that lithium may induce a mild therapeutic antidepressive response in some bipolar depressions. For a conclusive statement further therapeutic trials of lithium versus tricyclics are needed in bipolar and unipolar depressed illness. Certainly severe depressive episodes respond best to tricyclic antidepressants or electroshock treatment. The value of lithium in reactive or neurotic depression or suicidal depression has not been determined.

Future studies must take into account characteristics of the syndrome (e.g., whether the episode is recurrent or solitary, the family history). In addition, no study to date has employed a placebo group as a control. The possibility thus remains that improvement reported may be due to natural remission rather than to drug treatment.

PROPHYLAXIS

In 1963 Hartigan reported that maintenance doses of lithium carbonate could effectively prevent recurrence of manic and depressive episodes in patients subject to frequent attacks. A similar report from Baastrup (1964) followed. In 1967 Baastrup and Schou, after reviewing the data compiled over a period of 6 years on 88 female manic-depressives and recurrent depressives, concluded "lithium is the first drug demonstrated as a clear-cut prophylactic agent against one of the major psychoses." Needless to say, these claims provoked considerable interest and controversy.

To begin with, prophylaxis in psychiatry differs from that in any other field of medicine (Laurell and Ottoson, 1968). In addition to actual prevention, it can imply early treatment or stabilization of a recent remission. Does lithium decrease the frequency of attacks or attenuate their severity? Secondly, how does one scientifically test the claims? Blackwell and Shepherd (1968) criticized Baastrup and Schou (1967) for faulty experimental design, citing poor patient selection, statistical errors, and observer bias, stating that they invalidated the conclusions. Prophylactic trials, in contrast to treatment periods, can span months and even years. The ethics of keeping a control group, members of which are often suicidal, on placebo for such extended periods without offering effective help is unreasonable.

In view of the semantic and methodological problems, an airtight case in favor of lifetime lithium prophylaxis has been slow in coming. Nevertheless, the use of lithium as a preventive measure in bipolar manic depression is now quite well established.

In 1970 a joint open study by three European psychiatric clinics (Angst, Weis, Grof, Baastrup, and Schou, 1970) reported that in more than half of over 22 cases lithium had curtailed the duration and frequency of attacks in patients with "recurrent endogenous affective disorders." This supported the finding of Angst, Dittrich, and Grof (1969) that lithium, more than imipramine, successfully altered the course of illness.

Double-blind trials by Melia (1970, 1971), covering 2 years in the lives of 18 patients with "recurrent affective disorder," resulted in inconclusive findings. Some patients improved with lithium, others did not. Fieve, Platman, and Plutchik (1968b), after studying 43 bipolar patients in a longitudinal, single-blind effort, concluded that lithium produced a decrease in intensity, although not in frequency, of future bipolar depressive attacks.

Baastrup and co-workers redesigned an earlier study in an attempt to satisfy later criticism that had arisen (Baastrup, Poulsen, Schou, Thomsen, and Amdisen, 1970). Fifty bipolar and 34 unipolar depressives, all on maintenance lithium for a year, were randomly assigned to placebo or lithium. Within 5 months 21 placebo patients had suffered relapses; no lithium patients were affected. [Blackwell (1970) suggested that the relapses were the result of adverse patient reactions to withdrawal of a drug to which they had become accustomed.] This study provided the first double-blind indication that lithium was effective in preventing episodes of unipolar as well as bipolar illness. Among the bipolar group, 55% of those on placebo relapsed. Similarly, 53% of the unipolar patients on placebo relapsed, but none of the unipolar patients on lithium suffered a setback.

Coppen's group achieved similar results (Coppen, Noguera, Bailey, Burns, Swani, Hare, Gardner, and Maggs, 1971). Sixty-five patients hospitalized with mania or depression were randomly assigned at discharge to lithium or placebo for up to 112 weeks in a double-blind study. Lithium was considerably more effective than placebo in preventing manic and depressive behavior in both bipolar and unipolar patients. Whereas 95% of the placebo patients relapsed severely enough to receive adjunctive drug therapy or electroshock, only 50% of those on lithium needed comparable treatment.

The Veterans Administration and the National Institute of Mental Health have jointly sponsored the largest project on lithium prophylaxis, a two-part study conducted at 18 public, private, and veterans' hospitals. In the first study (Prien, Klett, and Caffey 1973), 122 acutely depressed patients (44 bipolar, 78 unipolar) were assigned at random to lithium, placebo, or imipramine regimens. Lithium was significantly better than imipramine and placebo in preventing bouts of illness in bipolar patients. Only 28% on lithium, compared to 77% on imipramine and 77% on placebo, had episodes. Unipolar patients responded equally well to lithium and imipramine; placebo was not effective. Episodes occurred in 92% of placebo patients compared to 48% of lithium and imipramine patients.

Another two-part prophylactic study was recently completed at the Lithium Clinic of the New York State Psychiatric Institute. The first part focused on a double-blind controlled investigation of lithium prophylaxis in bipolar illness (Fieve and Mendlewicz, 1972; Stallone, Shelley, Mendlewicz, and Fieve, 1973). A total of 52 manic depressives, symptom-free and not receiving antidepressants or tranquilizers, were assigned at random to lithium or placebo for up to 28 months. Results show lithium unequivocally more effective than placebo in combating mania. Lithium prophylaxis of bipolar depression, although not as dramatically clear, was also evident.

These double-blind findings are consistent with those of earlier investigations (Baastrup et al. 1970; Coppen et al. 1971). In addition, our study indicates that family history and previous lithium treatment may be critical factors in determining lithium response. A genetic history of mania appeared more frequently in lithium responders. This is consistent with the findings by Mendlewicz, Fieve, Rainer, and Fleiss (1972) that manic-depressives with a genetic background of mania tend to have more severe attacks. The findings of this study underscore the need to relate lithium response to depression subtype and family history.

The second part of the double-blind study examined lithium prophylaxis in unipolar depression (Fieve, Dunner, Stallone, and Kumbaraci, *unpublished observations*). Beginning in December 1969, 52 unipolar outpatients were assigned at random to lithium (25 subjects) or placebo (27 subjects) treatment. Each patient had had at least two depressive episodes during the previous 5 years and no history of hypomania. However, four patients in the lithium group and five in the placebo group appeared hypomanic during clinic visits and were dropped from the trial. Seven members of the placebo group whose depression lasted 6 months or longer were dropped and reclassified as chronic depressives; none from the lithium group was so excluded. By February 1974 evaluations concerning only 28 patients could be made, 14 in each group. Lithium patients tended to remain well for longer periods of time; they had relatively fewer ratings of depression (3.4% for lithium, 15.4% for placebo), and the frequency of depressive attacks per patient-year was considerably less in the lithium group than in the placebo group.

MECHANISM OF LITHIUM ACTION

Although the effectiveness of lithium in the treatment of manic-depressive disorders is well documented, the precise mechanism of action, as well as the site of action, has yet to be elucidated. Despite the widespread attention lithium has received during the last quarter-century, there have been only a handful of attempts to lay out a unified mechanism of action for this drug. As one of the alkali metals, lithium shares with sodium and potassium such physical and chemical properties as high ionization potential and water solubility. Lithium salts are almost totally absorbed through the gastrointestinal tract, and lithium is excreted through renal metabolism.

According to Singer and Rotenberg (1973), lithium can be thought of in two interrelated ways: (1) as an imperfect substitute for the potassium and sodium cations which normally participate in ion distribution and transfer, helping to maintain and produce electrochemical gradients and osmotic steady states; and (2) as a perhaps critical factor in the cellular microenvironment that determines structure, energy supply, or the timing of cellular processes. Because of these properties, lithium can exert an important influence on many different organ systems, particularly those involved with ion transport and polypeptide hormone action.

It is known that lithium suppresses the morning peak plasma cortisol levels in normal subjects (Halmi, Noyes, and Millard, 1972) and increases the level toward normal in manic patients (Schou, 1957; Davis and Fann, 1971). It is unclear, however, whether these lithium-induced changes in cortisol level actually control the manic state or reflect another mechanism of action, e.g., abnormal monoamine metabolism. Manic episodes are sometimes accompanied by a marked rise in urinary catecholamine levels. It is unclear whether alterations in catecholamine or corticosteroid metabolism are the cause or effect of the increased psychomotor activity typical of mania. Studies have sought to link lithium to the changes it induces in central nervous system (CNS) monoamine metabolism, e.g., accelerating presynaptic destruction of norepinephrine, inhibiting neuronal release of norepinephrine and serotonin, and increasing neuronal uptake of norepinephrine. Although it is well established that lithium acts on biogenic amine metabolism, it is not clear if these actions are directly linked to the treatment of mania.

Singer and Rotenberg (1973) suggest two mechanisms of action by which lithium might exert an effect on the CNS. The first relies on the ability of lithium to substitute for sodium in cation transport processes. Like sodium, lithium enters neurons along concentration gradients; but unlike the sodium ion, lithium is not as easily removed. Neurophysiological processes depending on ion transport may thus be altered. Experiments with giant squid axons have shown that substitution of lithium for sodium in perfused axons supports nerve excitation. Nerve conduction is inhibited in unperfused axons, however. Reversible changes have also been noted in the encephalograms of patients on lithium.

A second mechanism of action is suggested by recent findings that lithium suppresses hormone-activated adenyl cyclase within the CNS in a way similar to that seen in thyroid and kidney. Neurotransmitters exert control of neurophysiological events at least partly by activating adenyl cyclase to produce cyclic adenosine-3'5'-monophosphate (cyclic AMP). Urinary cyclic AMP levels may be high in manic patients. The restoration of normal behavior following treatment with lithium is sometimes accompanied by a drop in cyclic AMP levels.

There is also a possibility that lithium interferes with neuronal carbohydrate metabolism. For example, lithium suppresses CNS uptake of myoinositol, glutamate, and γ-aminobutyric acid. The questions remain whether these effects are direct or indirect and if they are relevant to the therapeutic action of lithium.

This is a fertile field for exploration. The mechanism of action of lithium remains a mystery. What is clear, however, is that lithium is the most effective agent yet discovered for treating mania and for preventing manic depression and some forms of unipolar depression. If we are successful in determining just how this ion exerts its effect, we may have the key to understanding the manic state itself.

BLOOD LEVELS OF LITHIUM

Blood levels of lithium can be monitored with relative ease. The instrumentation necessary to measure blood lithium—a flame photometer—is common apparatus in clinical chemistry laboratories. Because of the potentially toxic effects of excessive lithium, it is wise to monitor blood levels of the drug when initiating treatment or attempting to establish a maintenance dosage. For the average patient therapeutic blood levels are 1.0 to 1.5 mEq/liter, and maintenance (or prophylactic) blood levels 0.8 to 1.3 mEq/liter. Regardless of whether lithium is being used therapeutically or prophylactically, it should not be allowed to exceed 2 mEq/liter except under very special circumstances. Once proper dosing has been established, and assuming that no troublesome adverse effects have emerged, the blood lithium can be assayed less frequently. Depending on the patient's history of compliance and periodicity of mood swings, the interval between determinations could range from 1 week to once every 1 to 2 months.

There are additional circumstances under which it is wise to monitor blood lithium levels. Whenever a patient is suffering from a disease or is being treated with a drug that might impair lithium excretion, constant monitoring is essential. For example, patients with altered renal function or renovascular disease require special attention. In addition, caution must be exercised when administering a diuretic agent or a natriuretic agent together with lithium, as these drugs slow the elimination of lithium. Therefore if there is not an appropriate change in the dosing regimen, toxic levels of lithium might accumulate. Needless to say, the possibility of toxicity is a strong argument for closely mointoring plasma levels of the ion.

ADVERSE SIDE EFFECTS

Adverse reactions to lithium can be grouped into two broad categories: (1) those which may occur at therapeutic blood levels of lithium and which although bothersome are not toxic; and (2) those that are toxic and which should be viewed as manifestations of poisoning.

Within the first category the reactions that patients most frequently report are gastrointestinal in nature, including nausea, abdominal distress, and diarrhea. Related complaints are polydipsia and polyuria. There may also be a spectrum of behavioral reactions, e.g., fatigue and general lassitude. Ordinarily none of these lithium-induced effects needs to be viewed as serious. An obvious exception would be that in which the adverse effect diminishes or abolishes compliance in drug taking by the patient. Otherwise the manic state should be judged as a greater peril than adverse reactions to the drug. Fortunately for the patient, the discomforts associated with lithium usage tend to wane with time.

Toxic reactions to lithium can involve essentially every organ in the body, but special attention should be focused on the nervous and cardiovascular systems. Moderately severe intoxication might produce slurred speech, dizziness, or mental confusion. Severe intoxication might manifest as epileptiform discharges, vertigo, coma, electroencephalographic and electrocardiographic changes, or circulatory collapse. If the toxic dose of lithium was ingested shortly prior to medical intervention, gastric lavage is indicated. If the interval has been too long to warrant lavage, then supportive measures should be used. Because of the possibility of cardiac arrest or circulatory failure, cardiovascular function must be monitored.

Besides the reactions listed above, there is a body of data which implicates lithium in endocrine dysfunction. Possible hypothyroidism and diminished glucose tolerance have both drawn attention. These and other endocrine effects were reviewed by Shopsin and Gershon (1973). As these authors point out, most of the untoward endocrine effects do not occur often enough or with sufficient intensity to impair the physiology of the healthy patient. By contrast, patients with compromised endocrine function may require careful drug supervision.

A final adverse reaction of note is tremor. The mechanism underlying this drug-induced effect is not established. However, β-adrenergic blockers are commonly used in the treatment of endogenous tremor. Therefore such drugs (e.g., propranolol) have been used, apparently to good advantage, in managing lithium-induced tremor (Kirk, Baastrup, and Schou, 1972).

HISTORY OF RUBIDIUM

In recent years rubidium, another member of the group 1A alkali metals, has attracted the interest of researchers in depression. Rubidium was discovered in 1861 by Bunsen and Kirchoff. Like lithium, it is widely distributed in mineral deposits and is extracted mainly from lepidolite and carnallite rocks. Found in virtually all biological systems, it most closely resembles potassium in physiological action; both elements exhibit a great degree of metabolic interchangeability.

Early animal and *in vitro* experiments laid the groundwork for the introduction of rubidium into clinical medicine during the 1880s. In 1864 Grandeau and Bernard compared the effects of intravenous infusion of sodium, potassium, and rubidium chlorides. Reports of animal studies in the laboratories of Ringer (1882) and Richet (1886) suggested that rubidium might play an important role in human therapy.

Rubidium was first used clinically by Botkin in St. Petersburg in 1877 to 1888 to treat acute cardiovascular disease. Botkin's doctoral dissertation on rubidium, supervised by the renowned physiologist Pavlov and presented to the Imperial Biomedical Academy in 1888, described the effect of rubidium chloride administered orally to 10 seriously ill cardiac patients. Patients exhibited decreased pulse rates and increased blood pressures. Of particular interest to modern-day investigators was the observation of notable improvement in several patients' subjective sense of well-being.

Rubidium received wider acceptance, however, as a replacement for potassium in the treatment of epilepsy and syphilis. In 1889 Laufenauer and Rottenbiller separately reported no untoward side effects with rubidium bromide in epileptics. In 1898 Colombini and Pasquini reported rubidium iodide to be as effective as potassium iodide in treating syphilis.

European literature of the late 1800s is surprisingly comprehensive regarding rubidium; at least 60 well-documented trials of human rubidium therapy were recorded. Eventually, however, rubidium was phased out of use (as was potassium) when more specific and effective treatments were developed. It should be emphasized, though, that no serious adverse reactions were ever reported. The literature records no deaths and no surprising or irreversible side effects. Rubidium research after 1918 concentrated exclusively on animal experiments. It was not until 1969 that the use of rubidium in human therapy was again postulated. By then, the focus had changed from questions of toxicity and comparisons with potassium to possible behavioral effects.

RECENT RESEARCH ON RUBIDIUM

In 1969 Meltzer, Taylor, Platman, and Fieve reported that rubidium and lithium have contrasting behavioral, electroencephalographic, and biochemical properties. In trials with monkeys it was noted that rubidium increased the prevalent frequency of the electroencephalogram and altered behavior in the direction of increased activity. Platman and Fieve (1969) and Mayfield and Brown (1966) had earlier shown that lithium, in contrast, slowed the electroencephalogram in manic and nonmanic patients. Meltzer and his associates conjectured that rubidium might have some application to psychiatric therapy, particularly the affective disorders. Since lithium is a proved antimanic agent, might not rubidium, with its "opposite" effects, be an equally potent antidepressant?

This hypothesis was further strengthened by the biogenic amine studies of Stolk, Conner, and Barchas (1971), which indicated that rubidium increased norepinephrine turnover in rats whose biosynthesis of norepinephrine was inhibited. These data suggested that rubidium could activate release of neuronally stored norepinephrine to central adrenergic receptors. Lithium studies demonstrated opposite results; lithium increased uptake of norepinephrine into synaptosomes (Colburn, Goodwin, and Bunney, 1967), reflecting a decrease in active norepinephrine concentration at postsynaptic receptors.

Stolk, Nowack, and Barchas (1970) also knew that rats receiving daily rubidium chloride demonstrate increased levels of shock-elicited aggressive behavior compared to controls. Lithium, on the other hand, decreased the incidence of such behavior (Sheard, 1970). In an independent study Eichelman, Thea, and Perez-Cruet (1972) confirmed the findings of Stolk and his associates.

Human studies of rubidium as an antidepressant have thus far been few. Researchers have been particularly hampered by difficulties in designing safe experimental trials. Considerable time over the last 5 years has been devoted to animal toxicology studies. Earlier investigations simply did not provide enough information to meet the legal and ethical requirements for drug investigation laid out by the Food and Drug Administration. Of particular importance in preparing a clinical trial are the studies of Relman, Lambie, and Burrows (1957), which indicate that rubidium replaces potassium intracellularly, milliequivalent for milliequivalent. When 40 to 50% of total body potassium was replaced by rubidium, the animals became aggressive and hyperactive, had convulsions, and eventually died. Since rubidium is known to be lethal to animals when it enters the bloodstream rapidly, doses larger than trace amounts must be given orally. A further complication results from the long biological half-life of rubidium, i.e., 50 to 60 days.

To date, chronic loading studies in human subjects have been directed primarily to administering a safe dose and only secondarily to determining the therapeutic dose level. Results of the few human trials have been promising but inconclusive. At the Metabolic Unit of the New York State Psychiatric Institute, a total of 14 patients, bipolar and unipolar, have received rubidium chloride (Fieve, Meltzer, and Taylor, 1971; Fieve, Meltzer, Dunner, Levitt, Mendlewicz, and Thomas, 1973). The highest level of retained rubidium in any subject was 480 mEq; the highest steady state concentration level was 0.40 mEq/liter. Half the patients showed some overall improvement, and half showed no change with dosages of over 250 mEq rubidium retained. There were no side effects, either psychological or physiological, although several years have passed since the first trials.

The results of these preliminary studies indicate that the loading dose has been much too small to produce significant and measurable antidepressive effects or accompanying side effects. Further trials with higher loading doses of rubidium (the Food and Drug Administration has approved raising the retained dosage to 750 mEq) are warranted.

TREATMENT SUMMARY

Generic name	Trade name	Daily dosage range (mg)[a]
Lithium carbonate	Eskalith, Lithane, Lithonate	1,500–2,400[b]
Lithium carbonate	Eskalith, Lithane, Lithonate	900–1,500[c]

[a] Ranges are approximate. A better estimate of proper dosages can be obtained by monitoring the blood lithium of levels.

[b] Dosage range for therapeutic use of lithium.

[c] Dosage range for maintenance or prophylactic use of lithium.

REFERENCES

Andreani, G., Caselli, G., and Martelli, G. (1958): Rilieve clinici ed electtroencefalografici durante il trattamento con sali di litio in malati psichiatrici. *G. Psichiat. Neuropat.*, 86:273–328.

Angst, J., Dittrich, A., and Grof, P. (1969): The course of endogenous affective psychoses and its modification by prophylactic administration of imipramine and lithium. *Int. Pharmacopsychiatry,* 2:1–11.

Angst, J., Weis, P., Grof, P., Baastrup, P. C., and Schou, M. (1970): Lithium prophylaxis in recurrent affective disorders. *Br. J. Psychiatry,* 116:604–614.

Baastrup, P. C. (1964): The use of lithium in manic depressive psychosis. *Compr. Psychiatry,* 5:396–408.

Baastrup, P. C., Poulsen, J. C., Schou, M., Thomsen, K., and Amdisen, A. (1970): Prophylactic lithium: Double-blind discontinuation in manic-depressive and recurrent-depressive disorders. *Lancet,* 2:326–329.

Baastrup, P. C., and Schou, M. (1967): Lithium as a prophylactic agent: Its effect against recurrent depressions and manic-depressive psychosis. *Arch. Gen. Psychiatry,* 16:162–172.

Blackwell, B. (1970): Lithium. *Lancet,* 2:875.

Blackwell, B., and Shepherd, M. (1968): Prophylactic lithium: Another therapeutic myth? *Lancet,* 1:968–971.

Botkin, S. S. (1888): The influence of the salts of rubidium and cesium upon the heart and circulation in connection with the laws of physiological action of alkali metals. Doctoral dissertation. St. Petersburg, St. Petersburg Military Academy.

Bunney, W. E., Jr., Goodwin, F. K., Davis, J. M., and Fawcett, J. A. (1968): A behavioral-biochemical study of lithium treatment. *Am. J. Psychiatry,* 125:499–512.

Cade, J. F. J. (1949): Lithium salts in the treatment of psychotic excitement. *Med. J. Aust.,* 36:349–352.

Cade, J. F. J. (1970): Story of lithium. In: *Discoveries in Biological Psychiatry,* edited by F. J. Ayd and B. Blackwell, pp. 218–229. Lippincott, Philadelphia.

Colburn, R., Goodwin, F., and Bunney, W. E., Jr. (1967): Effect of lithium on the uptake of noradrenaline by synaptosomes. *Nature (Lond.),* 215:1395–1397.

Colombini, P., and Pasquini, P. (1898): The action of rubidium iodide on syphilitic blood. *Reforma Med.,* 3:387–389, 399–405, 411–415.

Coppen, A., Noguera, R., Bailey, J., Burns, B. H., Swani, M. S., Hare, E. H., Gardner, R., and Maggs, R. (1971): Prophylactic lithium in affective disorders: Controlled trial. *Lancet,* 2:275–279.

Culbreth, D. M. R. (1917): *A Manual of Meteria Medica and Pharmacology,* Ed. 6. Lea & Febiger, Philadelphia.

Davis, J. M., and Fann, W. E. (1971): Lithium. *Annu. Rev. Pharmacol.,* 11:285–302.

Dyson, W. L., and Mendels, J. (1968): Lithium and depression. *Curr. Ther. Res.,* 10: 601–608.

Eichelman, B., Thea, N. B., and Perez-Cruet, J. (1972): Rubidium and cesium: Effects on aggression, adrenal enzymes and amine turnover. *Fed. Proc.,* 31:289.

Fieve, R. R. (1970): Lithium in psychiatry. *Int. J. Psychiatry,* 9:375–412.

Fieve, R. R., Meltzer, H., Dunner, D. L., Levitt, M., Mendlewicz, J., and Thomas, A. (1973): Rubidium: Biochemical, behavioral and metabolic studies in humans. *Am. J. Psychiatry,* 130:1, 55–61.

Fieve, R. R., Meltzer, H., and Taylor, R. M. (1971): Rubidium chloride ingestion by volunteer subjects: Initial experience. *Psychopharmacologia,* 20:307–314.

Fieve, R. R. and Mendlewicz, J. (1972): Lithium prophylaxis in bipolar manic depressive illness. *Psychopharmacologia,* 26 (Supp): 93.

Fieve, R. R., Platman, S. R., and Plutchik, R. R. (1968*a*): The use of lithium in affective disorder. I. Acute endogenous depression. *Am. J. Psychiatry,* 125:487–491.

Fieve, R. R., Platman, S. R., and Plutchik, R. R. (1968*b*): The use of lithium in affective disorder. II. Prophylaxis of depression in chronic recurrent affective disorder. *Am. J. Psychiatry,* 125:492–498.

Goodwin, F. K., Murphy, D. L., and Bunney, W. E., Jr. (1969): Lithium in depression and mania. *Arch. Gen. Psychiatry,* 21:486–496.

Grandeau, L. (1864): Experiments on the physiological action of the salts of potassium, sodium and rubidium injected into veins. *J. Anat. Physiol.,* 1:378–385.

Halmi, K. A., Noyes, R., Jr., and Millard, S. A. (1972): Effect of lithium on plasma cortisol and adrenal response to adrenocorticotropin in man. *Clin. Pharmacol. Ther.,* 13:699–703.

Hartigan, G. P. (1963): The use of lithium salts in affective disorders. *Br. J. Psychiatry,* 109:810–814.

Johnson, G., Gershon, S., and Hekimian, L. J. (1968): Controlled evaluation of lithium and chlorpromazine in the treatment of manic states: An interim report. *Compr. Psychiatry,* 9:563–573.

Kirk, L., Baastrup, P. C., and Schou, M. (1972): Propranolol and lithium-induced tremor. *Lancet,* 1:839.

Klein, D. F., and Davis, J. M. (1969): *Diagnosis and Drug Treatment of Psychiatric Disorders.* Williams & Wilkins, Baltimore.

Laufenauer, K. (1889): On the therapeutic action of rubidium ammonium bromide. In: *Comptes Rendus: Congres Internationale de Medicine Mentale,* pp. 183–192.

Laurell, B., and Ottoson, J-O. (1968): Prophylactic lithium? *Lancet,* 2:1245.

Maggs, R. (1963): Treatment of manic illness with lithium carbonate. *Br. J. Psychiatry,* 109:56–65.

Mayfield, D., and Brown, R. G. (1966): The clinical, laboratory and encephalographic effects of lithium. *J. Psychiatr. Res.,* 4:207–219.

Melia, P. I. (1970): Prophylactic lithium: A double-blind trial in recurrent affective disorders. *Br. J. Psychiatry,* 116:621–624.

Melia, P. I. (1971): Lithium prophylaxis in recurrent affective disorders. *Br. J. Psychiatry,* 118:135.

Meltzer, H. L., Taylor, R. M., Platman, S. R., and Fieve, R. R. (1969): Rubidium: A potential modifier of affect and behavior. *Nature (Lond.),* 223:321–322.

Mendels, J., Secunda, S. K., and Dyson, W. L. (1972): A controlled study of the anti-depressant effects of lithium carbonate. *Arch. Gen. Psychiatry,* 26:154–157.

Mendlewicz, J., Fieve, R. R., Rainer, J. D., and Fleiss, J. L. (1972): Manic depressive illness: A comparative study of patients with and without a family history. *Br. J. Psychiatry,* 120:523–530.

Platman, S. R. (1970): A comparison of lithium carbonate and chlorpromazine in mania. *Am. J. Psychiatry,* 127:351–353.

Platman, S. R., and Fieve, R. R. (1969): The effect of lithium carbonate on the electro-encephalogram of patients with affective disorders. *Br. J. Psychiatry,* 115:1185–1188.

Prien, R. F., Caffey, E. M., and Klett, C. J. (1972): Comparison of lithium carbonate and chlorpromazine in the treatment of mania. *Arch. Gen. Psychiatry,* 26:146–153.

Prien, R. F., Caffey, E. M., Jr., and Klett, C. J. (1973): Prophylactic efficacy of lithium carbonate in manic-depressive illness. *Arch. Gen. Psychiatry,* 28:337–341.

Prien, R. F., Klett, C. J., and Caffey, E. M., Jr. (1973): Lithium carbonate and imipramine in prevention of affective episodes. *Arch. Gen. Psychiatry,* 29:420–425.

Relman, A. S., Lambie, A. T., and Burrows, B. A. (1957): Cation accumulation by muscle tissue: The displacement of K by Rb and Cs in the living animal. *J. Clin. Invest.,* 36:1249–1256.

Richet, C. (1886): The physiological action of rubidium salts. *Arch. Physiol. Pathol.,* 3:101–151.

Ringer, S. (1882): An investigation concerning the action of rubidium and cesium salts compared with the action of potassium salts on the ventricle of the frog's heart. *J. Physiol. (Lond.),* 4:370–378.

Rottenbiller, J. (1889): The curative effects of rubidium ammonium bromide. *Gyogyaszat,* 43:505.

Schou, M. (1957): Biology and pharmacology of the lithium ion. *Pharmacol. Rev.,* 9:17–58.

Schou, M., Juel-Nielsen, N., Stromgren, E., and Voldby, H. (1954): The treatment of manic psychoses by the administration of lithium salts, *J. Neurol. Neurosurg. Psychiatry,* 17:250–260.

Sheard, M. H. (1970): Effect of lithium on foot shock aggression in rats. *Nature (Lond.),* 228:284–285.

Shopsin, B., and Gershon, S. (1973): Pharmacology-toxicology of the lithium ion. In: *Lithium: Its Role in Psychiatric Research and Treatment,* edited by S. Gershon and B. Shopsin. Plenum Press, New York.

Shull, W. K., and Sapira, J. D. (1970): Critique of studies of lithium salts in the treatment of mania. *Am. J. Psychiatry,* 127:218–222.

Singer, I., and Rotenberg, D. (1973): Mechanisms of lithium action. *N. Engl. J. Med.,* 289:254–260.

Spring, G. K. (1971): Some current thoughts on lithium carbonate in manic depressive illness, based on a double-blind comparison with chlorpromazine. *Psychosomatics,* 12:336–340.

Squire, P. (1908): *Squire's Companion to the Latest Edition of the British Pharmacopoeia,* Ed. 18. Churchill, London.

Stallone, F., Shelley, E., Mendlewicz, J., and Fieve, R. R. (1973): Part III. Lithium prophylaxis in manic depressive illness (double-blind study). *Am. J. Psychiatry,* 130:1006–1010.

Stokes, P. E., Stoll, P. M., Shamoian, C. A., and Patton, M. J. (1971): Efficacy of lithium as acute treatment of manic depressive illness. *Lancet,* 2:1319–1325.

Stolk, J. M., Conner, R. L., and Barchas, J. D. (1971): Rubidium-induced increase in shock-elicited aggression in rats. *Psychopharmacologia,* 22:250–260.

Stolk, J. M., Nowack, W. J., and Barchas, J. D. (1970): Brain norepinephrine: Enhanced turnover after rubidium treatment. *Science,* 168:501–503.

Warick, L. H. (1970): Lithium carbonate in the treatment and prophylaxis of recurrent affective disorders, long-term follow-up. *Bull. Los Angeles Neurol. Soc.,* 35:169–180.

Wharton, R. N., and Fieve, R. R. (1966): The use of lithium in the affective psychoses. *Am. J. Psychiatry,* 123:706–712.

Vojtechovsky, M. (1957): Zkŭsenosti s léčbou solemi litlia. In: *Problemy Psychiatrie v Praxia ve Vyskumu,* pp. 216–218. Czechoslovak Medical Press, Prague.

Chapter 14

The Use of Psychotherapeutic Drugs in Pediatrics

M. Campbell and A. M. Small

Experience has shown that drug therapy can be a valuable addition or an essential modality of the total treatment of moderately to severely disturbed children. These categories include psychotic, disturbed-retarded, or brain-damaged children, as well as hyperactive children with minimal brain dysfunction (MBD).

In our present state of knowledge, there is no specific drug or class of drugs for any of the psychiatric disorders of childhood, although the stimulants are clearly effective in many MBD children. In addition, the problem of classification is harassing child psychiatry (Group for the Advancement of Psychiatry, 1966; Eisenberg, 1967; Rutter, Lebovici, Eisenberg, Sneznevskij, Sadoun, Brooke, and Lin, 1969). The young, particularly the preschool, child's behavioral repertoire is very small, undifferentiated, and nonspecific. The child may respond with the same symptom(s) and behavior to a variety of causes: to his own slow maturation and development due to intrinsic factors; to the frustration of being a late talker, an aphasic, or a poor reader; to having a depressed and unstimulating or a rejecting mother with nevertheless high expectations; or to gross neglect, boredom, central nervous system (CNS) pathology, etc. To any of these and many more conditions, a frequent reaction is excessive irritability, hyperactivity, temper tantrums, withdrawal, aggressiveness, or even self-mutilation. Thus various environmentally evoked responses or etiologically different brain dysfunctions can be manifested in similar overt behaviors of various severity. On the other hand, the same underlying pathology may be manifested in different overt behaviors at different chronological or mental ages. Thus the choice of drug depends on factors other than just the diagnosis; age, intellectual functioning, and severity and duration of illness are variables which also must be taken into account (Fish, 1968a).

Except for the specificity of lithium in the treatment of mania, currently available drugs are thought to be most effective in reducing "target symptoms" (Freyhan, 1959). However, perhaps a more rational approach to selecting drugs would be to meet the specific needs of the patient and modify "target functions" of the disturbed behavior, as suggested by Irwin (1968, 1974a). It is known that drugs affect and interact with enzymes, neurotransmitters, and other systems; these biochemical alterations at the cellular level affect organ functions resulting in both physiological and behavioral changes. There is some evidence that this is taking place in a subgroup of hyperkinetic children with MBD (Conners, 1972a; Satterfield, Cantwell, Saul, Lesser, and Podosin, 1973; Satterfield, Cantwell, and Satterfield, 1974), and pharmacotherapy at an early developmental stage has been suggested (Mandell, 1975). Drugs themselves do not create learning or normal cognitive or adaptive behavior, nor do they necessarily alter parental attitude when administered to the child. However, a therapeutically effective drug can make a child more amenable to environmental variables or manipulations, such as remedial work, special education, individual psychotherapy, or parental counseling. The same variables in conjunction with the psychoactive agent hopefully produce a more lasting effect on the child.

The hyperactive, distractible child may be able to acquire some reading and writing skills when calmed by a drug, since he is then able to focus his attention on a task. The excessively aggressive, assaultive, or self-mutilating child, when this symptom is abolished or reduced, hopefully will be able to develop more positive and adaptive social interactions, which in turn helps to improve learning. Such children fail to respond, or do so only minimally, to an educational, remedial milieu and/or psychotherapy without drug treatment.

On the other hand, certain conditions (e.g., delinquency and reactive aggressiveness) respond less favorably or not at all to pharmacotherapy. Drug administration to a child whose symptoms stem from correctable social, familial, biological, or intrapersonal disturbances, without attempting to alter the factors causing the symptoms, is poor medicine (Eisenberg, 1964, 1968).

DRUG ADMINISTRATION AND SPECIAL CONSIDERATIONS IN CHILDREN

Since a child is dependent on an adult for the administration of drugs, the parent should be informed regarding the expected therapeutic effects as well as the possible side effects of the medication. Because major tranquilizers (antipsychotic drugs) and tricyclic antidepressants can be potentially harmful, these drugs should be prescribed on an outpatient basis only if the child is under the care of a responsible and cooperative parent. Unfortunately, parents might use the drug for controlling and sadistic purposes, or they may want to see a quick drug cure rather than work out some interpersonal problems with the child. The child's interpretation of taking the drug is also extremely important: Some children fear a loss of control, and others fear being poisoned or weakened. Conversely, some children feel stronger and better with the medication, and to some the drug may represent a substitute for object need.

Observation of the child on a daily basis is essential to ascertain at what dosage positive effects occur or adverse effects develop. This can be accomplished without much difficulty within an inpatient setting. However, on an outpatient basis the physician's observation must be supplemented by parents' and teachers' observations. Therefore, in addition to a cooperative parent, one needs a cooperative teacher. Since learning is an important part of a child's adjustment to life, it is necessary to determine if the child is excessively sedated in school or, at the other end of the spectrum, if the drug is failing to exert its therapeutic effect.

Dosages in children bear little relationship to those in adults. Weight and age are not reliable guidelines. A more accurate method is to determine the dosage for a child by body surface. However, since there are great individual differences in drug sensitivity and tolerance, one must again rely on careful clinical observation of each child. Starting with a very low, possibly ineffective dose and increasing it with stepwise increments is recommended for all psychopharmacological agents. The drug should be increased slowly at regular intervals until optimal therapeutic levels are reached or untoward effects observed. It is very important to explore the full dose range.

Untoward effects include behavioral and/or neurological changes, among others. There is some inconclusive evidence that chlorpromazine and the imipramine-like drugs may have epileptogenic properties in some susceptible individuals (Tarjan, Lowery, and Wright, 1957; Campbell, Fish, Shapiro, and Floyd, 1971b; Fromm, Amores, and Thies, 1972; Brown, Winsberg, Bialer, and Press, 1973; Petti and Campbell, 1975). The younger the child, the more likely it is that he will express his discomfort due to excess drug on an affectomotor level (irritability, changes in motor activity, loss of appetite, etc.) rather than on a verbal one. Behavioral side effects seen in children might be an increase in the symptoms one is trying to eradicate, i.e., irritability, excitement, or hyperactivity. Certain side effects (e.g., extrapyramidal signs and dystonic reactions) occur less often in children than in adults. Drug-induced jaundice, impaired liver function, and changes in cardiovascular or hematopoietic parameters are not frequently seen in children. Untoward effects caused by psychotropic agents in children are thoroughly reviewed by DiMascio, Soltys, and Shader (1970).

Common clinical errors are to maintain a child on an ineffectually small dose, on an excessively high dose, or to continue medication when it is no longer necessary. It is recommended that drug-free periods be instituted to determine whether the child has acquired new adaptive behavior or development and therefore no longer needs the medication. Psychotherapeutic agents currently in use do not appear to have addictive qualities or to promote psychological dependence in a child. Of greater importance are the long-term effects of drugs on the growth, weight, and certain endocrine systems and functions, including those of the CNS. Knowledge in this area is still limited. Recent reports indicate that chlorpromazine suppresses secretion of growth hormone in adults (Sherman, Kim, Benjamin, and Kolodny, 1971), and that administration of methylphenidate and dextroamphetamine over a period of 2 yr decreases the growth (height and weight) of hyperactive schoolchildren (Safer and Allen, 1973), whereas L-DOPA serves as a stimulus for growth hormone secretion (Boyd, Lebowitz, and Pfeiffer, 1970; Root and Russ,

1972). When pemoline treatment was given to 288 schoolchildren for up to 18 months, initial weight loss returned to the normal curve of weight gain after 3 to 6 months of continuous drug administration (Page, Bernstein, Janicki, and Michelli, 1974). The actual height gain was 94.4% of the expected gain, with the difference not being statistically significant. However, there is some evidence that growth might be retarded in mentally subnormal, brain-damaged, and psychotic children who never received psychoactive drugs (Dutton, 1964; Simon and Gillies, 1964; Bailit and Whelan, 1967). To our knowledge there are no reports on the effect of drugs on puberty. It is known, though, that many psychoactive agents affect the neurotransmitters and the hypothalamus, which is implicated in the initiation of puberty.

The effects of drugs on learning and intelligence are still controversial, although recent studies indicate that stimulants improve the general attention span and performance in hyperkinetic nonretarded children (Knights and Hinton, 1969; Sprague, Barnes, and Werry, 1970; Cohen, Douglas, and Morgenstern, 1971; Conners, 1971, 1972a; Sprague and Sleator, 1973). It appears that the sedative type of neuroleptics (e.g., chlorpromazine and thioridazine) decrease cognitive functions in psychotic and retarded children, as well as in hyperactive children of normal intelligence, although not all findings are in agreement (Bair and Herold, 1955; Freed and Pfeifer, 1956; Ison, 1957; Helper, Wilcott, and Garfield, 1963; Freeman, 1966, 1970; Werry, Weiss, Douglas, and Martin, 1966; Alexandris and Lundell, 1968). On the basis of her clinical experience, Fish emphasized that these drugs cause excessive sedation at doses which control some of the psychotic symptoms, and that the sedation results in decreased functioning (Fish, 1960, 1970; Campbell, Fish, Korein, Shapiro, Collins, and Koh, 1972b).

There are a few recent reports on the occurrence of a neurological syndrome resembling tardive dyskinesia in children treated with antipsychotic agents (Schiele, Gallant, Simpson, Gardner, and Cole, 1973). In a retrospective investigation McAndrew, Case, and Treffert (1972) found that after withdrawal of phenothiazines 10 (seven schizophrenics and three with behavior disorders, ages 8 to 15 years) of 125 hospitalized children had developed akathisia and involuntary movements of upper extremities. In addition, six of the 10 children had facial tics. The symptoms were first noted 3 to 10 days after discontinuation of drugs and ceased within 3 to 12 months. The children who developed this syndrome had been on phenothiazines for a longer time and on higher doses than those who were asymptomatic after drug withdrawal.

In a study involving 34 schizophrenics 6 to 12 years of age, 14 children showed neurological withdrawal emergent symptoms (involuntary movements of the extremities, trunk, and head, with ataxia; one child had oral dyskinesia) after 6 to 15 months of treatment with antipsychotic agents (Polizos, Engelhardt, Hoffman, and Waizer, 1973). The relationship of this probably reversible syndrome to persistent tardive dyskinesia in adults has not been established (Engelhardt, 1974).

Clearly it is of great importance to weigh the beneficial effects of the psychoactive drugs on severe behavior disorders or psychoses against the possible adverse effects on growth, development, and endocrine systems of children.

PSYCHOMOTOR STIMULANTS

The superiority of stimulants over placebo in the treatment of hyperactive MBD children has been confirmed. Included in this category are those children with behavior and/or learning disorders whose poor attention span and distractibility are usually associated with hyperactivity. Since Bradley's report in 1937 on the effects of benzedrine in children with a variety of behavioral disorders, stimulant drugs have been accepted as therapeutic for hyperactive children with MBD. The early reports by Bradley (1937; Bradley and Bowen, 1941) and later by Bender and Cottington (1942) were basically uncontrolled clinical impressions. More recently, however, many of their conclusions have been corroborated and refined by several authors using controlled studies in clinically homogeneous populations. In fact, of all the psychoactive agents used in child psychiatry, the best documented are the effects of this class of drugs.

Fish (1971) cautions that there are many causes of hyperactivity in children and that stimulant drugs are useful in only some of them. Furthermore, stimulants may be equally effective in certain nonhyperactive children. She makes a plea for careful diagnosis prior to drug administration, since giving a stimulant drug to children diagnosed as psychotic generally causes worsening of their mental disorganization (Fish, 1971; Campbell, Fish, David, Shapiro, Collins, and Koh, 1972a).

As a general rule, dextroamphetamine can be started at 2.5 mg/day and methylphenidate at 5 mg/day, given at breakfast and at noon (O'Malley and Eisenberg, 1973); maximum dosages of 80 mg dextroamphetamine and 200 mg methylphenidate have been reported before beneficial results were seen (Millichap and Fowler, 1967; Solomons, 1971). Anorexia and insomnia are the most frequent side effects. No habituation or addiction has been reported during childhood, even after several years of use (O'Malley and Eisenberg, 1973). A federally sponsored report (Freedman, 1971) concludes that several scientific studies have failed to reveal an association between the medical use of stimulants in preadolescents and later drug abuse. Nevertheless, drugs should not be used longer than necessary. Sleator, VonNeumann, and Sprague (1974) suggest that physicians treating hyperactive children with stimulants should try drug-free periods. In a 2-year follow-up of 42 hyperactive children, Sleator et al. showed that although 40% of the sample still required methylphenidate 26% functioned well without drug. They maintained that spontaneous remissions could develop and the clinician should watch for them. Sprague and Werry (1973) demonstrated that a 0.30 mg/kg dose of methylphenidate was as effective as higher dosages. In fact, side effects increased with dosage increase until at 1.00 mg/kg over 50% of the children had some untoward effects, mainly weight loss and worsening of behavior.

Response to stimulant medication can be rapidly obtained if adequate dosages are given. Drug administration can be promptly discontinued if improvement does not occur after a trial of several weeks. Treatment is usually terminated after age 11 or 12.

Precisely how stimulants work on the CNS is not known, although the literature contains several interesting theories about their mode of action (Laufer, Denhoff, and Solomons, 1957; Small, Hibi, and Feinberg, 1971; Wender, 1971). Gittelman-Klein and Klein (1973b) suggest that stimulants enhance attentional processes, which then enable the child to focus and attend. Secondary to improved attention, the child's behavior is more controlled and he is less impulsive and distractible. Schacter and Singer (1962) suggest that stimulants potentiate available cognitions. Another theory indicates that the stimulants appear to mobilize and increase the child's ability to focus on meaningful stimuli and to organize bodily movements more purposefully (Freedman, 1971). Satterfield et al. (1974) presented evidence that stimulants raise low CNS arousal and inhibitory control in a subgroup of hyperkinetic children, resulting in behavioral improvement. Additional reviews on the stimulant drugs can be found in Conners (1972b) and Gittelman-Klein (1975).

Amphetamines

Eisenberg, Conners, and their group have consistently reported significant drug-induced improvement in children with learning and/or behavioral problems. In a double-blind crossover study involving 52 children whose average age was 11.6 years, a statistically significant improvement was reported with 10 mg dextroamphetamine as compared with placebo based on teacher ratings of the children's behavior (Conners, Eisenberg, and Barcai, 1967). Furthermore, reliable increases were noted on a factor thought to reflect assertiveness and drive, while a factor measuring primarily intellectual ability was unaffected by the drug. Conners, Rothschild, Eisenberg, Schwartz, and Robinson (1969) reported on the beneficial effects of dextroamphetamine on a group of 42 children referred for learning and behavior problems in school. The average age of these children was 12 years. Dextroamphetamine (in doses up to 25 mg/day) was significantly superior to placebo as evaluated by achievement tests, Porteus mazes, some visual perception tests, auditory synthesis, and rote learning. In addition, "hyperkinetic" symptoms were statistically significantly reduced, according to the parents' symptom ratings. The drug showed no effects on intelligence test scores, oral reading, copying of Bender designs, drawing of a man, and auditory discrimination of memory. Denhoff, Davids, and Hawkins (1971) found that dextroamphetamine was significantly superior to placebo in reducing hyperactivity, as measured by a teacher rating scale in a sample of 42 children. Similar results were reported by other investigators (Finnerty, Soltys, and Cole, 1971; Steinberg, Troshinsky, and Steinberg, 1971).

More recently levoamphetamine has been found to be effective in some children with behavior disorders, particularly with reference to decreasing hyperactivity and aggressiveness (Arnold, Wender, McCloskey, and Snyder, 1972; Arnold, Kirilcuk, Corson, and Corson, 1973).

Methylphenidate

Methylphenidate has been shown to be as effective as dextroamphetamine in the same population of children. In a controlled double-blind study of methylphenidate (up to 60 mg/day) in 81 children ages 7 to 15 in residential care institutions, Conners and Eisenberg (1963) showed significant behavioral improvement on the basis of symptom ratings. Creager and Van Riper (1967) reported a statistically significant improvement in speech development in a group of 30 children 8 to 10 years of age diagnosed as having cerebral dysfunction. In a double-blind study of 76 hyperactive grade school boys ages 6 to 12 years, Rapoport, Quinn, Bradbard, Riddle, and Brooks (1974) demonstrated that methylphenidate (30 mg/day) and imipramine were superior to placebo, but the former was more effective. Hoffman, Engelhardt, Margolis, Polizos, Waizer, and Rosenfeld (1974) reported on 62 hyperkinetic children of low socioeconomic background referred from public schools. Methylphenidate in dosages up to 80 mg/day was effective in decreasing hyperactivity and in improving performance on a variety of psychological test parameters. Satterfield, Cantwell, Lesser, and Podosin (1972) found significant correlation between the degree of evidence of brain dysfunction—obtained from electroencephalographic (EEG) abnormalities, skin conduction levels, and neurological findings—and response to methylphenidate treatment in a controlled double-blind study of 31 hyperactive boys. In this study baseline low arousal was associated with a good clinical response, whereas pretreatment measures of the children who had a poor clinical response indicated a high arousal state. Knights and Hinton (1969) reported a double-blind study comparing methylphenidate (40 mg/day) to placebo on the motor skills and behavior of 40 children with learning problems. Teachers and parents rated the drug group as less distractible and more attentive. The psychological test data indicated that methylphenidate was associated with improved attention span, and that this was the basis for better motor coordination and performance skills.

Pemoline

More recently magnesium pemoline has been shown to be promising in hyperactive children with behavior disorders (Plotnikoff, 1971). One of its advantages is that it is given in a single morning dose. Conners, Taylor, Meo, Kurtz, and Fournier (1972) investigated pemoline in 81 hyperactive children who were having school difficulties. There was a decrease of symptoms in both the pemoline and dextroamphetamine groups as compared to the placebo group, although improvement with dextroamphetamine was greater. Pemoline was given in a single dose, in dosages of 25 to 125 mg/day.

In a collaborative study involving a well-defined population of 413 schoolchildren, 238 patients were assigned in random fashion to pemoline or placebo for 9 weeks (Page et al., 1974). The maximum daily (single) dose was 112.5 mg (mean daily dose 2.69 mg/kg); maximum effectiveness was at 6 weeks. Pemoline was found to be clinically and statistically significantly superior to placebo by all raters on the various measures. Impressive improvement in gross behavior was accompanied by improvement in cognitive and perceptual functions with minimal side effects. Pemoline was investigated for safety in 407 of the 413 children; blood pressure and pulse remained stable in both drug and placebo groups. When data analysis was performed on all 413 patients (some of whom failed to meet certain inclusion criteria), the level of improvement of the pemoline group was almost identical to that of the 238 children who met all protocol criteria. Among a total of 288 children the efficacy of pemoline remained stable on long administration up to 18 months (mean daily dosage range 1.91 to 2.51 mg/kg). Page and his co-investigators concluded that this drug is a "highly useful clinical alternative to the amphetamines and methylphenidate as an adjunct in the management of hyperkinetic behavior due to minimal brain dysfunction."

Deanol

During the past two decades more than a dozen controlled studies and open trials were reported on the use of deanol (a precursor of acetylcholine) in a variety of behavioral disorders of childhood and in mental retardation (Conners, 1973). It appears that deanol's efficacy and full dose range should be explored in hyperkinetic, nonretarded children; its therapeutic action and possible effect on performance with apparently mild side effects warrant such testing.

Caffeine

Casual reports concerning the possible efficacy of caffeine in hyperactive children are currently being followed up with placebo-controlled clinical trials.

ANTIDEPRESSANTS

Although the imipramine-like drugs are effective in adults, particularly in those with psychomotor retardation, such effects in "depressed" children cannot be evaluated easily since controlled studies are lacking. In addition, depressive states in children are poorly defined conditions; manic-depressive illness is perhaps nonexistent under 10 to 12 yr of age (*The Nervous Child,* 1952; Anthony and Scott, 1960; Annell, 1972; Graham, 1974).

Tricyclic Antidepressants

Anecdotal reports are available on the usage of tricyclic antidepressants in "depressed" children, some as young as 2.5 years of age (Frommer, 1967, 1968, 1972; Stack, 1972). In a heterogeneous sample of depressed children, the efficacy of amitriptyline was explored in a placebo-controlled double-blind study (Lucas, Lockett, and Grimm, 1965). Nortriptyline was tried in retarded, autistic children whose symptoms were refractory to previously applied medications, including major tranquilizers. It was found to be effective in decreasing hyperactivity, aggressiveness, and destructiveness (Kurtis, 1966).

In a double-blind study of 10 autistic schizophrenic inpatients 2 to 6 years of age (intellectual functioning was low average to severely retarded), imipramine in doses of 6 to 75 mg/day (mean 34.5) was infrequently therapeutic, and the beneficial effects were usually outweighed by untoward effects (Campbell et al., 1971*b*). In general, this drug produced a mixture of stimulating, tranquilizing, and disorganizing actions.

The effects of imipramine were also explored in hyperkinetic disorders of childhood. A diagnostically heterogeneous group of 41 private outpatients ages 5 to 21 years, was treated with imipramine in doses up to 20 to 40 mg/day (Rapoport, 1965). Difficulties varied "from temper tantrums to frank delinquency, or daydreaming, to poor grades in school." The EEGs showed some abnormalities in most cases, often suggestive of those seen in epilepsy. On drug maintenance "all symptoms diminished" with particular improvement in learning skills, and there was a "marked progress in alertness and attention span." Rapoport felt that imipramine "helped to establish a consistent rhythmic pattern of sleep and arousal in these children who, previously, because of some central nervous system dysfunction, had been poorly patterned individuals." In another clinical trial of 52 hyperkinetic children of normal intelligence (ages 3 to 14 years), 67% showed clinically marked improvement on dosages of 25 to 125 mg/day given in a single dose (Huessy and Wright, 1970).

In a double-blind procedure, imipramine, dextroamphetamine, and placebo were compared in a heterogeneous population of 32 hyperkinetic and aggressive children (most with MBD) 5 to 13 years of age (Winsberg, Bialer,

Kupietz, and Tobias, 1972). All subjects were receiving the drugs assigned in one of two counterbalanced orders. As assessed by parents, significant decreases in both aggressiveness and hyperactivity were obtained on imipramine (75 to 150 mg/day) and on dextroamphetamine, whereas a significant decrease in inattentiveness occurred only with imipramine. Sixty-nine percent of the sample responded to imipramine, whereas 44% responded to dextroamphetamine. Imipramine was therapeutic in a diagnostically homogeneous group of 19 hyperactive schoolchildren 6 to 12 years of age (Waizer, Hoffman, Polizos, and Engelhardt, 1974). The patients, diagnosed as "hyperkinetic reaction" (*DSM-II*) and having scored 1.5 or greater on the hyperactivity factor of the Teacher Rating Scale developed by Conners, were placed on increasing doses of drug (optimal dose 100 to 200 mg/day) for 8 weeks. The drug condition was preceded by a washout period of at least 1 week and was followed by a period of 4 weeks on placebo. The patients were evaluated on a variety of behavioral rating scales and psychometric measures; statistical analysis of ratings showed a significant decrease of hyperactivity and other symptoms on imipramine. However, there was a statistically significant deterioration of recall, which subsequently improved on placebo. Except for some weight loss, there were no serious untoward effects on imipramine treatment. In a well-designed double-blind study using a variety of rating scales and other measures in a well-defined population, imipramine was compared to methylphenidate and placebo (Rapoport et al., 1974). The patients were 76 middle class hyperactive schoolboys, ages 6 to 12 years, with IQs of 80 or above. Both drugs were statistically significantly superior to placebo; all measures favored methylphenidate. It was suggested that the dosage of imipramine (50 to 150 mg/day) was perhaps not adequately explored.

In another well-designed and controlled study, imipramine was demonstrated to be an effective drug in nonpsychotic children ages 6 to 14 years with school phobia, in conjunction with other therapeutic modalities (Gittelman-Klein and Klein, 1971, 1973a). Eighty-one percent of the 16 patients treated with imipramine (100 to 200 mg/day) attended school after 6 weeks, whereas only 47% of the 19 children who received placebo did so; the difference was statistically significant. Other measures too reflected the superiority of the drug. Side effects were minor.

At present the psychomotor stimulants are the drugs of choice in the treatment of hyperkinetic nonpsychotic children. The role of imipramine in this clinical picture remains to be elucidated.

Reports indicate that the tricyclic amines are promising in the treatment of enuresis. In a double-blind placebo-controlled study of 47 nonretarded children 5 to 16 years of age, imipramine (in doses of 25 to 50 mg/day) was clinically and statistically superior to placebo in decreasing enuresis (Poussaint and Ditman, 1965). Side effects were minimal, and insomnia was not reported. In another double-blind placebo-controlled study, 12 psychiatric inpatients (nine diagnosed as having character disorders), age 6 to 12 years, responded to the drug (25 mg/day) in a similar fashion (Alderton, 1965). The use of imipramine in enuretic retardates was critically reviewed by Sprague and Werry (1971).

Monoamine Oxidase Inhibitors

Phenelzine and isocarboxazid were used in the treatment of depressed children by the same investigators who had used tricyclic antidepressants (Frommer, 1967, 1968, 1972; Stack, 1972). Reportedly, monoamine oxidase (MAO) inhibitors are more effective in phobic and anxious types of childhood depressions than imipramine (Frommer, 1967, 1972). However, the same contraindications as for adults apply to children, and in addition these drugs may cause disorganization of behavior.

SEDATIVES

Chloral hydrate, a sedative and hypnotic, remains an important agent in emergency situations and in the treatment of insomnia in doses of 50 mg/kg. It appears that diphenhydramine, an antihistaminic, has not been sufficiently explored and that the cause of such failure may be traced to dosages that are usually neither individualized nor sufficiently high. Diphenhydramine is a safe and effective drug and is easy to regulate. As such, it merits exploration in behavioral and organic disorders associated with hyperactivity (Fish, 1960). Prior to placing a schizophrenic child on a major tranquilizer, it is worthwhile to try this drug as a first stage of drug therapy.

In an open trial involving 85 private patients 1 to 12 years of age (after a thorough psychiatric, neurological, and psychological examination), diphenhydramine was among a variety of psychoactive agents Fish evaluated (1960). Among the sample of 48 children with behavior disorders, diphenhydramine had a beneficial effect in 57% under 10 years of age, decreasing anxiety and hyperactivity. In patients over age 10, it acted mainly as a bedtime sedative. In the 28 schizophrenics with IQs of 70 to 135 who comprised part of the report, this drug was therapeutic in doses of 2 to 10 mg/kg/day (average 4 mg/kg/day). In the more retarded autistics, it evoked only excessive sedation or decreased hyperactivity. In general, diphenhydramine was most effective in the immature and the less severely disturbed children. Other reports too indicate that this drug may be of value in schizophrenic children with normal intellectual functioning (Effron and Freedman, 1953; Silver, 1955).

In a controlled double-blind study of school-age hospitalized children (Fish and Shapiro, 1964, 1965; Korein, Fish, Shapiro, Gerner, and Levidow, 1971), diphenhydramine (in daily doses of 200 to 800 mg/day, 3 to 26 mg/kg/day) was therapeutic in 50% of types I and II (autistic-dysjunctive and immature-labile) with borderline to defective IQs, whereas it was ineffective in all type III and IV patients (anxious-neurotic and sociopathic-paranoid). However, in the same populations, it was less effective than chlorpromazine and only minimally superior to placebo.

Diphenhydramine is a valuable agent for the relief of acute dystonic reactions caused by neuroleptics.

HYPNOTICS AND ANTICONVULSANTS

With the advent of major tranquilizers, barbiturates and diphenylhydantoin should now be used only as antiepileptics in children. The usefulness of diphenylhydantoin in the treatment of behavioral disorders has not been demonstrated in controlled double-blind studies. Placebo was shown to be statistically superior to it in alleviating disruptive and disturbed behavior, including impulsivity and hyperactivity, in delinquent boys (Lefkowitz, 1969). In this study the 50 institutionalized patients, 13 to 16 years of age and of normal intelligence, were randomly assigned to the treatment conditions. In another study of 43 aggressive and disturbed, delinquent, institutionalized boys ages 9 to 14 years, neither diphenylhydantoin nor methylphenidate yielded positive change when behavioral ratings and other measurements were subjected to statistical analysis (Conners, Kramer, Rothschild, Schwartz, and Stone, 1971). Looker and Conners (1970) found no statistically significant group change on diphenylhydantoin when this drug was investigated with placebo in a crossover design. The sample consisted of 17 nonretarded MBD children ages 5.5 to 14.5 years with severe temper tantrums. In another study adult chronic schizophrenics were randomly assigned to either diphenylhydantoin or placebo; the drug reduced hostility, but there was worsening of most other symptoms (Simopoulos, Pinto, Uhlenhuth, McGee, and DeRosa, 1974).

ANTIANXIETY DRUGS (MINOR TRANQUILIZERS)

Although the minor tranquilizers are frequently prescribed to children with anxiety and neurotic symptoms, their value has not yet been critically assessed in these populations. Chlordiazepoxide was reported to be of some value in certain depressed, inhibited children (Fish, 1968b). In a double-blind crossover trial involving a heterogeneous group of 16 nonpsychotic children ages 7 to 14 years, chlordiazepoxide (20 mg/day) was less effective than dextroamphetamine (10 mg/day) in reducing hyperkinesis, and both were superior to placebo (Zrull, Westman, Arthur, and Bell, 1963).

In a trial of 130 outpatients ages 2 to 17 years with a variety of behavioral disorders, chlordiazepoxide (30 to 130 mg/day in divided doses) was most effective in children with school phobia, while those with brain damage or epilepsy and abnormal EEGs responded poorly (Kraft, Ardali, Duffy, Hart, and Pearce, 1965). It would be important to know the ages of patients, since in school phobia both the response to treatment and the prognosis in younger children differ from those in adolescents. Thirteen children aged 6 to 14 years developed a "paradoxical reaction" which included loss of control (on doses of 30 to 70 mg/day); some of these children had abnormal EEG patterns. This drug, with its stimulating actions, may worsen the pre-existing psychosis or even create a florid psychosis in children with border-line schizophrenic features (Fish, 1968b; Campbell and Fish, 1975). There is evidence that it is not therapeutic, or that it is even contraindicated, in certain diagnostic categories or behavioral profiles (LaVeck and Buckley, 1961; Pilkington, 1961; Skynner, 1961; LeVann, 1962). Data from studies with adults, including normals, suggest that chlordiazepoxide and some other antianxiety agents should not be given to individuals with poor impulse control or aggressiveness (Gardos, DiMascio, Salzman, and Shader, 1968; DiMascio, Shader, and Harmatz, 1969; Irwin, 1974b), although others have not confirmed these findings (Rickels and Downing, 1974).

ANTIPSYCHOTIC DRUGS (MAJOR TRANQUILIZERS, NEUROLEPTICS)

While the role of sedatives and anticonvulsants was only to facilitate the management of disturbed and agitated children, the advent of antipsychotic drugs created hope for a more efficacious pharmacotherapy. It was expected that by virtue of their antipsychotic effect the psychotic process would be arrested or at least alleviated, and that symptoms of anxiety, hyperactivity, or aggressiveness would be diminished.

Phenothiazines

Clinical experience has shown that chlorpromazine is of great value as an adjunct in the total treatment of psychotic, disturbed-retarded, and brain-damaged children, and particularly in schizophrenic adolescents with acute symptomatology. However, well-designed and controlled studies in homogeneous populations of children are sparse (Freeman, 1970; Lipman, 1970; Sprague and Werry, 1971; Conners, 1972b; Werry, 1972); therefore no definite conclusions can be made, particularly about the long-term outcome. Neuroleptics generally seem to affect the illness in adult schizophrenics in the long run (WHO, 1967).

Fish (1960) found chlorpromazine (dose range 1 to 4 mg/kg/day, average 2 mg/kg/day) to be a useful drug in schizophrenic and organic children and in those with behavior disorders, although hypoactive and apathetic children tended to become sedated. In a subsequent controlled study, a heterogeneous sample of 45 hospitalized children 6 to 12 years of age, matched for age and symptom severity, were treated with either chlorpromazine, diphen-hydramine, or placebo (Fish and Shapiro, 1964, 1965; Korein et al., 1971).

The children had a detailed diagnostic work-up that included EEG; their psychopathologies ranged from mild neuroses and behavior disorders to schizophrenia. While none of the more severely disturbed and impaired children improved on placebo, 80% demonstrated positive changes on chlorpromazine. Forty-three percent of the children with less severe psychopathology showed improvement on placebo, and 60% responded to chlorpromazine. The difference in efficacy was statistically significant. Positive behavioral or toxic changes, or both, often were associated with EEG changes (Korein et al., 1971). Maintenance levels of chlorpromazine ranged from 100 to 200 mg/day (2 to 9 mg/kg/day).

In a group of hyperactive children with IQs over 85, chlorpromazine was statistically significantly superior to placebo in reducing hyperactivity, while distractibility, excitability, and aggressiveness were less affected by the drug (Werry et al., 1966). In this controlled double-blind study, 24 children (mean age 8.58 years) were treated with chlorpromazine (mean daily dosage 106 mg) and 15 (mean age 8.13 years) were given placebo (mean daily dosage 140 mg). A history for organicity or an abnormal EEG did not seem to influence the behavioral response. Evaluation was based on rating scales and psychometric measures which were subjected to statistical analysis.

Thioridazine, along with chlorpromazine, is the most widely used drug in retarded-hyperactive and/or brain-damaged children (Lipman, 1970). Alexandris and Lundell (1968) investigated thioridazine in hyperkinetic children 7 to 12 years of age (IQ 55 to 85). In this double-blind study, the 21 inpatients were randomly assigned to either thioridazine, amphetamine, or placebo. Thioridazine (30 to 150 mg/day) was shown superior to both amphetamine (7.5 to 75 mg/day) and placebo based on symptom ratings and psychometric measures. Decreased aggressiveness and increased concentration span, comprehension, sociability, and work interest and capacity were among the improvements noted.

Fish and her associates found that the prepuberty schizophrenic child is often excessively sedated by chlorpromazine at doses which decrease certain symptoms (often only minimally), and this interferes with the child's learning and functioning (Fish, 1960, 1970; Campbell et al., 1972b). Trifluoperazine, a less sedative and more potent phenothiazine, proved to be somewhat better than chlorpromazine, especially in hypoactive, under-responsive, retarded schizophrenic children. In a clinical trial (Fish, 1960) 13 outpatients received this drug in doses of 0.005 to 0.4 mg/kg/day (average 0.02 mg/kg/day). Subsequently this drug was explored in a controlled, double-blind study involving 22 hospitalized retarded, autistic schizophrenics 2 to 6 years of age (Fish, Shapiro, and Campbell, 1966). After a 3-week placebo washout, the treatment group was given increasing doses of trifluoperazine up to maximum individual tolerance (dose range 0.11 to 0.69 mg/kg/day), and the control group (matched for severity of illness, including impairment of language function) was receiving increasing doses of amphetamine. Amphetamine was substituted by placebo when side effects (i.e., irritability) were noted. The children were rated by the psychiatrist on a symptom severity scale developed by the senior author (Fish, 1968a). Trifluoperazine produced statistically significant changes only in the most severely impaired children who had no speech. The same subgroup of children required higher doses of drug than the less-impaired children, who were also responsive to the milieu therapy. Therapeutic changes on the drug included increases in language production, alertness, social responsiveness, and motor initiation. One patient, a 2-year-old apathetic, anergic girl, showed a dramatic improvement on trifluoperazine. In these authors' experience this is one of the few schizophrenic children who showed such a response to any treatment modality, including psychoactive agents.

Fluphenazine is probably useful in the behavior disorders of mentally retarded children (Waites and Keele, 1963). Its efficacy was investigated in a double-blind fashion in 30 schizophrenic outpatients (19 autistics) 6 to 12 years of age (Engelhardt, Polizos, Waizer, and Hoffman, 1973). After a 1- to 2-week placebo washout, the children were given fluphenazine or haloperidol in increasing doses until a maximum therapeutic response was noted. Ninety-three percent of the patients showed "much" or "very much" improvement on fluphenazine (mean dose 10.4 mg/day), whereas 87% of those on haloperidol (mean dose 10.4 mg/day) showed the same change. There was no statistical difference between responses to the two drugs. On a 19-item symptom rating scale, there was a statistically significant decrease in severity on both drugs. With fluphenazine there was significant improvement in self-awareness, constructive play, compulsive acts, and self-mutilation, whereas with haloperidol significant changes occurred in coordination, self-care, affect, and exploratory behavior. Side effects, which included extrapyramidal symptoms (mainly increased salivation), were infrequent and usually mild.

In another double-blind study the same drugs were assigned randomly to 60 severely impaired inpatients 5 to 12 years of age, 52 of whom were schizophrenics (Faretra, Dooher, and Dowling, 1970). The dose range for both agents was 0.75 to 3.75 mg/day; over 50% of the children showed some degree of improvement in both treatment conditions. Both fluphenazine and haloperidol decreased anxiety but failed to reduce assaultiveness. There was no difference in drug efficacy when considering overall improvement.

Butyrophenones

Trifluperidol is an antipsychotic agent with stimulating properties; it is more effective in the treatment of young autistic schizophrenic children than either chlorpromazine or trifluoperazine (Fish, Campbell, Shapiro, and Floyd, 1969a; Campbell, Fish, Shapiro, and Floyd, 1972c). However, its relatively narrow therapeutic index, with extrapyramidal symptoms appearing at doses 1.3 to two times higher than the therapeutic range (Fish et al., 1969a; Campbell et al., 1972a), limited trifluperidol to investigational use and resulted in its subsequent withdrawal in the United States.

As noted above, haloperidol (in doses up to 16 mg/day) was said to be a therapeutically effective agent in schizophrenic children, and it produced a low incidence of side effects (Faretra, Dooher, and Dowling, 1970; Engelhardt et al., 1973). Faretra and her associates found that haloperidol was successful in reducing autism and provocative behavior, but failed to reduce assaultiveness; others, however, found this drug particularly effective in decreasing or controlling hyperactivity, assaultiveness, and self-injury in retarded and nonretarded children (Burk and Menolascino, 1968; LeVann, 1969; Ucer and Kreger, 1969; Grabowski, 1973; Serrano and Forbis, 1973). The superiority of haloperidol over phenothiazines in schizophrenics or patients with certain behavioral profiles has not been demonstrated or even sufficiently explored (Claghorn, 1972). The efficacy of this drug in the treatment of Gilles de la Tourette's disease has not been documented, although anecdotal reports are available (Lucas, 1967; Shapiro, Shapiro, and Wayne, 1973).

Thioxanthenes

Thiothixene appears to be a safe, effective drug for schizophrenic children. It possesses both stimulating properties and a wide therapeutic margin. In a double-blind study, 10 hospitalized preschoolers were given thiothixene after a 4-week washout period (Campbell, Fish, Shapiro, and Floyd, 1970). The optimal doses ranged from 1 to 6 mg/day (mean 2 mg/day). Positive changes included lessening of withdrawal, excitability, stereotypy, psychotic speech, and an increase in verbal production. The change in mean pathological scores for the group was statistically significant, but the changes in the scores for single symptoms were not. It was felt that this drug with its nonsedative antipsychotic activity is superior to chlorpromazine in the severely impaired young psychotic child (Fish, Campbell, Shapiro, and Weinstein, 1969c).

In a single-blind study, after 2 weeks of placebo washout thiothixene was given in increasing doses up to 10 to 24 mg/day (mean 16.9 mg/day) to 18 schizophrenic outpatients 5 to 13 years of age (Waizer, Polizos, Hoffman, Engelhardt, and Margolis, 1972). The change of mean scores on the symptom rating scale developed for this population showed a statistically significant improvement with this drug. On single symptoms, significant improvement occurred in motor activity, stereotypies, coordination, sleep, affect, exploratory behavior, concentration, and eating habits. No child was rated unchanged or worse. Simeon, Saletu, Saletu, Itil, and DaSilva (1973) administered thiothixene to 10 psychotic boys 5 to 15 years of age. On the optimal dosage (6 to 30 mg/day; mean 14 mg/day) statistically significant improvements occurred in global ratings as well as decreases in symptoms of motor activity, speech abnormality, social relationship to adults, anger, mood lability, emotional unresponsiveness, feeding difficulties, and attention disorders. The positive behavioral effects were associated with changes in visual evoked potentials and the EEG.

In a double-blind study 16 school-age schizophrenic children were assigned randomly to a thiothixene or a trifluoperazine group. According to the global impressions of the raters, four children improved on thiothixene (13 to 20 mg/day) and three on trifluoperazine; the positive changes were in the area of autism, socialization, stereotypies, and appetite. Unfortunately the pretreatment washout (3 days) was insufficient, and valid conclusions cannot be drawn (Wolpert, Hagamen, and Merlis, 1967).

Indoles

There is only one report on the use of molindone in children (Campbell, Fish, Shapiro, and Floyd, 1971a). In a double-blind study of 10 severely disturbed (eight schizophrenic) inpatients 3 to 5 years of age, this drug (1 to 2.5 mg/day; mean 1.5 mg/day) seemed to be a potential therapeutic agent. On the global rating of change, two children were markedly improved, four slightly improved, two unchanged, and two worse.

LITHIUM

Lithium therapy in adults has a well-established role in the manic phase of manic-depressive illness and in the prevention of recurrent depressive episodes; its place has not been established in the treatment of psychiatric disturbances of childhood (Schou, 1972). In addition, mood disorders in children present a diagnostic problem, and even their existence is questioned by some investigators in the field.

Van Krevelen and Van Voorst (1959) found lithium effective in the treatment of a 14-year-old retarded boy with alternating hypomanic and depressive states. The child failed to respond to other drugs, including chlorpromazine. Subsequently lithium has been given to children with "depressive" and "manic" conditions with reportedly good results (Frommer, 1968, 1972; Annell, 1969a,b; Dyson and Barcai, 1970). However, the populations were not well defined, and the reports are anecdotal.

In clinical trials of hyperactive children, lithium was ineffective in reducing the hyperactivity (Whitehead and Clark, 1970; Greenhill, Rieder, Wender, Buchsbaum, and Zahn, 1973).

Rifkin, Quitkin, Carillo, Blumberg, and Klein (1972) conducted a study in adolescents with emotionally unstable character disorder (EUCD) characterized by chronic maladaptive behavior patterns and usually nonreactive depressive and hypomanic mood swings. The 21 hospitalized patients were randomly assigned to lithium or placebo in a double-blind crossover design. Lithium, at blood levels of 0.6 to 1.5 mEq/liter, was found therapeutically effective and statistically significantly superior to placebo. Rifkin and associates concluded on the basis of the patients' drug response that EUCD is related to affective illness. They also feel that lithium is as valuable as chlorpromazine in the treatment of this condition, particularly because it lacks the sedative effect that is objectionable to adolescents. Schou (1972) also suggested that lithium maintenance may have a "stabilizing and normalizing action" in children and adolescents with "undulating and periodic disturbances of mood and behavior."

Two controlled, double-blind crossover studies indicate that lithium administration is effective in some retarded autistic schizophrenic children, resulting in a moderate decrease of hyperactivity, aggressiveness, and stereotypies, among other symptoms (Campbell et al., 1972b; Gram and Rafaelsen, 1972). There is evidence that lithium has a specific antiaggressive effect in retarded and psychotic children when the aggressiveness is associated with explosiveness and excitability (Campbell et al., 1972b; Dostal, 1972). Assessment of the efficacy of lithium is awaiting further exploration: it might prove of value in certain behavioral profiles of severe treatment-resistant disturbances of childhood (Campbell, 1973a).

L-DOPA

Because of the biochemical and some behavioral effects of L-DOPA, this drug was administered by Ritvo and associates to four autistic children over a period of 6 months in doses up to 2,000 to 4,000 mg/day (Ritvo, Yuwiler, Geller, Kales, Rashkis, Schicor, Plotkin, Axelrod, and Howard, 1971). L-DOPA interacts with brain serotonin, and abnormalities of this neurotransmitter were found in the blood and platelets of some autistic and schizophrenic children (Boullin, Coleman, and O'Brien, 1970; Ritvo, Yuwiler, Geller, Ornitz, Saeger, and Plotkin, 1970; Coleman, 1973; Campbell, Friedman, DeVito, Greenspan, and Collins, 1974; Campbell, Friedman, Green, Collins, Small, and Breuer, 1975). The lowering of blood serotonin in three of the four children was not accompanied by clinical improvement in Ritvo's study. Administration of L-DOPA to schizophrenic adults resulted in worsening of symptoms (Angrist, Sathananthan, and Gershon, 1973), although several investigators reported that, in Parkinson's disease and depression, awakening-alerting effects and improvement in cognitive functions were noted (Campbell, 1973b). It was because of these positive stimulating effects that Fish and associates explored L-DOPA in the treatment of preschool schizophrenic children with autistic features. In a double-blind crossover study involving 12 patients, five showed global improvement, five no change, and two became worse on doses of 900 to 2,500 mg/day (Campbell, Korein, Small, Collins, Friedman, David, Genieser, Carroll, and Fish, 1975b). A comparison of the means of the symptom scores for pre- and optimum ratings on the symptoms severity scale developed by Fish (1968a) showed five subjects improving on total symptomatology, three with no change, and four with a slight worsening. The greatest improvements were in the rating of decreased negativism, and increases in play, energy, and motor initiation in hypoactive children. L-DOPA merits further exploration in a larger population of young psychotic children because of its stimulating properties.

HALLUCINOGENS

Both acute and maintenance clinical trials were carried out with d-lysergic acid diethylamide (LSD-25) and a methylated derivative of LSD, L-methyl-D-lysergic acid butalamide bimaleate in schizophrenic and autistic children. The reported results are inconclusive: In some patients, presumably in the most retarded ones, these drugs acted as effective therapeutic stimulants, leading to improvement in behavior with a decrease in withdrawal; whereas in others stimulation resulted in an increase in anxiety and disorganization (Bender, Goldschmidt, and Sankar, 1962; Freedman, Ebin, and Wilson, 1962; Bender, Faretra, and Cobrinik, 1963; Rolo, Krinsky, Abramson, and Goldfarb, 1965; Bender, Cobrinik, Faretra, and Sankar, 1966; Simmons, Leiken, Lovaas, Schaeffer, and Perloff, 1966; Fish, Campbell, Shapiro, and Floyd, 1969b).

MEGAVITAMINS

Hoffer (1970) reported that niacinamide and ascorbic acid proved superior to placebo in some schizophrenic children, but others could not confirm these findings. In a double-blind study, 57 schizophrenics 4 to 12 years of age were placed into three groups, each receiving niacinamide, niacinamide plus a tranquilizer, or placebo for a period of 6 months (Greenbaum, 1970). Statistical analysis showed no significant difference in the average scores of the three groups, and it was thought that maturation was probably the most significant cause of improvement. The Forum School arrived at similar conclusions after conducting an open trial for 12 months in a population of 19 severely disturbed children, including 16 who were psychotic (Roukema and Emery, 1970).

In a preliminary report Rimland (1973) detailed the results of a study of 190 outpatient psychotic children receiving megadoses of vitamins over 24 weeks. The subgroup of 37 children identified as having classic infantile autism showed the greatest improvement, but the author considers the results only "encouraging."

An American Psychiatric Association task force came to the conclusion that megavitamin therapy was of no value in the treatment of adult schizophrenia (Lipton, Ban, Kane, Levine, Mosher, and Wittenborn, 1973).

TRIIODOTHYRONINE

Triiodothyronine (T_3), a thyroid hormone, has been tested in a small number of very young, euthyroid schizophrenic, autistic, and nonpsychotic severely disturbed children (Sherwin, Flach, and Stokes, 1958; Campbell, Fish, David, Shapiro, Collins and Koh, 1972*a*, 1973; Campbell and Fish, 1974). In these studies T_3 had both stimulating and antipsychotic effects and was viewed as an agent potentially effective in the treatment of this population of children. Further investigations are required under more controlled conditions in a homogeneous group of patients.

CONCLUDING REMARKS

1. The superiority of psychomotor stimulants over placebo has been demonstrated in hyperactive nonretarded (MBD) children.
2. The neuroleptics comprise an important treatment modality in the total therapy of many psychotic children and brain-damaged and retarded children with behavioral problems. By decreasing certain symptoms, these drugs can make the child more amenable to other therapies and thus hopefully facilitate learning and development. Drugs should never be used as chemical straight-jackets.
3. The superiority of one neuroleptic over another has not been documented with controlled studies in homogenous populations, although clinical experience suggests that the less-sedative agents are more therapeutic for young children.
4. Polypharmacy, frequent change of drugs, or unnecessary dose escalation are bad practices.
5. Possible hazards of drug use must be weighed against the hazards of the untreated illness itself.
6. Pharmacotherapy versus other treatment modalities has not yet been critically assessed.
7. Drug treatment is not indicated in all diagnostic categories of childhood, and even when required it should never be the sole treatment modality.
8. Until the diagnostic entities in childhood are more precisely defined by both behavioral and biological criteria, children's psychopharmacology will remain on an empirical basis.

ACKNOWLEDGMENTS

This work was supported in part by U.S. Public Health Service Grant MH-04665 from the National Institute of Mental Health.

The authors wish to thank Mrs. Nancy Polevoy and Miss Barbara Drosins for their technical assistance.

REFERENCES

Alexandris, H., and Lundell, F. (1968): Effect of thioridazine, amphetamine and placebo on the hyperkinetic syndrome and cognitive area in mentally deficient children. *Can. Med. Assoc. J.,* 98:92–96.

Alderton, M. B. (1965): Imipramine in the treatment of nocturnal enuresis of childhood. *Can. Psychiatr. Assoc. J.,* 10:141–151.

Angrist, B., Sathananthan, G., and Gershon, S. (1973): Behavioral effects of L-Dopa in schizophrenic patients. *Psychopharmacologia,* 31:1–12.

Annell, A. L. (1969a): Manic-depressive illness in children and effect of treatment with lithium carbonate. *Acta Paedopsychiatr. (Basel),* 36:292–361.

Annell, A. L. (1969b): Lithium in the treatment of children and adolescents. *Acta Psychiatr. Scand. [Suppl.],* 207:19–30.

Annell, A. L., editor (1972): *Depressive States in Childhood and Adolescence.* Almquist & Wiksell, Stockholm.

Anthony, J., and Scott, P. (1960): Manic-depressive psychosis in childhood. *J. Child. Psychol. Psychiatry,* 1:53–72.

Arnold, L. E., Kirilcuk, V., Corson, S. A., and Corson, E. O'L. (1973): Levoamphetamine and dextroamphetamine: Differential effect on aggression and hyperkinesis in children and dogs. *Am. J. Psychiatry,* 130:165–170.

Arnold, L. E., Wender, P. W., McCloskey, K., and Snyder, S. H. (1972): Levoamphetamine and dextroamphetamine: Comparative efficacy in the hyperkinetic syndrome. *Arch. Gen. Psychiatry,* 27:816–822.

Bailit, H. L., and Whelan, M. A. (1967): Some factors related to size and intelligence in an institutionalized mentally retarded population. *J. Pediatr.,* 71:897–909.

Bair, H. V., and Herold, W. (1955): Efficacy of chlorpromazine in hyperactive mentally retarded children. *Arch. Neurol. Psychiatry,* 74:363–364.

Bender, L., Cobrinik, L., Faretra, G., and Sankar, D. V. S. (1966): The treatment of childhood schizophrenia with LSD and UML. In: *Biological Treatment of Mental Illness,* edited by M. Rinkel. Page & Co., New York.

Bender, L., and Cottington, F. (1942): The use of amphetamine sulfate (benzedrine) in child psychiatry. *Am. J. Psychiatry,* 99:116–121.

Bender, L., Faretra, G., and Cobrinik, L. (1963): LSD and UML treatment of hospitalized disturbed children. In: *Recent Advances in Biological Psychiatry,* edited by J. Wortis. Plenum Press, New York.

Bender, L., Goldschmidt, L., and Sankar, D. V. S. (1962): Treatment of autistic schizophrenic children with LSD-25 and UML-491. In: *Recent Advances in Biological Psychiatry,* edited by J. Wortis. Plenum Press, New York.

Boullin, D. J., Coleman, M., and O'Brien, R. A. (1970): Abnormalities in platelet 5-hydroxytryptamine efflux in patients with infantile autism. *Nature (Lond.),* 226:371–372.

Boyd, A. E., Lebovitz, H. E., and Pfeiffer, J. B. (1970): Stimulation of human-growth-hormone secretion by L-dopa. *N. Engl. J. Med.,* 282:1425–1429.

Bradley, C. (1937): The behavior of children receiving benzedrine. *Am. J. Psychiatry,* 94:577–585.

Bradley, C., and Bowen, M. (1941): Amphetamine (benzedrine) therapy of children's behavior disorders. *Am. J. Orthopsychiatry,* 11:92–103.

Brown, D., Winsberg, B. G., Bialer, I., and Press, M. (1973): Imipramine therapy and seizures: Three children treated for hyperactive behavior disorders. *Am. J. Psychiatry,* 130:210–212.

Burk, H. W., and Menolascino, F. J. (1968): Haloperidol in emotionally disturbed mentally retarded individuals. *Am. J. Psychiatry,* 124:1589–1591.

Campbell, M. (1973a): A psychotic boy with self-mutilating behavior and the anti-aggressive effect of lithium. Presented at the twentieth Annual Meeting of the American Academy of Child Psychiatry, Washington, D.C., Oct. 18–21.

Campbell, M. (1973b): Biological interventions in psychoses of childhood. *J. Autism Child. Schizo.,* 3:347–373.

Campbell, M., and Fish, B. (1974): Triiodothyronine in schizophrenic children. In:
    Thyroid Axis and Behavior, edited by A. J. Prange, Jr. Raven Press, New York.
Campbell, M., and Fish, B. (1975): A study of chlordiazepoxide in disturbed children
    (*in preparation*).
Campbell, M., Fish, B., David, R., Shapiro, T., Collins, P., and Koh, C. (1972*a*):
    Response to triiodothyronine and dextroamphetamine: A study of preschool schizo-
    phrenic children. *J. Autism Child. Schizo.,* 2:343–358.
Campbell, M., Fish, B., David, R., Shapiro, T., Collins, P., and Koh, C. (1973):
    Liothyronine treatment in psychotic and nonpsychotic children under 6 years. *Arch.
    Gen. Psychiatry,* 29:602–608.
Campbell, M., Fish, B., Korein, J., Shapiro, T., Collins, P., and Koh, C. (1972*b*):
    Lithium-chlorpromazine: A controlled crossover study in hyperactive severely dis-
    turbed young children. *J. Autism Child. Schizo.,* 2:234–263.
Campbell, M., Fish, B., Shapiro, T., and Floyd, A., Jr. (1970): Thiothixene in young
    disturbed children: A pilot study. *Arch. Gen. Psychiatry,* 23:70–72.
Campbell, M., Fish, B., Shapiro, T., and Floyd, A., Jr. (1971*a*): Study of molindone
    in disturbed preschool children. *Curr. Ther. Res.,* 13:28–33.
Campbell, M., Fish, B., Shapiro, T., and Floyd, A., Jr. (1971*b*): Imipramine in pre-
    school autistic and schizophrenic children. *J. Autism Child. Schizo.,* 1:267–282.
Campbell, M., Fish, B., Shapiro, T., and Floyd, A., Jr. (1972*c*): Acute responses of
    schizophrenic children to a sedative and "stimulating" neuroleptic: A pharmacologic
    yardstick. *Curr. Ther. Res.,* 14:759–766.
Campbell, M., Friedman, E., DeVito, E., Greenspan, L., and Collins, P. J. (1974):
    Blood serotonin in psychotic and brain damaged children. *J. Autism Child. Schizo.,*
    4:33–41.
Campbell, M., Friedman, E., Green, W. H., Collins, P. J., Small, A. M., and Breuer,
    H. (1975*a*): Blood serotonin in schizophrenic children. A preliminary study. *Int.
    Pharmacopsychiatry* (*in press*)
Campbell, M., Korein, J., Small, A. M., Collins, P. J., Friedman, E., David, R., Genie-
    ser, N. B., Carroll, P., and Fish, B. (1975*b*): L-Dopa and L-amphetamine: A cross-
    over study in schizophrenic children (*submitted for publication*).
Claghorn, J. L. (1972): A double-blind comparison of haloperidol (Haldol) and thio-
    ridazine (Mellaril) in outpatient children. *Curr. Ther. Res.,* 14:785–789.
Cohen, N. J., Douglas, V. I., and Morgenstern, G. (1971): The effect of methylpheni-
    date on attentive behavior and autonomic activity in hyperactive children. *Psycho-
    pharmacologia,* 22:282–294.
Coleman, M. (1973): Serotonin and central nervous system syndromes in childhood: A
    review. *J. Autism Child. Schizo.,* 3:27–35.
Conners, C. K. (1971): The effect of stimulant drugs on human figure drawings in
    children with minimal brain dysfunction. *Psychopharmacologia,* 19:329–333.
Conners, C. K. (1972*a*): II. Psychological effects of stimulant drugs in children with
    minimal brain dysfunction. *Pediatrics,* 49:702–708.
Conners, C. K. (1972*b*): Pharmacotherapy of psychopathology in children. In: *Psycho-
    pathological Disorders of Childhood,* edited by H. C. Quay and J. S. Werry. Wiley,
    New York.
Conners, C. K. (1973): Deanol and behavior disorders in children: A critical review
    of the literature and recommended future studies for determining efficacy. *Psycho-
    pharmacol. Bull.* (*Special Issue*): *Pharmacotherapy of Children,* pp. 188–195.
Conners, C. K., and Eisenberg, L. (1963): The effects of methylphenidate on symp-
    tomatology and learning in disturbed children. *Am. J. Psychiatry,* 120:458–464.
Conners, C. K., Eisenberg, L., and Barcai, A. (1967): Effect of dextroamphetamine on
    children. *Arch. Gen. Psychiatry,* 17:478–485.
Conners, C. K., Kramer, R., Rothschild, G. H., Schwartz, L., and Stone, A. (1971):
    Treatment of young delinquent boys with diphenylhydantoin sodium and methylphen-
    idate: A controlled comparison. *Arch. Gen. Pyschiatry,* 24:156–162.
Conners, C. K., Rothschild, G., Eisenberg, L., Schwartz, L. S., and Robinson, E.
    (1969): Dextroamphetamine sulfate in children with learning disorders. *Arch. Gen.
    Psychiatry,* 21:182–190.
Conners, C. K., Taylor, E., Meo, G., Kurtz, M. A., and Fournier, M. (1972): Mag-

nesium pemoline and dextroamphetamine: A controlled study in children with minimal brain dysfunction. *Psychopharmacologia,* 26:321–336.

Creager, R. O., and Van Riper, C. (1967): The effect of methylphenidate on the verbal productivity of children with cerebral dysfunction. *J. Speech Hear. Res.,* 10:623–628.

Denhoff, E., Davids, A., and Hawkins, R. (1971): Effects of dextroamphetamine on hyperkinetic children. *J. Learn. Disorders,* 4:491–498.

DiMascio, A., Shader, R. I., and Harmatz, J. (1969): Psychotropic drugs and induced hostility. *Psychosomatics,* 10:46–47.

DiMascio, A., Soltys, J. J., and Shader, R. I. (1970): Psychotropic drug side effects in children. In: *Psychotropic Drug Side Effects,* edited by R. I. Shader and A. DiMascio. William & Wilkins, Baltimore.

Dostal, T. (1972): Antiaggressive effect of lithium salts in mentally retarded adolescents. In: *Depressive States in Childhood and Adolescence,* edited by A. L. Annell. Almquist & Wiksell, Stockholm.

Dutton, G. (1964): The growth pattern of psychotic boys. *Br. J. Psychiatry,* 110:101–103.

Dyson, W. L., and Barcai, A. (1970): Treatment of children of lithium-responding parents. *Curr. Ther. Res.,* 12:286–290.

Effron, A. S., and Freedman, A. M. (1953): The treatment of behavior disorders in children with benadryl. *J. Pediatr.,* 42:261–266.

Eisenberg, L. (1964): Role of drug in treating disturbed children. *Children,* 2:167–173.

Eisenberg, L. (1967): The role of classification in child psychiatry. *Int. J. Psychiatry,* 3:179–181.

Eisenberg, L. (1968): Psychopharmacology in childhood: a critique. In: *Foundations in Child Psychiatry,* edited by E. Miller. Pergamon Press, Oxford.

Engelhardt, D. M. (1974): CNS consequences of psychotropic drug withdrawal in autistic children: a follow-up report. Presented at the Annual ECDEU Meeting, Key Biscayne, Fla., May 23–25.

Engelhardt, D. M., Polizos, P., Waizer, J., and Hoffman, S. P. (1973): A double-blind comparison of fluphenazine and haloperidol. *J. Autism Child. Schizo.,* 3:128–137.

Faretra, G., Dooher, L., and Dowling, J. (1970): Comparison of haloperidol and fluphenazine in disturbed children. *Am. J. Psychiatry,* 126:1670–1673.

Finnerty, R. J., Soltys, J. J., and Cole, J. O. (1971): The use of D-amphetamine with hyperkinetic children. *Psychopharmacologia,* 21:302–308.

Fish, B. (1960): Drug therapy in child psychiatry: Pharmacological aspects. *Compr. Psychiatry,* 1:212–227.

Fish, B. (1968*a*): Methodology in child psychopharmacology. In: *Psychopharmacology, Review of Progress,* 1956–1967, edited by D. H. Efron, J. O. Cole, J. Levine, and J. R. Wittenborn. Public Health Service Publication No. 1836. Government Printing Office, Washington, D. C.

Fish, B. (1968*b*): Drug use in psychiatric disorders of children. *Am. J. Psychiatry (Suppl.),* 124:31–36.

Fish, B. (1970): Psychopharmacologic response of chronic schizophrenic adults as predictors of responses in young schizophrenic children. *Psychopharmacol. Bull.,* 6:12–15.

Fish, B. (1971): The "one child, one drug" myth of stimulants in hyperkinesis: Importance of diagnostic categories in evaluating treatment. *Arch. Gen. Psychiatry,* 25:193–203.

Fish, B., Campbell, M., Shapiro, T., and Floyd, A., Jr. (1969*a*): Comparison of trifluperidol, trifluoperazine and chlorpromazine in preschool schizophrenic children: The value of less sedative antipsychotic agents. *Curr. Ther. Res.,* 11:589–595.

Fish, B., Campbell, M., Shapiro, T., and Floyd, A., Jr. (1969*b*): Schizophrenic children treated with methysergide (Sansert). *Dis. Nerv. Syst.,* 30:534–540.

Fish, B., Campbell, M., Shapiro, T., and Weinstein, J. (1969*c*): Preliminary findings on thiothixene compared to other drugs in psychotic children under five years. In: *The Thioxanthenes: Modern Problems of Pharmacopsychiatry,* edited by H. E. Lehmann and T. A. Ban. Karger, Basel.

Fish, B., and Shapiro, T. (1964): A descriptive typology of children's psychiatric disorders. II. A behavioral classification. *Psychiatr. Res. Rep.,* 18:75–86.

Fish, B., and Shapiro, T. (1965): A typology of children's psychiatric disorders. I. Its application to a controlled evaluation of treatment. *J. Am. Acad. Child Psychiatry,* 4:32–52.

Fish, B., Shapiro, T., and Campbell, M. (1966): Long-term prognosis and the response of schizophrenic children to drug therapy: A controlled study of trifluoperazine. *Am. J. Psychiatry,* 123:32–39.

Freed, H., and Pfeifer, C. (1956): Treatment of hyperkinetic emotionally disturbed children with prolonged administration of chlorpromazine. *Am. J. Psychiatry,* 113:22–26.

Freedman, A. M., Ebin, E. V., and Wilson, E. A. (1962): Autistic schizophrenic children: An experiment in the use of D-lysergic acid diethylamide (LSD-25). *Arch. Gen. Psychiatry,* 6:203–213.

Freedman, D. X. (1971): *Report of the Conference on the Use of Stimulant Drugs in the Treatment of Behaviorally Disturbed Young School Children.* Office of Child Development and the Office of the Assistant Secretary for Health and Scientific Affairs, U.S. Department of Health, Education, and Welfare, Washington, D.C.

Freeman, R. D. (1966): Drug effects on learning in children: A selective review of the past thirty years. *J. Spec. Ed.,* 1:17–44.

Freeman, R. D. (1970): Psychopharmacology and the retarded child. In: *Psychiatric Approaches to Mental Retardation,* edited by F. Menolascino. Basic Books, New York.

Freyhan, F. A. (1959): Clinical and Investigative Aspects. In: *Psychopharmacology Frontiers,* edited by N. S. Kline. Little Brown, Boston.

Fromm, G. H., Amores, C. Y., and Thies, W. (1972): Imipramine in epilepsy. *Arch. Neurol.,* 27:198–204.

Frommer, E. A. (1967): Treatment in childhood depression with antidepressant drugs. *Br. Med. J.,* 1:729–732.

Frommer, E. A. (1968): Depressive illness in childhood. *Br. J. Psychiatry (Special Publication No. 2): Recent Development in Affective Disorders: A symposium,* edited by A. Coppen and A. Walk.

Frommer, E. A. (1972): Indications for antidepressant treatment with special reference to depressed preschool children. In: *Depressive States in Childhood and Adolescence,* edited by A. L. Annell. Almquist & Wiksell, Stockholm.

Gardos, G., DiMascio, A., Salzman, C., and Shader, R. I. (1968): Differential actions of chlordiazepoxide and oxazepam on hostility. *Arch. Gen. Psychiatry,* 18:757–760.

Gittelman-Klein, R. (1975): Review of clinical psychopharmacological treatment of hyperkinesis. In: *Biennial Review of Psychiatric Drug Treatment,* edited by D. F. Klein and R. Gittelman-Klein. Brunner/Mazel, New York *(in press).*

Gittelman-Klein, R., and Klein, D. F. (1971): Controlled imipramine treatment of school phobia. *Arch. Gen. Psychiatry,* 25:204–207.

Gittelman-Klein, R., and Klein, D. F. (1973a): School phobia: Diagnostic considerations in the light of imipramine effects. *J. Nerv. Ment. Dis.,* 156:199–215.

Gittelman-Klein, R., and Klein, D. F. (1973b): The relationship between behavioral and psychological test changes in hyperkinetic children. Presented at the 12th Annual Meeting of the American College of Neuropsychopharmacology, Palm Springs, Calif.

Grabowski, S. W. (1973): Safety and effectiveness of haloperidol for mentally retarded behaviorally disordered and hyperkinetic patients. *Curr. Ther. Res.,* 15:856–861.

Graham, P. (1974): Depression in pre-pubertal children. *Dev. Med. Child. Neurol.,* 16:340–349.

Gram, L. F., and Rafaelsen, O. J. (1972): Lithium treatment of psychotic children and adolescents: A controlled clinical trial. *Acta Psychiatr. Scand.,* 48:253–260.

Greenbaum, G. H. (1970): An evaluation of niacinamide in the treatment of childhood schizophrenia. *Am. J. Psychiatry,* 127:129–132.

Greenhill, L. L., Rieder, R. O., Wender, P. H., Buchsbaum, M., and Zahn, T. P. (1973): Lithium carbonate in the treatment of hyperactive children. *Arch. Gen. Psychiatry,* 28:636–640.

Group for the Advancement of Psychiatry (1966): *Report No. 62: Psychopathological Disorders in Childhood: Theoretical Considerations and a Proposed Classification.* New York City.

Helper, M., Wilcott, R. C., and Garfield, S. L. (1963): Effects of chlorpromazine on learning and related processes in emotionally disturbed children. *J. Consult. Psychol.,* 27:1–9.

Hoffer, A. (1970): Childhood schizophrenia: A case treated with nicotinic acid and nicotinamide. *Schizophrenia,* 2:43–53.

Hoffman, S. P., Engelhardt, D. M., Margolis, R. A., Polizos, P., Waizer, J., and Rosenfeld, R. (1974): Response to methylphenidate in low socioeconomic hyperactive children. *Arch. Gen. Psychiatry,* 30:354–359.

Huessy, H. R., and Wright, A. L. (1970): The use of imipramine in children's behavior disorders. *Acta Paedopsychiatr. (Basel),* 37:194–199.

Irwin, S. (1968): A rational framework for the development, evaluation, and use of psychoactive drugs. *Am. J. Psychiatry (Suppl.),* 124:1–19.

Irwin, S. (1974a): How to prescribe psychoactive drugs. *Bull. Menninger Clin.,* 38:1–13.

Irwin, S. (1974b): The uses and relative hazard potential of psychoactive drugs. *Bull. Menninger Clin.,* 38:14–48.

Ison, G. M. (1957): The effect of "thorazine" on Wechsler scores. *Am. J. Ment. Defic.,* 62:543–547.

Knights, R. M., and Hinton, G. (1969): The effects of methylphenidate (Ritalin) on the motor skills and behavior of children with learning problems. *J. Nerv. Ment. Dis.,* 148:643–653.

Korein, J., Fish, B., Shapiro, T., Gerner, E. W., and Levidow, L. (1971): EEG and behavioral effects on drug therapy in children: Chlorpromazine and diphenhydramine. *Arch. Gen. Psychiatry,* 24:552–563.

Kraft, I. A., Ardali, C., Duffy, J. H., Hart, J. T., and Pearce, P. (1965): A clinical study of chlordiazepoxide used in psychiatric disorders of children. *Int. J. Neuropsychiatry,* 1:433–437.

Kurtis, L. B. (1966): Clinical study of the response to nortriptyline on autistic children. *Int. J. Neuropsychiatry,* 2:298–301.

Laufer, M., Denhoff, E., Solomons, G. (1957): Hyperkinetic impulse disorder in children's behavior problems. *Psychosom. Med.,* 19:38–49.

LaVeck, G. D., and Buckley, P. (1961): The use of psychopharmacologic agents in retarded children with behavior disorders. *J. Chronic Dis.,* 13:174–183.

Lefkowitz, M. M. (1969): Effects of diphenylhydantoin on disruptive behavior. *Arch. Gen. Psychiatry,* 20:643–651.

LeVann, L. J. (1962): Chlordiazepoxide, a tranquilizer with anticonvulsant properties. *Can. Med. Assoc. J.,* 86:123–126.

LeVann, L. J. (1969): Haloperidol in the treatment of behavioural disorders in children and adolescents. *Can. Psychiatr. Assoc. J.,* 14:217–220.

Lipman, R. S. (1970): The use of psychopharmacological agents in residential facilities for the retarded. In: *Psychiatric Approaches to Mental Retardation,* edited by F. Menolascino. Basic Books, New York.

Lipton, M. A., Ban, T. A., Kane, F. J., Levine, J., Mosher, L. R., and Wittenborn, R. (1973): *Megavitamin and Orthomolecular Therapy in Psychiatry.* American Psychiatric Association, Washington, D.C.

Looker, A., and Conners, C. K. (1970): Diphenylhydantoin in children with severe temper tantrums. *Arch. Gen. Psychiatry,* 23:80–89.

Lucas, A. R. (1967): Gilles de la Tourette's disease in children: Treatment with haloperidol. *Am. J. Psychiatry,* 124:243–245.

Lucas, A. R., Lockett, H. J., and Grimm, F. (1965): Amitriptyline in childhood depressions. *Dis. Nerv. Syst.,* 26:105–110.

Mandell, A. J. (1975): Neurobiological mechanisms of adaptation in relation to models of psychobiological development. In: *Proceedings of the First International Leo Kanner Colloquium on Child Development, Deviations, and Treatment,* edited by R. Reichler and E. Schopler.

McAndrew, J. B., Case, Q., and Treffert, D. (1972): Effects of prolonged phenothiazine intake on psychotic and other hospitalized children. *J. Autism Child. Schizo.,* 2:75–91.

Millichap, J. G., and Fowler, G. W. (1967): Treatment of "minimal brain dysfunction" syndromes: Selection of drugs for children with hyperactivity and learning disabilities. *Pediatr. Clin. North Am.,* 14:767–777.

O'Malley, J. E., and Eisenberg, L. (1973): The hyperkinetic syndrome. *Semin. Psychiatry,* 5:95–103.

Page, J. G., Bernstein, J. E., Janicki, R. S., and Michelli, F. A. (1974): A multi-clinic trial of pemoline in childhood hyperkinesis. In: *Clinical Use of Stimulant Drugs in Children,* edited by C. K. Conners. Excerpta Medica, The Hague.

Petti, T. A., and Campbell, M. (1975): Imipramine and seizures. *Am. J. Psychiatry, (in press).*

Pilkington, T. L. (1961): Comparative effects of Librium and Taractan on behavior disorders of mentally retarded children. *Dis. Nerv. Syst.,* 22:573–575.

Plotnikoff, N. (1971): Pemoline: Review of performance. *Tex. Rep. Biol. Med.,* 29:467–479.

Polizos, P., Engelhardt, D. M., Hoffman, S. P., and Waizer, J. (1973): Neurological consequences of psychotropic drug withdrawal in schizophrenic children. *J. Autism Child Schizo.,* 3:247–253.

Poussaint, A. F., and Ditman, K. S. (1965): A controlled study of imipramine (Tofranil) in the treatment of childhood enuresis. *J. Pediatr.,* 67:283–290.

Rapoport, J. (1965): Childhood behavior and learning problems treated with imipramine. *Int. J. Neuropsychiatry,* 1:635–642.

Rapoport, J. L., Quinn, P. O., Bradbard, G., Riddle, D., and Brooks, E. (1974): Imipramine and methylphenidate treatments of hyperactive boys. *Arch. Gen. Psychiatry,* 30:789–793.

Rickels, K., and Downing, R. W. (1974): Chlordiazepoxide and hostility in anxious outpatients. *Am. J. Psychiatry,* 131:442–444.

Rifkin, A., Quitkin, F., Carrillo, C., Blumberg, A. G., and Klein, D. F. (1972): Lithium carbonate in emotionally unstable character disorder. *Arch. Gen. Psychiatry,* 27:519–523.

Rimland, B. (1973): High-dosage levels of certain vitamins in the treatment of children with severe mental disorders. In: *Orthomolecular Psychiatry,* edited by D. Hawkins and L. Pauling. Freeman, San Francisco.

Ritvo, E. R., Yuwiler, A., Geller, E., Ornitz, E. M., Saeger, K., and Plotkin, S. (1970): Increased blood serotonin and platelets in early infantile autism. *Arch. Gen. Psychiatry,* 23:566–572.

Ritvo, E. R., Yuwiler, A., Geller, E., Kales, A., Rashkis, S., Schicor, A., Plotkin, S., Axelrod, R., and Howard, C. (1971): Effects of L-dopa in autism. *J. Autism Child. Schizo.,* 1:190–205.

Rolo, A., Krinsky, L., Abramson, H., and Goldfarb, L. (1965): Preliminary method study of LSD with children. *Int. J. Neuropsychiatry,* 1:552–555.

Root, A. W., and Russ, R. D. (1972): Effect of l-dihydroxyphenylalanine upon serum growth hormone concentrations in children and adolescents. *J. Pediatr.,* 81:808–813.

Roukema, R. W., and Emery, L. (1970): Megavitamin therapy with severely disturbed children. *Am. J. Psychiatry,* 127:167.

Rutter, M., Lebovici, S., Eisenberg, L., Sneznevskij, A. V., Sadoun, R., Brooke, E., and Lin, T-Y. (1969): A tri-axial classification of mental disorders in childhood. *J. Child. Psychol. Psychiatry,* 10:41–61.

Safer, D. J., and Allen, R. P. (1973): Factors influencing the suppressant effects of two stimulant drugs on the growth of hyperactive children. *Pediatrics,* 51:660–667.

Satterfield, J. H., Cantwell, D. P., Lesser, L. I., and Podosin, R. L. (1972): Physiological studies of the hyperkinetic child. I. *Am. J. Psychiatry,* 128:1418–1424.

Satterfield, J. H., Cantwell, D., Saul, R. E., Lesser, L. I., and Podosin, R. L. (1973): Response to stimulant drug treatment in hyperactive children: Prediction from EEG and neurological findings. *J. Autism Child. Schizo.,* 3:36–48.

Satterfield, J. H., Cantwell, D. P., and Satterfield, B. T. (1974): Pathophysiology of the hyperactive child syndrome. *Arch. Gen. Psychiatry,* 31:839–844.

Schachter, S., and Singer, J. E. (1962): Cognitive, social and physiological determinants of emotional state. *Psychol. Rev.,* 69:379–399.

Schiele, B. C., Gallant, D., Simpson, G., Gardner, E. A., and Cole, J. O. (1973): Tardive dyskinesia. *Am. J. Orthopsychiatry,* 43:506, 688.

Schou, M. (1972): Lithium in psychiatric therapy and prophylaxis. a review with special regard to its use in children. In: *Depressive States in Childhood and Adolescence,* edited by A. L. Annell. Almquist & Wiksell, Stockholm.

Serrano, A. C., and Forbis, O. L. (1973): Haloperidol for psychiatric disorders in children. *Dis. Nerv. Syst.,* 34:226–231.

Shapiro, A. K., Shapiro, E., and Wayne, H. (1973): Treatment of Tourette's syndrome. *Arch. Gen. Psychiatry,* 28:92–97.

Sherman, L., Kim, S., Benjamin, F., and Kolodny, H. D. (1971): Effect of chlorpromazine on serum growth-hormone in man. *N. Engl. J. Med.,* 284:72–74.

Sherwin, A. C., Flach, F. F., and Stokes, P. E. (1958): Treatment of psychoses in early childhood with triiodothyronine. *Am. J. Psychiatry,* 115:166–167.

Silver, A. A. (1955): Management of children with schizophrenia. *Am. J. Psychother.,* 9:196–215.

Simeon, J., Saletu, B., Saletu, M., Itil, T. M., and DaSilva, J. (1973): Thiothixene in childhood psychoses. Presented at the Third International Symposium on Phenothiazines. Rockville, Md.

Simmons, J. Q., III, Leiken, S. J., Lovaas, O. I., Schaeffer, B., and Perloff, B. (1966): Modification of autistic behavior with LSD-25. *Am. J. Psychiatry,* 122:1201–1211.

Simon, G. B., and Gillies, S. M. (1964): Some physical characteristics of a group of psychotic children. *Br. J. Psychiatry,* 110:104–107.

Simopoulos, A. M., Pinton, A., Uhlenhuth, E. H., McGee, J. J., and DeRosa, E. R. (1974): Diphenylhydantoin effectiveness in the treatment of chronic schizophrenics. *Arch. Gen. Psychiatry,* 30:106–111.

Skynner, A. C. R. (1961): Effect of chlordiazepoxide. *Lancet,* 1:1110.

Sleator, E. K., VonNeumann, A., and Sprague, R. L. (1974): Hyperactive children: A continuous long-term placebo-controlled follow-up *J.A.M.A.,* 229:316–317.

Small, A., Hibi, S., and Feinberg, I. (1971): Effects of dextroamphetamine sulfate on EEG sleep patterns of hyperactive children. *Arch. Gen. Psychiatry,* 25:369–380.

Solomons, G. (1971): The role of methylphenidate and dextroamphetamine in hyperactivity in children. *J. Iowa Med.,* 61:658–661.

Sprague, R. L., Barnes, K. R., and Werry, J. S. (1970): Methylphenidate and thioridazine: Learning, reaction time, activity and classroom behavior in disturbed children. *Am. J. Orthopsychiatry,* 40:615–628.

Sprague, R. L., and Sleator, E. K. (1973): Effects of psychopharmacologic agents on learning disorders. *Pediatr. Clin. North Am.,* 20:719–735.

Sprague, R. L., and Werry, J. S. (1971): Methodology of psychopharmacological studies with the retarded. In: *International Review of Research in Mental Retardation,* edited by N. R. Ellis. Academic Press, New York.

Sprague, R. L., and Werry, J. S. (1973): Pediatric psychopharmacology. *Psychopharmacol. Bull. (Special issue): Pharmacotherapy of Children,* pp. 21–23.

Stack, J. J. (1972): Chemotherapy in childhood depression. In: *Depressive States in Childhood and Adolescence.* Almquist & Wiksell, Stockholm.

Steinberg, G. S., Troshinsky, C., and Steinberg, H. C. (1971): Dextroamphetamine-responsive behavior disorder in school children. *Am. J. Psychiatry,* 128:174–179.

Tarjan, G., Lowery, V. E., and Wright, S. W. (1957): Use of chlorpromazine in two hundred seventy-eight mentally deficient patients. *J. Dis. Child.,* 94:294–300.

The Nervous Child (1952): Vol. 9.

Ucer, E., and Kreger, K. C. (1969): A double-blind study comparing haloperidol with thioridazine in emotionally disturbed, mentally retarded children. *Curr. Ther. Res.,* 11:278–283.

Van Krevelen, D. A., and Van Voorst, J. A. (1959): Lithium in the treatment of a cryptogenetic psychosis in a juvenile. *Z. Kinderpsychiatr.,* 26:148–152.

Waites, L., and Keele, D. K. (1963): Fluphenazine in management of disturbed mentally retarded children. *Dis. Nerv. Syst.,* 24:113–114.

Waizer, J., Hoffman, S. P., Polizos, P., and Engelhardt, D. M. (1974): Outpatient treatment of hyperactive school children with imipramine. *Am. J. Psychiatry,* 131:587–591.

Waizer, J., Polizos, P., Hoffman, S. P., Engelhardt, D. M., and Margolis, R. A. (1972):

A single-blind evaluation of thiothixene with outpatient schizophrenic children. *J. Autism Child Schizo.*, 2:378–386.

Wender, P. H. (1971): *Minimal Brain Dysfunction in Children.* Wiley Interscience, New York.

Werry, J. S. (1972): Childhood psychosis. In: *Psychopathological Disorders of Childhood,* edited by H. C. Quay and J. S. Werry. Wiley, New York.

Werry, J. S., Weiss, G., Douglas, V., and Martin, J. (1966): Studies on the hyperactive child. III. The effect of chlorpromazine upon behavior and learning ability. *J. Am. Acad. Child Psychiatry,* 5:292–312.

Whitehead, P. L., and Clark, L. D. (1970): Effect of lithium carbonate, placebo and thioridazine on hyperactive children. *Am. J. Psychiatry,* 127:824–825.

WHO Scientific Group on Psychopharmacology (1967): *Research in Psychopharmacology.* WHO Technical Report Series No. 371. World Health Organization, Geneva.

Winsberg, B. G., Bialer, I., Kupietz, S., and Tobias, J. (1972): Effects of imipramine and dextroamphetamine on behavior of neuropsychiatrically impaired children. *Am. J. Psychiatry,* 128:1425–1431.

Wolpert, A., Hagamen, M. B., and Merlis, S. (1967): A comparative study of thiothixene and trifluoperazine in childhood schizophrenia. *Curr. Ther. Res.,* 9:482–485.

Zrull, J. P., Westman, J. C., Arthur, B., and Bell, W. A. (1963): A comparison of chlordiazepoxide, D-amphetamine, and placebo in the treatment of the hyperkinetic syndrome in children. *Am. J. Psychiatry,* 120:590–591.

Chapter 15

Psychopharmacology of the Aged

Murray Raskind and Carl Eisdorfer

Persons age 65 years or older comprise one of the most rapidly growing segments of the population. In the United States the number and proportion of older persons has increased steadily throughout the twentieth century. A comparison of census data from 1900 to 1970 indicates that although the population of the United States grew by 2.5-fold during these years the number of persons age 65 or older increased sevenfold (Brotman, 1973). Projections indicate that the trend is continuing; and from the current level of 10% of the population (20 million aged persons), it is estimated that by 1990 the population of the United States will include 13% older persons, or more than 27 million (Brotman, 1973).

The older portion of the population (i.e., those 75 yr and older) are increasing at a somewhat accelerated rate. Of more than passing consequence is the fact that these increases have been the results of improving the mortality pattern for infants and children, as well as the fact that up to now there has been relatively little increase in longevity for adults. Changes in the mortality figure for diseases such as cancer and cardiovascular illness are likely to occur with current advances in medical and health information. These changes will have their impact on human longevity during later life, and this should yield further increases in the population.

Using the anchor point of 65 years of age, the aged are a population at high risk for a variety of physical and psychiatric disorders. Comprising as they do 10% of the population, they account for 14% of the outpatient visits to health care facilities in the United States and are admitted to general hospitals at about 2.5 times the rate of young adults. In addition, older persons have longer hospital stays and more days of incapacity per year. In long-term care facilities older persons occupy 85% of the 1.2 million nursing home and extended-care facility beds.

The data for psychiatric illness are no less impressive. Kramer, Tauber, and Redick (1973) documented the heightened risk for psychiatric disorders among the elderly. Pasamanick, Roberts, Lemkau, and Krueger (1959) suggested that the risk for organic psychoses goes up significantly with age, but that the prevalence for neuroses diminishes. This finding is open to some question, however, in view of the often reported data that a rather small proportion of psychiatric outpatient attention is devoted to the

aged (Kramer et al., 1973). The reluctance of older persons and physicians
to identify disorders as psychiatric problems in the aged, as well as the propensity to tolerate deviance in older persons for longer periods of time
(Lowenthal and Berkman, 1967), presents some difficulties in assessing the
prevalence of psychiatric disease for this group. It has been suggested that
the prevalence of emotional disorders significant enough to be labeled
psychiatric disease probably ranges from 20 to 45% among aged persons in
the community (Busse and Pfeiffer, 1969). If one actually examines elderly
patients residing in nursing homes, the prevalence of psychiatric illness
appears quite high. Stotsky (1967) reported symptoms of significant psychiatric disorders in 91% of a group of allegedly nonpsychiatric nursing home
patients, and the symptoms clusters were remarkably similar to those found
in elderly patients with longstanding "functional" psychoses.

Physicians have responded to this pervasive problem by prescribing
psychopharmacological agents liberally to their aged patients, especially to
those in supervised residential settings. Surveys (Special Committee on
Aging, U.S. Senate, 1974) indicate that 75% of all nursing home patients
are receiving at least one (and often several) standard psychotropic medications. In addition, various hormones, vasodilators, vitamins, cerebral stimulants, and other agents purported to improve behavioral disturbance by cor-
recting alleged physiological deficits accompanying the aging process are
being administered. Unfortunately, reliable data generated from well-designed
clinical psychopharmacological studies in elderly populations are rare.
Furthermore, the elderly often present a bewildering array of behavioral signs
and symptoms complicated by physical illness, sensory deficits, prescribed
and nonprescribed drugs, emotional losses, and social deprivation. This
chapter reviews studies available in geriatric psychopharmacology, identifies
issues in pharmacokinetics which involve the elderly, and discusses the special
problems encountered in the use of psychotropic drugs for older patients.

In accord with Hollister (1973), Eisdorfer (1975) suggested that a simpli-
fied nomenclature of psychotropic drugs be adopted. For the aged population the following categories have been proposed:
1. Antipsychotic
2. Antidepressant
3. Antimanic
4. Antianxiety and hypnotic
5. Cognitive acting

ADVERSE SIDE EFFECTS

The widespread clinical impression that aged patients are more susceptible
than the young to adverse drug reactions (side effects) from most classes
of drugs has been confirmed by several studies. In a large survey of both
psychiatric and general medical inpatients, Hurwitz (1969) found side

effects in 21.3% of patients ages 70 to 79, compared to 7.5% for patients 40 to 49 and 3.0% for those 20 to 29. Women had a higher risk of side effects than did men. Seidl, Thornton, Smith, and Cluff (1966) observed adverse reactions in 24.9% of medical patients over age 80, compared to 11.8% in those 41 to 50 and 9.9% in those 21 to 30. These figures are consistent with the high incidence of adverse effects of psychotropic drugs in an elderly population described by Learoyd (1972). Of patients admitted to his psychogeriatric ward, 16% presented disorders directly attributed to undesirable side effects of the psychoactive drugs they had received prior to admission. Among the major categories of adverse effects were drug intoxications with increased lethargy, confusion, and disorientation; "paradoxical" behavioral reactions, e.g., restlessness, agitation, and aggression; and medical effects, e.g., hypotension, respiratory depression, and urinary retention. Common offenders included various antipsychotic, antidepressant, and antianxiety agents, often prescribed in a multiple-drug regimen.

PHARMACOKINETICS

The pharmacokinetics of any drug is a function of absorption, distribution, metabolism, receptor state activity, and elimination. For most drugs we are only beginning to develop an understanding of these factors in clinical use with the elderly. Identical doses of digoxin result in a higher blood concentration and a longer blood half-life in an elderly than in a young patient (Ewy, Kapadia, and Yao, 1969). Similar results have been found for penicillin (Hansen, Kampmann, and Laursen, 1970), tetracycline, and dihydrostreptomycin (Vartia and Leikola, 1960). The highly lipid-soluble drug phenylbutazone, analogous in this respect to many of the psychotropic drugs, shows a similar pattern of increased half-life with advancing age (O'Malley, Crooks, Duke, and Stevenson, 1971). These age-related changes are probably secondary to both decreased drug metabolism and decreased drug elimination in the elderly (Bender, 1974). The replacement of lean body mass by fat as one ages (Gregerman and Bierman, 1974) affects distribution and acts further to increase retention of lipid-soluble psychotropic drugs.

On clinical grounds, Salzman, Shader, and Pearlman (1970) and Bendkowski (1970) suggested absorption difficulties to be a problem in older patients. If poor absorption is suspected and patients fail to respond to appropriate doses of medication in tablet or capsule form, the use of liquid concentrate or parenteral administration should be considered.

Changes in receptor site activity with age have been suggested (Eisdorfer, 1972; Bender, 1974). As demonstrated with analgesics (Bellville, Forrest, and Miller, 1971), age-dependent changes in drug activity can occur as a result of altered receptor sensitivity without change in the drug level in blood or tissue. Frolkis performed a number of studies indicating that electrical thresholds are elevated in the older end organ, at least so far as autonomic and hypothalamic end-organ response is concerned. There is greater sensitivity to neurotransmitters, and as much as 20 to 50% less neurotransmitter substance is required to initiate an end-organ response (Frolkis, Bezrukov, Duplenko, and Genis, 1972).

The clinician can therefore expect a high incidence of side effects, often at a relatively low dosage level, in the elderly patient. Although therapeutic effects also occur at lower dosage levels in the elderly, the margin of safety often shrinks drastically. It is advisable to start treatment with very low doses of psychotropic medication, increasing the dosage gradually until either therapeutic success occurs or prohibitive side effects appear. Unfortunately appearance of the latter before achieving the former is quite common.

ANTIPSYCHOTIC DRUGS

Therapeutic Effects

Although some data from clinical trials of antipsychotic agents in elderly patients do exist, interpretation of these data in terms of direct patient care is often confused by the operational definition of the term "psychosis" in the elderly population. The *Diagnostic and Statistical Manual,* or *DSM-II* (American Psychiatric Association, 1968), defines "psychosis" broadly, and the term is applied equally to the elderly patient with an acute schizophreniform illness and no evidence of dementia, and the patient with a chronic dementia (organic brain syndrome) without delusions, hallucinations, or illogical thinking but whose function in society is crippled by memory loss, disorientation, and general intellectual impairment. Compounding the problem are three further groups of elderly patients classified as psychotic: those whose chronic schizophrenia has persisted into later life; those with chronic dementia who have developed schizophreniform symptoms; and those with chronic dementia whose nonschizophreniform behavioral symptoms (agitation, irritability, assaultiveness, etc.) have become severe enough to cause marked distress to themselves or to those in their environment.

Uncontrolled, impressionistic reports of efficacy for many of the antipsychotic drugs have appeared in the literature, claiming striking success for the relief of almost any imaginable behavioral symptom of elderly patients. Fortunately some controlled studies are also available, although many otherwise well-designed studies have intermingled diagnostic groupings in their subject populations, often making generalizations from these studies to daily clinical practice difficult. A Veteran's Administration cooperative project (Honigfeld, Rosenblum, Blumenthal, Lambert, and Roberts, 1965) in geriatric psychiatry studied 308 chronically schizophrenic men treated for 24 weeks with either acetophenazine (average dose 120 mg/day), trifluoperazine (average dose 12 mg/day), imipramine (average dose 150 mg/day), or placebo. Both of the phenothiazines were decidedly superior to placebo in such areas as motor disturbances, conceptual disorganization, manifest psychosis, and personal neatness. Acetophenazine was superior to trifluoperazine in reducing irritability and increasing social competence, and acetophenazine alone was significantly effective in reducing excitement. The large (10:1) dosage ratio of acetophenazine to trifluoperazine may have biased results in favor of the former drug. Imipramine was not significantly effective for relieving any measurable symptom in this population. Depression, however, was not specifically evaluated. Interestingly, a weekly group therapy session, which was provided for half the patients in each drug treatment group, appeared effective in decreasing motor disturbance and irritability, and increasing cooperation and personal neatness.

Tsuang, Lu, Stotsky, and Cole (1971) compared haloperidol (average dose 2.0 mg/day) to thioridazine (average dose 113 mg/day) in a group of "acutely psychotic" geriatric patients which included both chronic schizophrenics and chronic organic brain syndrome (OBS) patients suffering from acute behavioral symptoms. The drugs were equally effective in reducing such "nonorganic" symptoms as hallucinations, mannerisms, grandiosity, hostility, excitement, and anxiety. No improvement in memory impairment, confusion, or other intellectual deficits was noted in the OBS patients. Both drugs induced drowsiness, tremor, and blurred vision in some patients. Dystonia occurred only in the haloperidol group, and tachycardia and depression only in the thioridazine group. This study did not include a placebo control.

Seager (1955) found chlorpromazine (average dose 150 to 200 mg/day) to exert a significantly beneficial effect (when compared to placebo) on the behavior of a mixed group of elderly chronic schizophrenics and acutely disturbed patients with chronic OBS. Ratings were global, and no breakdown of differential drug efficacy in the two diagnostic groups was attempted. In a double-blind placebo-controlled study, Sugerman, Williams, and Adlerstein (1964) found haloperidol to be significantly effective in alleviating agitation, overactivity, and hostility in patients with chronic OBS. Altman, Mehta, Evenson, and Sletten (1973a) compared chlorpromazine to thioridazine in a mixed group of elderly chronic schizophrenics and elderly chronic OBS patients. They also investigated divided dosage versus once-nightly dosage schedules and evaluated differences between total daily dosages of 30, 60, 90, and 120 mg. A placebo control was not used in this study. Patient response did not differ significantly between drugs or between divided versus once-nightly dosage. There was a trend toward greater efficacy of both drugs as dosage increased. An interesting and unexpected finding (not formally documented) was a rapid clinical improvement in many patients during the "clearance period" following discontinuation of previous maintenance psychotropic medications. Barton and Hurst (1966) made a similar observation and questioned the wisdom of maintenance antipsychotic medication in many elderly patients.

There have been several studies that found the antipsychotic drugs to be ineffective in a psychogeriatric population. Abse and Dahlstrom (1960) compared chlorpromazine (75 mg/day) to placebo and to no drug in a group of elderly OBS patients with both schizophreniform and nonschizophreniform behavioral symptoms. Chlorpromazine was not significantly superior to placebo in that study. The chlorpromazine group did show a trend toward decreased hostility, but the placebo group showed a trend toward improved mood and spontaneity compared to active drug. The group which received no capsule at all did most poorly, suggesting the power of placebo effect on this population. Danto (1969) found triflupromazine (30 mg/day for 2 weeks) ineffective in significantly alleviating behavior disorders (e.g., agitation, confusion, and uncooperativeness) in chronic OBS patients newly admitted to a psychiatric inpatient service. Robinson (1959) found chlorpromazine no better than placebo for the control of nonschizophreniform behavioral symptoms in female elderly patients with chronic OBS, and the chlorpromazine group actually deteriorated at a significantly higher rate than did the placebo group, with most of this deterioration attributed to increased inertia in the active drug group. Williams, Csalany, and Misevic (1967) found chlorprothixene (average dose 100 to 300 mg/day) no better than placebo in improving behavior of a group of geriatric patients in a mental hospital, but these patients were predominantly chronic schizophrenics. Sheppard, Bhattacharyya, DiGiacomo, and Merlis (1964) compared acetophenazine (79 mg/day) to chlorpromazine (98 mg/day) and placebo in a group of elderly female patients with chronic paranoid schizophrenia. This study focused on improvement in paranoid symptomatology and found that neither drug was significantly superior to placebo. Acetophenazine showed a statistical trend toward better results, but the proposed specificity of acetophenazine for treatment of paranoid symptomatology was not confirmed. Also, chlorpromazine may have been used in a too-low dose, given the higher potency of acetophenazine. Lehmann, Ban, and Suxena (1972) found thioridazine (75 to 150 mg/day) not statistically superior to placebo in a group of elderly predominantly chronic schizophrenics. Interestingly, thioridazine did attain statistical superiority when fluoxymesterone, an anabolic steroid, was given with it.

On balance, it appears that the antipsychotic drugs in adequate dosage are probably effective for symptom relief in both elderly chronic schizophrenics and behaviorally disturbed patients with chronic OBS, especially if the patients are acutely disturbed. Such effects, however, are less consistently positive than in younger patients. The paranoid schizophreniform psychoses of later life—"paraphrenia" (Kay and Roth, 1961)—are allegedly (Post, 1965) responsive to antipsychotic drugs, but no clinical studies with this difficult group of patients have been reported. There is no evidence that these drugs are effective for reversal of memory impairment, confusion, or intellectual deterioration in the patient with a chronic OBS, even if one follows standard nomenclature and labels the patient "psychotic."

There is also no evidence at this time that one antipsychotic agent is more effective than another in this age group, a finding analogous to the lack of any drug specificity for particular subgroups of young functionally psychotic patients (Caffey, Kaim, Hollister, and Pokorny, 1970). Although chlorpromazine appears prominently in the negative clinical studies reviewed above, this showing may have been partially a function of suboptimal dosage levels. The clinician thus must choose the specific antipsychotic drug least likely to produce deleterious effects in the individual elderly patient.

Adverse Effects

The adverse effects of antipsychotic medications can be described as relating to short- and long-term drug use. Short-term use may lead to side effects including peripheral and central anticholinergic effects, as well as undesirable medical and neurological effects. Paradoxically, increased confusion in patients treated with antipsychotic agents, especially if an antiparkinsonian agent is administered concurrently, is secondary to central anticholinergic toxicity (El-Yousef, Janowsky, Davis, and Sekerke, 1973). This phenomenon is common in the elderly patient, particularly if some degree of organic dementia is present. Snyder, Greenberg, and Yamamura (1974) measured the central anticholinergic activity of various antipsychotic agents. Thioridazine, a piperidine phenothiazine, has the highest such activity; chlorpromazine and promazine among the aliphatic phenothiazines, intermediate activity; and the low-dose piperazine phenothiazines and butyrophenones the lowest activity of all. Given that central anticholinergic activity counteracts the parkinsonism-inducing action of these drugs, it follows that thioridazine should be the least and the butyrophenones and piperazines the most parkinsonism-inducing of these agents. This prediction is confirmed in clinical practice and has earned thioridazine a favored place in the psychogeriatric pharmacopeia. However, the same reasoning predicts a high incidence of central anticholinergic confusion from thioridazine. This prediction has yet to be widely tested; and, in fact, comparison of thioridazine with haloperidol did not indicate a higher incidence of increased confusion for either drug (Tsuang et al., 1971). It is crucial for the clinician to realize that increased confusion in a patient receiving antipsychotic agents may well be an adverse drug effect, and temporarily discontinuing all medications with anticholinergic activity (antipsychotic agents, antiparkinsonian agents other than L-DOPA, and tricyclic antidepressants) should be considered.

Although a number of the phenothiazines have been associated with electrocardiographic (ECG) changes (Ban and St. Jean, 1964), clinical cardiac toxicity has been most prominently reported with thioridazine, and to a lesser extent with chlorpromazine (Alexander and Nino, 1969). Thioridazine, usually in larger than normal doses, has been implicated in the production of supraventricular arrhythmias and conduction defects (Fletcher and Wenger, 1969) as well as ventricular arrhythmias, including ventricular tachycardia with fatal outcome (Kelly, Fay, and Laverty, 1963; Schoonmaker, Osteen, and Greenfield, 1966). Thioridazine commonly produces apparently benign ECG T-wave disturbances in psychiatric patients free of heart disease, the severity of which are directly related to chronological age (Thornton and Wendkos, 1971). Although thioridazine has not been associated with striking cardiotoxicity in elderly patients, this and other antipsychotic agents must be administered with caution to elderly patients with documented or suspected cardiac disease.

The recent recognition of tardive dyskinesia as a not uncommon adverse effect of prolonged (and sometimes relatively brief) administration of antipsychotic drugs is especially pertinent to the elderly patient (Crane, 1968; Greenblatt, Dominick, Stotsky, and DiMascio, 1968). This syndrome of buccofaciolingual involuntary movement occasionally accompanied by choreoathetoid movements of the extremities and trunk is especially common in elderly psychiatric patients, because of both a high incidence of extended antipsychotic administration in the elderly chronic schizophrenic and the physiognomic relationship that ill-fitting dentures or the edentulous state bears to this syndrome (Pryce and Edwards, 1966). Although physicians may tend to dismiss cosmetic factors as unimportant to the elderly patient, advanced age is often accompanied by a heightened self-consciousness of physical appearance, especially in our youth-oriented society. This self-consciousness can lead to social withdrawal and despondency if a prominent and disfiguring tardive dyskinesia develops. Steps can be taken to lower the incidence of this phenomenon in elderly patients who require antipsychotic medication. Dosage should be kept as low as is clinically possible, and the patient should occasionally be tested without medicine to assess the necessity of drug treatment. Second, anticholinergic antiparkinsonian medications should be avoided if possible, for anticholinergics may increase the intensity, duration, and perhaps the appearance of tardive dyskinesia (Crane, 1968; Klawans, 1973). Also, the antipsychotic drug with the lowest central anticholinergic effect is theoretically preferable if dyskinesia is present and antipsychotic medication cannot be discontinued.

The clinician must also consider if an antipsychotic agent is actually needed to control target symptoms. In the patient with chronic OBS and behavioral disturbances (especially tension and anxiety) of a nonschizophreniform and nonbelligerent type, the benzodiazepines are probably as efficacious as the antipsychotics (Feigenbaum, 1971; Kirven and Montero, 1973) and carry less risk of long-term toxicity. Unfortunately there is no evidence that the antianxiety agents are effective in chronic schizophrenia, paraphrenia, or schizophreniform symptoms superimposed on a chronic OBS.

ANTIDEPRESSANT DRUGS

Therapeutic Effects

Depression is the most common psychiatric illness of the elderly, both in populations of elderly persons attending psychiatric treatment facilities and among those residing in their communities (Pfeiffer and Busse, 1973). Unfortunately many of these treatable depressive illnesses are overlooked or accepted as "just growing old" because of the similarity of depressive symptomatology to the common stereotype of the withdrawn, listless, pessimistic elderly person. To complicate diagnosis further, depression can mimic dementia in the older patient (Post, 1965), with transient confusion, disorientation, and impaired intellectual function accompanying the affective episode. This picture of "pseudodementia" clears as the depression responds to treatment. Another common fallacy is the belief that depression in the elderly patient is prodromal to dementia, even when signs of organicity are absent. Careful follow-up studies have demonstrated that elderly patients with depression develop dementia (chronic OBS) no more frequently than do a control group of nondepressed elderly (Post, 1972). Although depression and dementia both occur with high frequency in the elderly, they appear to be distinct and separate illnesses, and any tendency to link depression with the prognostically discouraging dementias must be avoided. There is a risk that untreated depression may lead to secondary nutritional deficiency disease, institutional placement, social isolation, and a deepening withdrawal syndrome.

Another obstacle to detection of depression in the elderly is the high incidence of "masked" depression presenting as somatic complaints or hypochondriasis. DeAlarcon (1964) found hypochondriacal symptoms to be the first manifestation of depression in 29.1% of 152 depressed patients over age 60 admitted to the Bethlem Royal Hospital. Somatic complaints typically preceded the appearance of overtly depressive symptoms in these patients by 2 to 3 months. Overall, 63.6% of the patients in this series had hypochondriacal symptoms at some time during their illness. Comparison with younger depressed patients confirmed the impression that hypochondriasis was far more common in elderly depressed patients. Furthermore, only 20% of these hypochondriacal depressed patients had a history of excessive bodily preoccupation during earlier life.

Depressive illnesses vary markedly in intensity and duration, from mild and transient disturbances of mood to severe and protracted psychotic disorders that can be life-threatening. Mild depressions characterized by saddened mood in the absence of eating disorder, sleep disturbance, or other physiological signs and symptoms are common in the elderly. They may be reactive to one of the frequent losses of later life or occur without obvious precipitant. These mild depressions respond to a supportive psychotherapeutic approach, with emphasis on promoting increased activity and interpersonal interaction, as well as providing regular opportunities for the patient to discuss his or her problems with an empathic physician. Somatic therapy is indicated when there is increased severity or persistence of illness despite supportive psychotherapy.

Antidepressant drugs include the monoamine oxidase (MAO) inhibitors, the tricyclics, and for our purposes in this context stimulant medications and estrogens.

Monoamine Oxidase Inhibitors

Of the classes of antidepressant drugs available, the MAO inhibitors appear least suitable for use in the elderly (Prange, 1973). Their capacity to produce both hypo- and hypertensive episodes, the latter usually precipitated by ingestion of foods rich in tyramine, is especially hazardous in elderly patients with already compromised cardiovascular systems. Although the risk of hypertensive crises can be controlled by careful dietary management (Goldberg, 1964), the frequent coexistence of poor nutrition and depression in the elderly makes any dietary restriction a complicating management problem. With the threat of drug-drug interactions, and until the efficacy of the MAO inhibitors is established to be greater than that of other effective antidepressant agents, they are best used judiciously with the aged.

Stimulants

Stimulants, especially methylphenidate and dextroamphetamine, have received some attention in antidepressant clinical drug trials in the elderly. Jacobson (1958) compared methylphenidate (30 to 90 mg/day) to placebo as an adjunct to outpatient psychotherapy in depressed patients aged 60 to 74. He found methylphenidate significantly superior to placebo, but ratings were not done blindly. Kastenbaum, Slater, and Aisenberg (1964) treated geriatric inpatients (diagnoses unspecified) with dextroamphetamine (2.5 mg t.i.d. for 6 weeks). Compared to placebo, dextroamphetamine produced deterioration in affect (comfort; happiness; and absence of complaints, worries, and fears) and vivacity at the end of the 6-week trial; moreover, patients became more likely to perceive themselves as "old." This study supports the clinical impression that although psychostimulants may initially improve mood this effect is often followed by dysphoria as treatment continues (Prange, 1973). There is evidence that the euphoriant effects of methylphenidate are decreased in the elderly, and the anorexiant effects are enhanced

(Bender, 1974). Methylphenidate potentiates the activity of several drugs (Ganettson, Perel, and Dayton, 1969) by decreasing the activity of microsomal enzymes. This effect must be considered if methylphenidate is prescribed to an elderly person receiving multiple medications. On balance, the role of the psychostimulants as antidepressant agents appears limited, although some clinicians have successfully used them over brief periods for the treatment of mild depression. Adverse effects of these agents include dysphoric mood, irritability, anorexia, and weight loss, as well as production or exacerbation of paranoid symptoms with extended use. These drugs should be avoided in patients with a history of paranoid ideation or drug abuse.

Tricyclic Antidepressants

The tricyclic antidepressants are effective agents (Morris and Beck, 1974) and are widely used with the elderly (Prien, Haber, and Caffey, 1975). Although few clinical studies have specifically examined their efficacy in the depressed geriatric patient, some data are available. Hordern, Burt, and Holt (1965) compared imipramine to amitriptyline in depressed female patients and specifically examined age-related effects. They found both drugs to be effective antidepressants, but amitriptyline was significantly more effective for the "middle aged" (50 to 59 years) and the "elderly" (60 to 70 years). Amitriptyline was more effective than imipramine for severely depressed patients. Neither drug was very useful for the severely depressed patient with delusions. Although side effects were described as "of little consequence," a 69-year-old woman died suddenly of a presumed myocardial infarct after 4 days of imipramine, and a 56-year-old woman developed acute glaucoma while receiving amitriptyline.

Kernohan, Chambers, Wilson, and Daugherty (1967) compared nortriptyline to placebo in 92 patients "with a variety of symptoms and diagnoses typical of geriatric mental hospital patients." Although the patients receiving active drug improved significantly in a few areas of self-care, the results were generally disappointing. Drowsiness, confusion, weakness, constipation, and urinary retention were problems in the drug group. Chesrow, Kaplitz, Breme, Sabatini, Vetra, and Marquardt (1964) compared nortriptyline to placebo in chronically medically ill patients of mixed age with symptoms of anxiety and depression. Although nortriptyline was significantly superior to placebo in relieving both anxiety and depression in the whole group, the drug was least effective in the subgroup of patients over 65. Since nortriptyline prolongs the half-life of antipyrine and bishydroxycoumarin by decreasing the activity of hepatic microsomal drug-metabolizing enzymes (Vesell, Passananti, and Greene, 1970), this effect must be considered in patients on oral anticoagulant therapy or other medical regimens.

Ayd (1971) used doxepin in an extended, open clinical trial in a group of 40 chronically depressed patients, 20 of whom were older adults (50 to 76 years old). Doxepin appeared to be an effective antidepressant and remarkably free of severe side effects. Orthostatic hypotension was not noted; and except for transient sinus tachycardia in five patients, no adverse cardiac effects were detected clinically or by ECG. Hollister (1974) questioned the antidepressant potency of doxepin compared to other tricyclics on theoretical grounds. Although his concerns have not been supported in human clinical trials, increased dosage levels may be necessary when using doxepin. Doxepin has been studied in geriatric nursing home patients (diagnoses not further specified) and was found to be of value (Chien, Stotsky, and Cole, 1973). However, these patients were not diagnosed as depressed. Grof, Saxena, Cantor, Daigle, Hetherington, and Haines (1974) compared doxepin and amitriptyline in depressed patients whose average age was 51 years. Although the two drugs were equally efficacious, doxepin had fewer side effects and was significantly superior for patients with hypochondriacal complaints. This latter finding, together with the low cardiac toxicity (Ayd, 1971) and relatively low anticholinergic activity (Prange, 1973), make doxepin an attractive tricyclic for use in elderly depressed patients.

Numerous studies (Overall and Hollister, 1971) have indicated that the antipsychotic drugs are effective in the treatment of agitated depressions, perhaps more so than the tricyclic antidepressants, which appear superior for the treatment of retarded depressions. Kiev (1972) found the antipsychotic agent thiothixene slightly superior to the tricyclic antidepressant protriptyline in a group of psychotically depressed patients, especially if agitation and anxiety were prominent. Because the tricyclic antidepressants often increase confusion in patients with a depression superimposed on an OBS, an antipsychotic agent such as thiothixene may be the drug of choice in elderly patients who present the latter two clinical syndromes. Controlled trials in elderly depressed patients of antipsychotic agents with demonstrated antidepressant potency are clearly needed.

Side Effects

A detailed discussion of tricyclic antidepressant side effects is contained elsewhere in this volume; therefore only the adverse reactions with special relevance for the elderly patient are discussed here. Orthostatic hypotension is a greater hazard to the elderly patient with possibly compromised cerebral circulation than to the younger patient; the elderly must be instructed to change from a supine to a sitting or standing position slowly and with careful attention to the onset of dizziness or unsteadiness. As is the case with some phenothiazines (Davis, 1974), tricyclic antidepressants block the action of guanethidine, a frequently used antihypertensive medication for the aged, and can thus complicate management of hypertension. The peripheral anticholinergic actions of the tricyclics can delay or halt micturition, produce constipation, or precipitate acute glaucoma. Implications are obvious for the elderly patient with prostatic hypertrophy, problems with bowel evacuation, or increased intraocular pressure. Although dryness of the mouth is usually benign, patients may drink excessive amounts of water to alleviate the discomfort. If a patient is already taking a thiazide diuretic or chlorpropamide, both of which are commonly prescribed to elderly patients, free water excretion may be impaired, and water intoxication can develop (Raskind, 1974).

The central anticholinergic toxicity of tricyclics has received less attention than peripheral anticholinergic toxicity but is a cause for concern in the elderly patient. Delirium as a complication of imipramine therapy in elderly patients has been recognized for more than a decade (Christe, 1961), but not until recently was this effect demonstrated to be secondary to central anticholinergic activity (El-Yousef et al., 1973). In a series of patients treated for depression with imipramine and amitriptyline, the incidence of delirium was 35% in those over 40 years of age, compared to only 13% in those under 40 (Davies, Tucker, Harrow, and Detre, 1971). Nineteen of the 20 patients who developed this confusional syndrome (nocturnal restlessness, pacing, forgetfulness, agitation, disorientation, illogical thoughts, and occasional delusional states) received imipramine. The risk of producing this anticholinergic confusion syndrome is especially high in elderly patients with a chronic OBS.

The cardiac toxicity of tricyclic antidepressants has received much more attention in the general medical than in the psychiatric literature. Frequent reports have documented the occurrence of serious arrhythmias, conduction disturbances, and cardiac death in young persons who had ingested large amounts of drug, usually as a self-induced overdose (Freeman, Mundy, Beattie, and Ryan, 1969). With the exception of doxepin, the commonly prescribed tricyclics have all produced cardiotoxicity in large doses. If supranormal doses can be cardiotoxic in young adults, will therapeutic doses produce serious cardiotoxity in elderly persons with clinical or subclinical heart disease? There are some data which indicate that the already damaged heart may in fact be more susceptible to the tricyclics. Williams and Sherter (1971) reported a man with hypertensive heart disease who developed fatal cardiac toxicity while receiving imipramine (75 mg/day). A large retrospective study found a significantly higher incidence of sudden, unexpected death in a population with pre-existing heart disease who had received amitriptyline than in a control group of cardiac patients who had not received tricyclics (Moir, 1973). Although retrospective studies and case reports present difficulties in interpretation, tricyclics must be administered cautiously to elderly patients, especially those with documented heart disease.

Estrogens

Estrogenic compounds have been widely advocated in the treatment of depression in menopausal and postmenopausal women on the assumption that gonadal hormone deficiency is responsible for depression and other behavioral symptoms in this group of middle-aged and elderly women (Wilson and Wilson, 1963; Rhoades, 1967; Kerr, 1968). Even though there is little factual support for a specific menopausal estrogen-deficiency behavioral syndrome (Eisdorfer and Raskind, 1975), early case reports (Danziger, 1942) claimed a definite degree of success with estrogen therapy of involutional melancholia.

A more careful study correlated psychiatric status in depressed menopausal and postmenopausal women with vaginal cytology as an index of estrogen effect (Ripley, Shorr, and Papanicolaou, 1940). These authors concluded that serious depressions with agitation, feelings of unreality, suspiciousness, hypochondriacal and nihilistic delusions, negativism, abusiveness, and combativeness showed little if any symptomatic response to estrogen therapy. They did find that the milder depressive reactions were more likely to be favorably influenced by estrogen therapy. In a group of menopausal women, however, Utian (1972) found no difference between estrogen and placebo in the relief of depressive symptoms.

Despite the absence of convincing studies, the efficacy of exogenous estrogen in promoting a sense of well-being in older women is widely accepted by clinicians. Data from estrogen administration in premenopausal women may help explain this clinical impression. After the oral contraceptive had been in use for several years, anecdotal reports appeared of patients noting a sense of well-being and "feeling better" while using estrogen-progesterone combinations (Glick, 1967). Hamburg, Moos, and Yalom (1968) correlated the increased sense of well-being with the estrogen phase of sequential pills and with the high estrogen follicular phase of the natural menstrual cycle, thus implicating estrogen as the agent producing the positive psychological effect.

Theoretical support for an estrogenic "antidepressant" effect comes from studies (Klaiber, Broverman, Vogel, Kobayashi, and Moriarity, 1972) demonstrating a lowered plasma MAO level following administration of conjugated equine estrogen to a group of endogenously depressed menstruating women (mean age 28.7 years). All of 14 endogenously depressed female patients reported improvement in mood ranging from moderate to marked, but a control group was not used. These data suggest that estrogens may exert a mood-elevating effect in certain patients regardless of whether a state of estrogen deficiency exists. Perhaps the sense of well-being noted by postmenopausal women given estrogen replacement is the same effect noted by young women receiving exogeneous estrogen as an oral contraceptive agent.

ANTIMANIC DRUGS

Lithium carbonate is effective in the treatment of acute mania and lowers the incidence of manic and probably depressive exacerbations of manic-depressive disease. This illness is often first detected in later life (Klerman and Barrett, 1974) and certainly continues into old age in patients who had developed the disease earlier. In a large collaborative study, Prien, Caffey, and Klett (1974) found lithium equally efficacious in elderly and young patients, supporting the clinical impression that lithium is useful in elderly manic patients, provided toxicity can be controlled.

Elderly patients tend to develop lithium central nervous system (CNS) and neuromuscular toxicity at lower serum levels than do young patients (Van Der Velde, 1971). Furthermore, the half-life of lithium increases from 24 hr for the middle-aged adult to 36 to 48 hr for the elderly person (Davis, 1974), and even longer if glomerular filtration rate is seriously impaired. The toxic level for certain older individuals may therefore be reached quickly, necessitating low dosage levels (600 to 900 mg/day for the acutely manic patient) and careful monitoring of serum levels and clinical status. It is sometimes helpful to add an antipsychotic agent to the regimen of the floridly manic elderly patient to speed recovery and prevent exhaustion while the more slowly acting lithium begins to exert its effect. Any of the antipsychotic drugs is probably effective for this purpose, although haloperidol, a commonly used agent in manic patients, has recently been implicated in a severe toxic reaction when used in combination with lithium. Cohen and Cohen (1974) described irreversible neurological sequelae in four female patients (two of whom were elderly) who received a combination of haloperidol and lithium for control of acute manic episodes. The two elderly women developed transient delirium, fever, leukocytosis, and hepatic enzyme elevations, as well as persistent dyskinesias and parkinsonian signs and symptoms. Serum lithium levels never exceeded 1.5 mEq/liter, and haloperidol was not given in excessive amounts. This unusual adverse reaction to the combination of lithium and haloperidol may prove to be rare but must still be considered if the drugs are used together.

The most common hazard of administering lithium to the elderly patient is the effect of body sodium depletion on lithium metabolism. Many elderly patients are on sodium-restricted diets as part of a treatment regimen for congestive heart failure, renal disease, or hypertension. As body sodium is depleted, the kidney avidly retains lithium, often rapidly leading to excessive serum lithium concentrations. This phenomenon may explain the deaths reported when lithium was used as a dietary salt substitute in sodium-free diets. The widespread use of thiazide diuretics, which enhance the proximal renal tubular absorption of lithium ion, poses a serious hazard. Giving a thiazide diuretic to a person on maintenance lithium can produce toxicity within 1 to 2 days (Baer, Platman, and Fieve, 1972). The distal tubule can more readily distinguish between sodium and lithium. Spironolactone (Aldactone®), an aldosterone antagonist that acts on the distal renal tubule, is unlikely to cause lithium retention. Thus if a diuretic is indicated for a patient on lithium, spironolactone may be the safest one with which to initiate therapy.

Lithium directly suppresses thyroid gland function and can produce both goiter and frank hypothyroidism, the latter often mimicking depression or dementia in the elderly patient (Eisdorfer and Raskind, 1975). Serum triio-dothyronine (T_3) levels decline significantly with age in the normal person, as opposed to a negligible decrease in serum thyroxine (T_4), as reported by Gregerman and Bierman (1974). Interestingly, lithium depresses T_3 production more than that of T_4 and could potentially magnify the natural age-related reduction in serum T_3. The physician monitoring thyroid function in the elderly patient on lithium should thus examine serum levels of both T_3 and T_4.

In summary, lithium is an effective drug for management of the elderly patient with an acute manic episode or recurrent episodes of mania. The toxicity of this drug, however, may be enhanced in the elderly patient, and management of concurrent illnesses which necessitate sodium restriction or diuretic administration can complicate lithium therapy tremendously.

ANTIANXIETY DRUGS AND HYPNOTICS

Although the barbiturates and nonbarbiturate hypnotics are generally prescribed for sleep, and the minor tranquilizers (benzodiazepines and propanediols) for the relief of daytime anxiety and agitation, the two groups have much in common. They are often prescribed for overlapping effects and hence are discussed together. Their use in elderly patients is widespread, with differential indications determined more by clinical opinion than by controlled studies.

Hypnotics

The barbiturates were without serious competition as hypnotic and sedative agents for many years, and clinical reports of excessive sedation, motor incoordination, and paradoxical excitement in elderly patients soon appeared. In a widely quoted article, Dawson-Butterworth (1970) stated that the barbiturates are "absolutely contraindicated in the geriatric population." Several clinical trials have suggested, however, that the alarm over barbiturates in the elderly was probably more a result of excessive dosage and prolonged use rather than a singular toxicity of barbiturates themselves.

Stotsky, Cole, Tang, and Gahm (1971) found butabarbital (50 mg h.s.) to be an effective and safe hypnotic but to be associated with some undesirable daytime sedation when the dose was increased to 100 mg h.s. Pattison and Allen (1972) found pentobarbital to be the best of four hypnotics (pentobarbital 100 mg, secobarbital 100 mg, ethchlorvynol 50 mg, methprylon 300 mg) in a group of elderly medical patients in a chronic disease hospital. Of these four hypnotics, only ethchlorvynol was not significantly superior to placebo. When Exton-Smith, Hodkinson, and Cranie (1963) compared amobarbital to placebo at the relatively large dose of 200 mg, morning drowsiness or "hangover" was a distressing problem and caused patients subjectively to rate the drug no better than placebo. Meprobamate 800 mg was judged superior to placebo in this study.

Benzodiazepines

The benzodiazepines, especially chlordiazepoxide, diazepam, and flurazepam, have received some scrutiny in clinical geriatric drug studies. Chesrow, Kaplitz, Breme, Musci, and Sabatini (1962) found diazepam effective in the relief of tremor, anxiety, restlessness, and somatic complaints in "nonschizophrenic elderly patients," but this study was neither blind nor controlled. DeLemos, Clement, and Nickels (1965) reported diazepam (7.5 mg/day) significantly better than placebo for improving sleep quality, and alleviating anxiety, hyperactivity, and confusion in 50 patients with chronic OBS. Side effects included oversedation in 12 patients and euphoria with impaired gait in one (a "paradoxical reaction"). All side effects were eliminated by adjusting the dose downward. Diazepam (average dose 8 mg/day) was compared to mesoridazine (average dose 42 mg/day), a phenothiazine antipsychotic agent, in chronic OBS patients with "nonpsychotic" symptoms such as anxiety, agitation, and irritability (Kirven and Montero, 1973). In this important study both drugs were judged effective, and although mesoridazine showed a slight trend toward increased efficacy, the most striking aspect of the data was the similarity of the two drugs in the treatment of nonschizophreniform behavioral signs and symptoms in demented patients.

In an open, uncontrolled study of chlordiazepoxide in elderly medical, surgical, and OBS patients, Jones (1962) found a dose of 10 mg t.i.d. effective in relieving anxiety, tension, and "behavioral crises." Chlordiazepoxide (average dose 21 mg/day) was compared to a phenothiazine (thioridazine, average dose 42 mg/day) in a group of OBS patients with behavioral disturbances. As in Kirven and Montero's study, the benzodiazepine was as effective as the phenothiazine in alleviating anxiety and tension over a 7-week period. Chlordiazepoxide was found less likely to produce significant hypotension in this group of patients (Feigenbaum, 1971).

Benzodiazepines have been compared directly to barbiturates in two studies using elderly subjects. Fisher and Gal (1969) compared the popular hypnotic flurazepam (15 mg) to amobarbital (50 mg) in a double-blind crossover study and found no significant difference between the two hypnotics. Stotsky and Borozne (1972) compared chlordiazepoxide (5 mg q.i.d.) to butabarbital (15 mg q.i.d.) for the treatment of anxiety and tension in geriatric patients and found the barbiturate equal or superior to the benzodiazepine.

As was found earlier for the barbiturates, benzodiazepines also have enhanced toxicity in the elderly. The percentage of patients who develop excessive drowsiness while receiving diazepam or chlordiazepoxide is significantly higher in the elderly than in persons less than 40 years of age (Boston Collaborative Drug Surveillance Program, 1973). Evans and Jarvis (1972) described a rapidly reversible syndrome of confusion, disorientation, and dysarthria in elderly patients receiving 5 mg nitrazepam per day. This syndrome did not occur at a lower dose of nitrazepam (2.5 mg/day) in these authors' extensive geriatric practice. Glasgow (1969) described reversible ataxia, apathy, and drowsiness in three elderly patients receiving 30 mg chlordiazepoxide daily. The syndrome was readily reproduced with administration of a challenge trial of chlordiazepoxide under controlled circumstances.

Despite the disappointing similarities between the side effects of benzodiazepines and barbiturates in the elderly, the former class of drugs has several practical and theoretical advantages. Foremost are the reportedly low incidence of drug dependence and addiction with benzodiazepines, and the low probability that an intentional or accidental overdose will prove fatal (Greenblatt and Shader, 1974). The clinician must keep in mind, however, that addiction can occur with chronic administration, and fatal overdose is possible, especially if benzodiazepines are combined with other depressant drugs. Also of importance to the elderly patient, who often receives multiple drugs, is the absence of documented significant effect on hepatic microsomal enzyme systems attributable to benzodiazepines. The barbiturates stimulate enzyme systems, thus enhancing metabolism of other drugs such as tricyclic antidepressants and oral anticoagulants (Conney, 1967). Flurazepam may be a more attractive hypnotic than barbiturates, glutethimide, chloral hydrate, or methaqualone because of superior persistence of hypnotic efficacy over time (Kales, Kales, Leo, and Bixlor, 1973) and possibly less interference with the normal sleep cycle (Kales, Allen, Scharf, and Kales, 1970). Flurazepam suppresses REM sleep only mildly if at all; and the undesirable REM rebound phenomenon seen with barbiturates and glutethimide is not a common problem (Greenblatt and Shader, 1974).

Some mention should be made concerning the usefulness in the elderly patient of the ancient antianxiety drug ethanol. Both beer and wine have been demonstrated to reduce disturbing behavioral symptoms and increase social interaction in institutional settings (Chien et al., 1973). Ethanol is also a useful and socially acceptable reinforcer in behavioral approaches to the treatment of behavioral disorders in the elderly (Mishara and Kastenbaum, 1974) and in changing role relationships in an inpatient setting, leading to more effective behavior on the part of older patients. In the outpatient, of course, the danger of alcoholism must be kept in mind.

A warning about the use of all the above agents, including the benzodiazepines, is necessary. They are most useful for short-term relief of anxiety and/or insomnia. Tolerance to them develops more or less rapidly, and the physician can expect decreasing therapeutic effectiveness and increasing risk of psychological dependence and/or physiological addiction with chronic administration of these antianxiety and hypnotic drugs.

COGNITIVE ACTING DRUGS

Intellectual impairment has always been regarded as an inevitable concomitant of normal aging. Recent longitudinal studies by Eisdorfer and his collaborators (Eisdorfer and Wilkie, 1973) as well as by others (Baltes and Labouvie, 1973) suggest that such decline is not as large as was thought, and for certain abilities may not occur at all until shortly before death (Jarvik and Cohen, 1973). Intellectual decline, when it does occur, may develop in the registration of information secondary to sensory deficits, response interference, or restrictions on retrieval. It may also be a function of environmental factors such as the speed of presentation of stimuli and of autonomic dysfunction (Granville-Grossman and Turner, 1966; Eisdorfer, Nowlin, and Wolkie, 1970).

Memory loss and intellectual impairment are among the hallmarks of senile brain syndrome regardless of etiology, and perhaps for this reason cognitive-acting drugs are often referred to as "geriatric" drugs. The search for drugs that may reverse or retard intellectual impairment and behavioral regression due to CNS impairment is intense, and a wide range of medications have been investigated for properties as "geriatric" drugs. The most promising and widely used are reviewed here.

Stimulants and Analeptics

The amphetamines, methylphenidate, deanol, pipradrol, pentylenetetrazol, and magnesium pemoline have been reported to increase activity level, alertness, and attention to stimuli; improve recall and recognition; counteract lethargy; and stimulate circulation and respiration. Promising early positive findings have not been supported by later controlled research, however (Gilbert, Donnelly, Zimmer, and Kubis, 1973).

The drug that is probably most widely used in geriatric studies is pentylenetetrazol. Equivocal or negative findings in recent controlled studies (Leckman, Ananth, Ban, and Lehmann, 1971; Lu, Stotsky, and Cole, 1971; Stotsky, Cole, Lu, and Smiflin, 1972) suggest that its effectiveness is limited, although individual patients seem to respond remarkably well. Symptomatic changes reportedly occur even in the absence of quantifiable improvement in intellectual functioning (La Brecque and Goldberg, 1967). The major side effects are few, though annoying: nausea, vomiting, dizziness, and headache. It is contraindicated in convulsive disorders.

Magnesium pemoline (Cylert®) was hailed as a possible breakthrough following positive findings in improving learning and memory in animal studies and in uncontrolled studies on humans. Follow-up studies were unable to confirm the initial encouraging reports, although the drug was found to have stimulant properties (Talland, Hagen, and James, 1967; Eisdorfer, Conner and Wilkie, 1968; Greenblatt, DiMascio, Messier, and Stotsky, 1969; Gilbert et al., 1973).

Vasodilators

Vasodilators (nicotinyl alcohol, papaverine, cyclandelate, isoxsuprine, hexobenidine) relax the smooth muscle of blood vessel walls in the peripheral circulation and possibly in the cerebral vessels. Hypothetically this effect would be to decrease ischemic changes in brain tissue by increasing cerebral blood flow and oxygenation of brain tissue. This presumed effect has not yet been convincingly demonstrated. Moreover, mental changes may not necessarily accompany increased cerebral blood flow and improved metabolism of glucose in hypoxic areas. At issue is the question of how much of the deficit is a function of primary degeneration and depletion of CNS tissue as opposed to degeneration secondary to reduced cerebral perfusion. Kety and Schmidt (1948) demonstrated reduced cerebral blood flow in aged patients, but Wang (1973) pointed out that reduced cerebral blood flow in the aged may occur "with or without neuropsychiatric disorder." Terry and Wisniewski (1972), among others, proposed that senile dementia is not different from Alzheimer's disease of later onset, and that neither disease is primarily of vascular origin. Thus the efficacy of vasodilator treatment for chronic OBS in the aged rests on questionable albeit logical clinical grounds.

Papaverine, an alkaloid derivative of opium with vasodilator properties, has been studied. Although general improvement in behavior and in the performance of activities of daily living, as well as increased cerebral blood flow and decreased arterial resistance, have been reported, significant intellectual improvement has not been consistently demonstrated (Jayne, Scheinber, and Rich, 1952; Stern, 1970; Lu et al., 1971). Reported side effects are drowsiness, dizziness, flushing, headache, and hypotension.

The action of cyclandelate is similar to that of papaverine (Karlsberg, Elliott, and Adams, 1963). Positive findings have been reported in both uncontrolled and controlled studies (Eichorn, 1965; Ball and Taylor, 1967; Birkett, 1971; Fine, 1971), including one (Smith, Lowrey, and Davis, 1968) in which patients improved on long-term memory, verbal expansiveness, reasoning, and orientation. The group consisted primarily of mildly impaired patients.

Hydergine

Hydergine®, consisting of three hydrogenated alkaloids of ergot, has been reported to increase cerebral blood flow and oxygen uptake by direct action on ganglion cell metabolism, without producing hypotension (Emmenegger and Meier-Ruge, 1968). The vast majority of controlled studies against placebo have been positive (Forster, Schultig, and Henderson, 1955; Freeman and Murray, 1966; Gerin, 1969; Triboletti and Ferri, 1969; Ditch, Kelly, and Resnick, 1971; Banen, 1972; Roubicek, Geiger, and Abt, 1972). In one study comparing it to papaverine, it was found to be clearly superior (Rao and Norris, 1972). Improvement has been noted in attitude, ward behavior, activities of daily living, and somatic complaints, but has not been demonstrated quantitatively in cognitive functions. The study of Roubicek et al. (1972) is of great interest in that improvement was most marked for symptoms commonly associated with depression (emotional withdrawal, depressive mood, motor retardation, blunted affect, activity, wakefulness), whereas cognitive function was not demonstrably improved. Perhaps the efficacy of Hydergine is a result of antidepressant activity. Pacha and Salzman (1970) found it to inhibit reuptake of norepinephrine *in vitro,* an action properly compatible with the antidepressant effect.

Anticoagulants

Walsh (1969) and Walsh and Walsh (1972), using bishydroxycoumarin in uncontrolled studies, claimed remarkable improvements in intellectual function, thus apparently confirming early clinical reports of such changes. The action is presumed to be due to decreased sludging and decreased tendency to thrombus formation. Better-controlled studies, however, have been less encouraging. Lukas, Hambacher, and Fullica (1973) compared an oral anticoagulant to papaverine over a 4-month period in small groups of patients with OBS. No significant differences were found between the two groups, and both groups showed significant deterioration in the Graham-Kendall test of organic abnormalities. There was an insignificant trend toward improvement on a mental status questionnaire in both groups. In a 1-yr placebo-controlled, double-blind study, Ratner, Rosenberg, Vojtech, and Engelsmann (1972) found no difference in 24 of 25 variables reflecting cognitive functions and mental changes. However, the anticoagulant group showed a trend toward less deterioration than the control group. The potential hazards of anticoagulation in aged subjects appear to be a legitimate deterrent to aggressive use of this approach.

RNA-Like Compounds

Tricyanoaminopropene precursors like magnesium pemoline and both RNA and DNA have been administered to patients with conflicting reports of significantly positive intellectual changes (Cameron and Solyom, 1961; Cameron, Sved, and Solyom, 1963).

Procaine Amide and Gerovital

For years a buffered form of procaine amide developed in Romania has been promoted enthusiastically as an antiaging medication. It is usually given intramuscularly three times a week for 12 weeks. Many uncontrolled studies, for the most part in Europe, found it effective for treating a broad spectrum of physical and mental disorders associated with aging. Procaine amide was studied intensively in England, Canada, and the United States by controlled studies, most of which were negative (Kral, Cahn, and Deutsch, 1962). For a time Gerovital ("European" procaine) was discredited. Recently, however, interest has been revived because the drug was found to be a reversible inhibitor of MAO (MacFarlane and Besbris, 1974). Sakalis, Oh, Gershon, and Shopsin (1974) found Gerovital to have a mild euphoriant effect in 10 senile-arteriosclerotic patients with features of depression, suggesting a possible antidepressant effect for the drug; and at this writing Kline and his collaborators (Kline, 1973) have initiated a series of open and controlled studies to evaluate its efficacy in the treatment of psychiatric disorders of aging, following procedures developed and clinically tested for many years in Romania (Aslan, 1956). In view of the data reported by Nies, Robinson, Davis, and Ravaris (1973), indicating increased levels of MAO in the aging CNS, the effectiveness of a mild reversible MAO inhibitor holds some promise.

Hyperbaric Oxygenation

Following remarkably positive findings by Jacobs and her associates (Jacobs, Winter, Alvis, and Small, 1969) of the effectiveness of pure oxygen administered under high pressure (100% at 2.5 atm absolute, 3 hr/day for 15 days) in improving memory and other cognitive functions, other investigators undertook to replicate their findings. Goldfarb's group (Goldfarb, Hochstadt, Jacobson, and Weinstein, 1972) were unable to confirm the findings, although some clinical reports are positive. Systematic studies are now underway to evaluate this phenomenon further. One serious problem is the transiency of such improvements and the elaborate procedures required for a relatively few patients.

Vitamins

Vitamin preparations are extensively administered to the elderly; Lehmann et al., (1972) suggest from clinical experience that the B vitamins and vitamin C may be helpful in demented patients and at least are nontoxic. Altman, Mehta, Evenson, and Sletten (1973b) found administration of a vitamin B complex-vitamin C combination strikingly effective in the reduction of excitement and agitation in patients with OBS. They hypothesized that institutionalized elderly may be vitamin C-deficient. Cognitive function *per se* was not tested. This interesting finding deserves further study. The therapeutic use of vitamins where medically indicated, particularly among the elderly with poor nutritional habits, should not be overlooked.

Gonadal hormones have also been suggested as therapeutic for elderly patients with cognitive deterioration. Michael (1970) administered conjugated equine estrogen to a group of elderly women in a nursing home in a 38-month placebo-controlled trial. The estrogen group showed significant behavioral improvement compared to placebo, but the dropout rate was very high. Lifshitz and Kline (1961) compared estrogen to placebo in a large group of chronically demented men for 15 months; the only significant difference between groups was a higher mortality in the estrogen-treated group. Further work in this area, however, may prove profitable.

β-Adrenergic Blockage

Eisdorfer et al. (1970) administered propranolol, a β-adrenergic receptor blocking agent, to aged patients and found that performance on serial rote learning improved and the level of serum free fatty acids decreased. These data suggest a facilitatory effect on cognitive function of decreased autonomic nervous system arousal. This finding warrants further investigation.

In summary, none of the cognitive-acting drugs has yet demonstrated significant retardation or reversal of intellectual impairment, although Hydergine, some of the vasodilators, and for some patients some of the stimulants have improved attitudes, moods, and performance of daily living activities.

CONCLUSIONS

It is clear that the therapeutic nihilism associated with the aged psychiatric patient is unwarranted. In addition to chemotherapy, a broad array of individual and group therapies, behavior modification strategies, sheltered workshops, and environmental manipulations are quite effective with this population (Gottesman, Quarterman, and Cohn, 1973). The recent trend toward moving the elderly psychiatric patient back into the community (i.e., nursing home) from the state psychiatric hospital has merit; but in consequence many aged patients with profound psychiatric problems are receiving no psychiatric evaluation, and their care is compromised as a result. Psychotropic medications may be used unwisely in this setting, especially in attempts to control recalcitrant individuals with excessive sedation. Such abuses are more likely to occur in the "hopeless and helpless" atmosphere of some custodial environments.

Psychopharmacological agents alone or in conjunction with other forms of treatment often produce gratifying therapeutic success among the aged. Results will be far more satisfactory, however, when more is known about the psychological and physiological bases for age-related changes, and for avenues of intervention into their more deleterious consequences.

REFERENCES

Abse, D. W., and Dahlstrom, W. G. (1960): The value of chemotherapy in senile mental disturbances. *J.A.M.A.,* 174:2036–2042.

Alexander, C. S., and Nino, A. (1969): Cardiovascular complications in young patients taking psychotropic drugs. *Am. Heart J.,* 78:757–769.

Altman, H., Mehta, D., Evenson, R., and Sletten, I. W. (1973*a*): Behavioral effects of drug therapy on psychogeriatric inpatients. I. Chlorpromazine and thioridazine. *J. Am. Geriatr. Soc.,* 21:241–248.

Altman, H., Mehta, D., Evenson, R., and Sletten, I. W. (1973*b*): Behavioral effects of drug therapy on psychogeriatric inpatients. II. Mutivitamin supplements. *J. Am. Geriatr. Soc.,* 21:249–252.

American Psychiatric Association (1968): *Diagnostic and Statistical Manual,* Ed. 2. American Psychiatric Association, Washington, D.C.

Aslan, A. (1956): A new method for prophylaxis and treatment of aging with Novocain—entrophic and rejuvenating effects. *Therapiewoche,* 7:14–24.

Ayd, F. J. (1971): Long term administration of doxepin (Sinequan). *Dis. Nerv. Syst.,* 32:617–622.

Baer, L., Platman, S., and Fieve, R. (1972): Lithium metabolism: its electrolyte actions and relationship to aldosterone. In: *Recent Advances in the Psychobiology of the Depressive Illnesses,* edited by T. A. Williams, M. M. Katz, and J. A. Shield. Department of Health, Education, and Welfare, Washington, D.C.

Ball, J. A. C., and Taylor, A. R. (1967): Effect of cyclandelate on mental function and cerebral blood flow in elderly patients. *Lancet,* 3:525–528.

Baltes, P. B., and Labouvie, G. V. (1973): Adult development of intellectual performance: description, explanation and modification. In: *The Psychology of Adult Development and Aging,* edited by C. Eisdorfer and M. P. Lawton. American Psychological Association, Washington, D.C.

Ban, T. A., and St. Jean, A. (1964): The effect of phenothiazines on the electrocardiogram. *Can. Med. Assoc. J.,* 91:537–541.

Banen, D. M. (1972): An ergot preparation (Hydergine) for relief of symptoms of cerebrovascular insufficiency. *J. Am. Geriatr. Soc.,* 20:22–24.

Barton, R., and Hurst, L. (1966): Unnecessary use of tranquilizers in elderly patients. *Br. J. Psychiatry,* 112:989–990.

Bellville, J. W., Forrest, W. H., and Miller, E. (1971): Influence of age on pain relief from analgesics. *J.A.M.A.,* 217:1835–1841.

Bender, A. D. (1974): Pharmacodynamic principles of drug therapy in the aged. *J. Am. Geriatr. Soc.,* 22:296–303.

Bendkowski, B. (1970): Choice of antibiotics for elderly patients. *Practitioner,* 205: 85–89.

Birkett, D. P. (1971): Vasodilators in geriatric psychiatry. *J. Med. Soc. N.J.,* 68:619–623.

Boston Collaborative Drug Surveillance Program (1973): Clinical depression of the central nervous system due to diazepam and chlordiazepoxide in relation to cigarette smoking and age. *N. Eng. J. Med.,* 288:277–280.

Brotman, H. B. (1973): Who are the aging? In: *Mental Illness in Later Life,* edited by E. W. Busse and E. Pfeiffer. American Psychiatric Association, Washington, D.C.

Busse, E. W., and Pfeiffer, E. (1969): Functional psychiatric disorders in old age. In: *Behavior and Adaptation in Late Life,* edited by E. W. Busse and E. Pfeiffer. Little Brown, Boston.

Caffey, E. M., Kaim, S. C., Hollister, L. E., and Pokorny, A. D. (1970): *Drug Treatment in Psychiatry.* Veterans Administration, Washington, D.C.

Cameron, D. E., and Solyom, L. (1961): Effects of ribonucleic acid on memory. *Geriatrics,* 16:74–81.

Cameron, D. E., Sved, S., and Solyom, L. (1963): Effects of ribonucleic acid on memory defects in the aged. *Am. J. Psychiatry,* 120:320–325.

Chesrow, E. J., Kaplitz, S. E., Breme, J. T., Musci, J., and Sabatini, R. (1962): Use of a new benzodiazepine derivative (Valium) in chronically ill and disturbed elderly patients. *J. Am. Geriatr. Soc.,* 10:667–670.

Chesrow, E. J., Kaplitz, S. E., Breme, J. T., Sabatini, R., Vetra, H., and Marquardt, G. H. (1964): Nortriptyline for the treatment of anxiety and depression in chronically ill and geriatric patients. *J. Am. Geriatr. Soc.,* 12:271–277.

Chien, C., Stotsky, B. A., and Cole, J. O. (1973): Psychiatric treatment for nursing home patients: Drug, alcohol and milieu. *Am. J. Psychiatry,* 130:543–548.

Christe, P. (1961): Experience with imipramine (Tofranil) in geriatrics. *Acta Psychiatr. Scand. [Suppl. 162]*, 37:118–120.

Cohen, W. J., and Cohen, N. H. (1974): Lithium carbonate, haloperidol, and irreversible brain damage. *J.A.M.A.,* 230:1283–1287.

Conney, A. H. (1967): Pharmacologic implications of microsomal enzyme induction. *Pharmacol. Rev.,* 19:317–366.

Crane, G. E. (1968): Tardive dyskinesias in patients treated with major neuroleptics: A review of the literature. *Am. J. Psychiatry. (Suppl.),* 124:40–48.

Danto, B. L. (1969): Triflupromazine versus pentylenetetrazol-nicotinic acid for treatment of chronic brain disease on a general-hospital psychiatric service. *J. Am. Geriatr. Soc.,* 17:414–420.

Danziger, L. (1942): Estrogen therapy of agitated depressions associated with the menopause, *Arch. Neurol. Psychiatry,* 49:305–310.

Davies, R. K., Tucker, G. J., Harrow, M., and Detre, T. P. (1971): Confusional episodes and antidepressant medication. *Am. J. Psychiatry,* 128:95–99.

Davis, J. M. (1974): Use of psychotropic drugs in geriatric patients. *J. Geriatr. Psychiatry,* 7:145–164.

Dawson-Butterworth, K. (1970): The chemopsychotherapeutics of geriatric sedation. *J. Am. Geriatr. Soc.,* 18:97–114.

DeAlarcon, R. (1964): Hypochondriasis and depression in the aged. *Gerontol. Clin.,* 6:266–277.

DeLemos, G. P., Clement, W. R., and Nickels, E. (1965): Effects of diazepam suspension in geriatric patients hospitalized for psychiatric illnesses. *J. Am. Geriatr. Soc.,* 13:355–359.

Ditch, M., Kelley, R. J., and Resnick, O. (1971): An ergot preparation (Hydergine) in the treatment of cerebrovascular disorders in the geriatric patient: Double blind study. *J. Am. Geriatr. Soc.,* 19:208–217.

Eichhorn, O. (1965): The effect of cyclandelate on cerebral circulation. *Vasc. Dis.,* 6:305–315.

Eisdorfer, C. (1972): Autonomic changes in aging: In: *Aging and the Brain,* edited by C. M. Gaitz. Plenum Press, New York.

Eisdorfer, C. (1975): Observations on the psychopharmacology of the aged. *J. Am. Geriatr. Soc.,* 23:53–57.

Eisdorfer, C., and Raskind, M. A. (1975): Endocrinologic bases of behavior in aging: In: *Hormonal Correlates of Behavior,* edited by R. L. Sprott and B. E. Eleftheriou. Jackson Laboratory, Bar Harbor.

Eisdorfer, C., Conner, J. F., and Wilkie, F. L. (1968): Effect of magnesium pemoline on cognition and behavior. *J. Gerontol.,* 23:283–288.

Eisdorfer, C., Nowlin, J., and Wilkie, F. (1970): Improvement of learning in the aged by modification of autonomic nervous system activity. *Science,* 170:1327–1329.

Eisdorfer, C., and Wilkie, F. (1973): Intellectual changes with advancing age. In: *Intellectual Functioning in Adults,* edited by L. F. Jarvik, C. Eisdorfer, and J. E. Blum. Springer, New York.

El-Yousef, M. K., Janowsky, D. S., Davis, J. M., and Sekerke, H. J. (1973): Reversal of antiparkinsonian drug toxicity by physostigmine: A controlled study. *Am. J. Psychiatry,* 130:141–145.

Emmenegger, H., and Meier-Ruge, W. (1968): The actions of Hydergine on the brain. *Pharmacology,* 1:65–78.

Evans, J. G., and Jarvis, E. H. (1972): Nitrazepam and the elderly. *Br. Med. J.,* 4:487–489.

Ewy, G. A., Kapadia, G. G., and Yao, L. (1969): Digoxin metabolism in the elderly. *Circulation,* 39:449–452.

Exton-Smith, A. N., Hodkinson, H. M., and Cranie, B. W. (1963): Controlled comparison of four sedative drugs in elderly patients. *Br. Med. J.,* 4:1037–1040.

Feigenbaum, E. M. (1971): Assessment of behavioral changes and emotional disturbance in a custodial geriatric facility. Presented at 124th Annual Meeting, American Psychiatric Association, Washington, D.C., May 3–7.

Fine, E. W. (1971): The use of cyclandelate in chronic brain syndrome with arteriosclerosis. *Curr. Ther. Res.,* 13:568–574.

Fisher, S., and Gal, P. (1969): Flurazepam versus amobarbital as a sedative-hypnotic for geriatric patients: Double-blind study. *J. Am. Geriatr. Soc.,* 17:397–399.

Fletcher, G. F., and Wenger, N. K. (1969): Cardiotoxic effects of Mellaril: Conduction disturbances and supraventricular arrhythmias. *Am. Heart J.,* 78:135–138.

Forster, W., Schultig, S., and Henderson, A. L. (1955): Combined hydrogenated alkaloids of ergot in senile and arteriosclerotic psychoses. *Geriatrics,* 10:26–30.

Freeman, J. W., Mundy, G. R., Beattie, R. R., and Ryan, C. (1969): Cardiac abnormalities in poisoning with tricyclic antidepressants. *Br. Med. J.,* 2:610–611.

Freeman, H., and Murray, P. (1966): Treatment of aged psychotic patients with Hydergine. *Gerontol. Clin.,* 8:279–284.

Frolkis, V. V., Bezrukov, V. V., Duplenko, Y. K., and Genis, E. D. (1972): The hypothalamus in aging. *Exp. Gerontol.,* 7:169–184.

Ganettson, L. K., Perel, J. M., and Dayton, P. G. (1969): Methylphenidate interactions with both anticonvulsants and ethyl biscoumacetate. *J.A.M.A.,* 207:2053–2056.

Gerin, J. (1969): Symptomatic treatment of cerebrovascular insufficiency with Hydergine. *Curr. Ther. Res.,* 11:539–546.

Gilbert, J., Donnelly, K. J., Zimmer, L. E., and Kubis, J. F. (1973): Effect of magnesium pemoline and methylphenidate on memory improvement and mood in normal aging subjects. *Aging Hum. Dev.,* 4:35–51.

Glasgow, J. F. T. (1969): A neurological disorder associated with chlordiazepoxide therapy. *Clin. Toxicol.,* 2:456–462.

Glick, I. D. (1967): Mood and behavioral changes associated with the use of the oral contraceptive agents. *Psychopharmacologia,* 10:363:373.

Goldberg, L. I. (1964): Monoamine oxidase inhibitors: Adverse reactions and possible mechanisms. *J.A.M.A.,* 190:456–462.

Goldfarb, A. I., Hochstadt, N. J., Jacobson, J. H., and Weinstein, E. A. (1972): Hyperbaric oxygen treatment of organic mental syndrome in aged person. *J. Gerontol.,* 27:212–217.

Gottesman, L. E., Quarterman, C. E., and Cohn, G. M. (1973): Psychosocial treatment of the aged. In: *The Psychology of Adult Development and Aging,* edited by C. Eisdorfer and M. P. Lawton. American Psychological Association, Washington, D.C.

Granville-Grossman, K. L., and Turner, P. (1966): The effect of propranolol on anxiety. *Lancet,* 1:788–790.

Greenblatt, D. J., DiMascio, A., Messier, M., and Stotsky, B. A. (1969): Magnesium pemoline and job performance in mentally handicapped workers. *Clin. Pharmacol. Ther.,* 10:530–533.

Greenblatt. D. J., Dominick, J. R., Stotsky, B. A., and DiMascio, A. (1968): Phenothiazine induced dyskinesia in nursing home patients. *J. Am. Geriatr. Soc.,* 16:27–34.

Greenblatt, D. J., and Shader, R. I. (1974): *Benzodiazepines in Clinical Practice.* Raven Press, N.Y.

Gregerman, R. I., and Bierman, E. L. (1974): Aging and hormones. In: *Textbook of Endocrinology,* edited by R. H. Williams. Saunders, Philadelphia.

Grof, P., Saxena, B., Cantor, R., Daigle, L., Hetherington, D., and Haines, T. (1974): Doxepin versus amitriptyline in depression: A sequential double-blind study. *Curr. Ther. Res.,* 16:470–476.

Hamburg, D. A., Moos, R. H., and Yalom, I. D. (1968): Studies of distress in the menstrual cycle and postpartum period. In: *Endocrinology and Human Behavior,* edited by R. P. Michael. Oxford University Press, London.

Hansen, J. M., Kampmann, J., and Laursen, H. (1970): Renal excretion of drugs in the elderly. *Lancet,* 1:1170.

Hollister, L. E. (1973): *Clinical Use of Psychotherapeutic Drugs.* Charles C Thomas, Springfield, Ill.

Hollister, L. E. (1974): Doxepin hydrochloride. *Ann. Intern. Med.,* 81:360–363.

Honigfeld, G., Rosenblum, M. P., Blumenthal, I. J., Lambert, H. L., and Roberts, A. J. (1965): Behavioral improvement in the older schizophrenic patient: Drug and social therapies. *J. Am. Geriatr. Soc.,* 13:57–71.

Hordern, A., Burt, C. G., and Holt, N. F. (1965): *Depressive States: A Pharmacotherapeutic Study.* Charles C Thomas, Springfield, Ill.

Hurwitz, N. (1969): Predisposing factors in adverse reactions to drugs. *Br. Med. J.,* 1:536–539.

Jacobs, E. A., Winter, P. M., Alvis, H. J., and Small, H. M. (1969): Hyperoxygenation effect on cognitive function in the aged. *N. Engl. J. Med.,* 281:753–758.

Jacobson, A. (1958): The use of Ritalin in psychotherapy of depression of the aged. *Psychiatr. Q.,* 32:475–483.

Jarvik, L. F., and Cohen, D. (1973): A biobehavioral approach to intellectual changes with aging. In: *The Psychology of Adult Development and Aging,* edited by C. Eisdorfer and M. P. Lawton. American Psychological Association, Washington, D.C.

Jayne, H. W., Scheinber, P., and Rich, M. (1952): The effect of intravenous papaverine hydrochloride on the cerebral circulation. *J. Clin. Invest.,* 31:111–114.

Jones, T. H. (1962): Chlordiazepoxide (Librium) and the geriatric patient. *J. Am. Geriatr. Soc.,* 10:259–263.

Kales, A., Allen, C., Scharf, M. B., and Kales, J. D. (1970): Hypnotic drugs and their effectiveness: All night EEG studies of insomniac patients. *Arch. Gen. Psychiatry,* 23:226–232.

Kales, A., Kales, J. D., Leo, L. A., and Bixlor, E. D. (1973): Evaluation of the effectiveness of hypnotic drugs under conditions of prolonged use. Presented at Annual Meeting of the Associations for the Psychophysiological Study of Sleep, San Diego, Calif., May 1973.

Karlsberg, P., Elliott, H. E., and Adams, J. E. (1963): Effect of various pharmacological agents on cerebral arteries. *Neurology (Minneap.),* 13:772–778.

Kastenbaum, R., Slater, P. E., and Aisenberg, R. (1964): Toward a conceptual model of geriatric psychopharmacology: An experiment with thioridazine and dextroamphetamine. *Gerontologist,* 4:68–71.

Kay, W. W. K., and Roth, M. (1961): Environmental and hereditary factors in the schizophrenias of old age ("late paraphrenia"). *J. Ment. Sci.,* 197:649–686.

Kelly, H. C., Fay, J. E., and Laverty, S. C. (1963): Thioridazine hydrochloride (Mellaril): Its effect on the electrocardiogram and a report of two fatalities with electrocardiographic abnormalities. *Can. Med. Assoc. J.,* 89:546–548.

Kernohan, W. J., Chambers, J. L., Wilson, W. T., and Daugherty, J. F. (1967): Effects of nortriptyline on the mental and social adjustment of geriatric patients in a mental hospital. *J. Am. Geriatr. Soc.,* 15:196–202.

Kerr, M. D. (1968): Psychohormonal approach to the menopause. *Mod. Treat.,* 5:587–593.

Kety, S. S., and Schmidt, C. F. (1948): The nitrous oxide method for the quantitative measurement of cerebral blood flow in man: Theory, procedure, and normal values. *J. Clin. Invest.,* 27:476–483.

Kirven, L. E., and Montero, E. F. (1973): Comparison of thioridazine and diazepam on the control of nonpsychiatric symptoms associated with senility: Double-blind study. *J. Am. Geriatr. Soc.,* 21:546–551.

Kiev, A. (1972): Double-blind comparison of thiothixene and protriptyline in psychotic depression. *Dis. Nerv. Syst.,* 33:811–816.

Klaiber, E. L. Broverman, D. M., Vogel, W., Kobayashi, Y., and Moriarity, D. (1972): Effects of estrogen on plasma MAO activity and EEG driving responses of depressed women. *Am. J. Psychiatry,* 128:1492–1498.

GERIATRIC PSYCHOPHARMACOLOGY

Klawans, L. K. (1973): The pharmacology of tardive dyskinesias. *Am. J. Psychiatry,* 130:82–86.

Klerman, G. L., and Barrett, J. E. (1974): The affective disorders: clinical and epidemiologic aspects. In: *Lithium: Its Role in Psychiatric Research and Treatment,* edited by S. Gershon and B. Shopsin. Plenum Press, New York.

Kline, N. S. (1973): Clinical studies using Gerovital H3. Paper presented at the 26th annual meeting of the Gerontological Society, Miami Beach, Fla., Nov. 9.

Kral, V. A., Cahn, C., and Deutsch, M. (1962): Procaine (Novocain) treatment of patients with senile and arteriosclerotic brain disease. *Can. Med. Assoc. J.,* 87: 1109–1113.

Kramer, M., Tauber, C. A., and Redick, R. W. (1973): Patterns of use of psychiatric facilities by the aged: past, present and future. In: *The Psychology of Adult Development and Aging,* edited by C. Eisdorfer and M. P. Lawton. American Psychological Association, Washington, D.C.

La Brecque, D. C., and Goldberg, R. I. (1967): A double blind study of pentylenetetrazol combined with niacin in senile patients. *Curr. Ther. Res.,* 9:611–617.

Learoyd, B. M. (1972): Psychotropic drugs and the elderly patient. *Med. J. Aust.,* 1:1131–1133.

Leckman, J., Ananth, J. W., Ban, T. A., and Lehmann, H. E. (1971): Pentylenetetrazol in the treatment of geriatric patients with disturbed memory function. *J. Clin. Pharmacol.,* 11:301–303.

Lehmann, H. F., Ban, T. A., and Suxena, B. M. (1972): Nicotinic acid, thioridazine, fluoxymesterone and their combinations in hospitalized geriatric patients. *Can. Psychiatr. Assoc. J.,* 17:315–320.

Lifshitz, K., and Kline, N. S. (1961): Use of an estrogen in the treatment of psychosis with cerebral arteriosclerosis. *J.A.M.A.,* 176:501–504.

Lowenthal, M. J., and Berkman, P. L. (1967): *Aging and Mental Disorder in San Francisco.* Jossey-Bass, San Francisco.

Lu, L. M., Stotsky, B. A., and Cole, J. O. (1971): A controlled study of drugs in long-term geriatric psychiatric patients. *Arch. Gen. Psychiatry,* 25:284–288.

Lukas, E. R., Hambacher, W. D., and Fullica, A. J. (1973): A note on the use of anticoagulant therapy in chronic brain syndrome. *J. Am. Geriatr. Soc.,* 21:224–225.

MacFarlane, D. M., and Besbris, H. (1974): Procaine (Gerovital H3) therapy: Mechanism of inhibition of monoamine oxidase. *J. Am. Geriatr. Soc.,* 22:365–371.

Michael, C. M. (1970): Further psychometric evaluation of older women: The effect of estrogen administration. *J. Gerontol.,* 25:337–341.

Mishara, B. L., and Kastenbaum, R. (1974): Wine in the treatment of long-term geriatric patients in mental institutions. *J. Am. Geriatr, Soc.,* 22:88–94.

Moir, D. C. (1973): Tricyclic antidepressants and cardiac disease. *Am. Heart J.,* 84:841–842.

Morris, J. B., and Beck, A. T. (1974): The efficacy of antidepressant drugs. *Arch. Gen. Psychiatry,* 301:667–674.

Nies, A., Robinson, D. S., Davis, J. M., and Ravaris, C. L. (1973): Changes in monoamine oxidase with aging. In: *Psychopharmacology and Aging,* edited by C. Eisdorfer and W. E. Fann. Plenum Press, New York.

O'Malley, K., Crooks, J., Duke, E., and Stevenson, I. H. (1971): Effect of age and sex on human drug metabolism. *Br. Med. J.,* 3:607–609.

Overall, J. E., and Hollister, L. E. (1971): Indications for tricyclic antidepressant drugs. *Dis. Nerv. Syst.,* 32:759–763.

Pacha, W., and Salzman, R. (1970): Inhibition of the reuptake of neuronally liberated noradrenaline and receptor blocking action of some ergot alkaloids. *Br. J. Pharmacol.,* 38:439–443.

Pasamanick, B., Roberts, D. W., Lemkau, P. W., and Krueger, D. B. (1959): A survey of mental disease in an urban population: prevalence by race and income. In: *Epidemiology of Mental Disorder,* edited by B. Pasamanick. American Association for the Advancement of Science, Washington, D.C.

Pattison, J. H., and Allen, R. P. (1972): Comparison of the hypnotic effectiveness of secobarbital, pentobarbital, methyprylon and ethchlorvynol. *J. Am. Geriatr. Soc.,* 22:398–402.

Pfeiffer, E., and Busse, E. W. (1973): Affective disorders. In: *Mental Illness in Later Life,* edited by E. W. Busse and E. Pfeiffer. American Psychiatric Association, Washington, D.C.

Post, F. (1965): *The Clinical Psychiatry of Late Life.* Pergamon Press, Oxford.

Post, F. (1972): The management and nature of depressive illnesses in late life: A follow-through study. *Br. J. Psychiatry,* 121:393–404.

Prange, A. J. (1973): The use of antidepressant drugs in the elderly patient. In: *Psychopharmacology and Aging,* edited by C. Eisdorfer and W. E. Fann. Plenum Press, New York.

Prien, R. F., Caffey, E. M., and Klett, J. (1974): Factors associated with treatment success in lithium carbonate prophylaxis. *Arch. Gen. Psychiatry,* 31:189–192.

Prien, R. F., Haber, P. A., and Caffey, E. M. (1975): The use of psychoactive drugs in elderly patients with psychiatric disorders: Survey conducted in twelve veterans administration hospitals. *J. Am. Geriatr. Soc.,* 23:104–112.

Pryce, I. G., and Edwards, H. (1966): Persistent oral dyskinesia in female mental hospital patients. *Br. J. Psychiatry,* 112:983–987.

Rao, D. B., and Norris, J. R. (1972): A double-blind investigation of Hydergine in the treatment of cerebrovascular insufficiency in the elderly. *Johns Hopkins Med. J.,* 130:317–324.

Raskind, M. A. (1974): Psychosis, polydipsia and water intoxication. *Arch. Gen. Psychiatry,* 30:112–114.

Ratner, J., Rosenberg, G., Vojtech, A. K., and Engelsmann, F. (1972): Anticoagulant therapy for senile dementia. *J. Am. Geriatr. Soc.,* 21:556–559.

Rhoades, F. P. (1967): Minimizing the menopause. *J. Am. Geriatr. Soc.,* 15:347–350.

Ripley, H. S., Shorr, E., Papanicolaou, G. N. (1940): The effect of treatment of depression in the menopause with estrogenic hormone. *Am. J. Psychiatry,* 96:905–913.

Robinson, D. B. (1959): Evaluation of certain drugs in geriatric patients. *Arch. Gen. Psychiatry,* 1:41–46.

Roubicek, J., Geiger, C. H., and Abt, K. (1972): An ergot alkaloid preparation (Hydergine) in geriatric therapy. *J. Am. Geriatr. Soc.,* 20:222–229.

Sakalis, G., Oh, D., Gershon, S., and Shopsin, B. (1974): A trial of Gerovital H3 in depression during senility. *Curr. Ther. Res.,* 16:59–63.

Salzman, C., Shader, R. I., and Pearlman, M. (1970): Psychopharmacology and the elderly. In: *Psychotropic Drug Side Effects,* edited by R. I. Shader and A. DiMascio. Williams & Wilkins, Baltimore.

Schoonmaker, F. W., Osteen, R. T., and Greefield, J. C. (1966): Thioridazine (Mellaril) induced ventricular tachycardia controlled with an artificial pacemaker. *Ann. Intern. Med.,* 65:1076–1078.

Seager, C. P. (1955): Chlorpromazine in treatment of elderly psychotic woman. *Br. Med. J.,* 1:882–884.

Seidl, L. G., Thornton, F., Smith, J. W., and Cluff, L. E. (1966): Studies on the epidemiology of adverse drug reactions. Ill. Reactions in patients on a general medical service. *Bull. Hopkins Hosp.,* 119:299–315.

Sheppard, C., Bhattacharyya, A., DiGiacomo, M., and Merlis, S. (1964): Effects of acetophenazine dimaleate on paranoid symptomatology in female geriatric patients. *J. Am. Geriatr. Soc.,* 12:884–888.

Smith, W. L., Lowrey, J. B., and Davis, J. A. (1968): The effects of cyclandelate on psychological test performance in patients with cerebral vascular insufficiency. *Curr. Ther. Res.,* 10:613–618.

Snyder, S., Greenberg, D., and Yamamura, H. I. (1974): Antischizophrenic drugs and brain cholinergic receptors. *Arch. Gen. Psychiatry,* 31:58–61.

Special Committee on Aging, United States Senate (1974): *Nursing Home Care in the United States: Failure in Public Policy.* Government Printing Office, Washington, D.C.

Stern, F. H. (1970): Management of chronic brain syndrome secondary to cerebral arteriosclerosis, with special reference to papaverine hydrochloride. *J. Am. Geriatr. Soc.,* 18:507–510.

Stotsky, B. A. (1967): Allegedly nonpsychiatric patients in nursing homes. *J. Am. Geriatr. Soc.,* 15:535–544.

Stotsky, B. B., and Borozne, J. (1972): Butisol sodium vs Librium among geriatric and younger outpatients and nursing home patients. *Dis. Nerv. Syst.*, 33:254–267.

Stotsky, B. A., Cole, J. O., Lu, L. M., and Smiflin, C. (1972): A controlled study of the efficacy of pentylenetetrazol in hard-core hospitalized psychogeriatric patients. *Am. J. Psychiatry,* 129:387–391.

Stotsky, B. A., Cole, J. O., Tang, Y. T., and Gahm, I. G. (1971): Sodium butabarbital (Butisol Sodium) as an hypnotic agent for aged psychiatric patients with sleep disorders. *J. Am. Geriatr. Soc.,* 19:860–870.

Sugerman, A. A., Williams, B. H., and Adlerstein, M. A. (1964): Haloperidol in the psychiatric disorders of old age. *Am. J. Psychiatry,* 120:1190–1192.

Talland, G. A., Hagen, D. Q., and James, M. (1967): Performance tests of amnesiac patients with Cylert. *J. Nerv. Ment. Dis.,* 144:421–429.

Terry, R. D., and Wisniewski, H. M. (1972): Ultrastructure of senile dementia and of experimental analogs. In: *Aging and the Brain,* edited by C. M. Gaitz. Plenum Press, New York.

Thornton, C. D., and Wendkos, M. H. (1971): EKG T-wave distortions among thioridazine treated psychiatric inpatients. *Dis. Nerv. Syst.,* 32:320–323.

Triboletti, F., and Ferri, H. (1969): Hydergine for treatment of symptoms of cerebrovascular insufficiency. *Curr. Ther. Res.,* 11:609–613.

Tsuang, M. M., Lu, L. M., Stotsky, B. A., and Cole, J. O. (1971): Haloperidol vs thioridazine for hospitalized psychogeriatric patients: Double-blind study. *J. Am. Geriatr. Soc.,* 19:593–600.

Utian, W. H. (1972): The true clinical features of postmenopause and oophorectomy, and their response to oestrogen therapy. *S. Afr. Med. J.,* 46:732–737.

Van Der Velde, C. D. (1971): Toxicity of lithium carbonate in elderly patients. *Am. J. Psychiatry,* 127:1075–1077.

Vartia, K. O., and Leikola, E. (1960): Serum levels of antibiotics in young and old subjects following administration of dihydrostreptomycin and tetracycline. *J. Gerontol.,* 15:392–395.

Vesell, E. S., Passananti, G. T., and Greene, F. E. (1970): Impairment of drug metabolism by allopurinol and nortriptyline. *N. Engl. J. Med.,* 283:1484–1488.

Walsh, A. C. (1969): Prevention of senile and presenile dementia by bishydroxycoumarin therapy. *J. Am. Geriatr. Soc.,* 17:447–487.

Walsh, A. C., and Walsh, B. H. (1972): Senile and presenile dementia: Further observations on the benefits of Dicumarol-psychotherapy regimen. *J. Am Geriatr. Soc.,* 20:127–131.

Wang, H. S. (1973): Evaluation of brain impairment. In: *Mental Illness in Later Life,* edited by E. W. Busse and E. Pfeiffer, p. 83. American Psychiatric Association, Washington, D.C.

Williams, J. R., Csalany, L., and Misevic, G. (1967): Drug therapy with or without group discussion. *J. Am. Geriatr. Soc.,* 15:34–40.

Williams, R. B., and Sherter, C. (1971): Cardiac complications of tricyclic antidepressant therapy. *Ann. Intern. Med.,* 74:395–398.

Wilson, R. A., and Wilson, T. A. (1963): The fate of the nontreated postmenopausal woman. *J. Am. Geriatr. Soc.,* 11:347–350.

Chapter 16

Adverse Reactions To Psychotherapeutic Drugs

Leo E. Hollister

Adverse reactions to drugs can generally be placed in one of three major categories: extensions of known and expected pharmacological effects of the drug (although sometimes manifesting in novel and unexpected ways); allergic or hypersensitivity reactions; and reactions of known or unknown mechanisms that are peculiar (idiosyncratic) to a patient.

Reactions to psychotherapeutic drugs have been of great interest, because some have provided remarkably good models for naturally occurring illnesses. For example, the amine hypothesis for endogenous depressions emanated from the observation that reserpine made patients depressed. The use of levodopa (L-DOPA) as a treatment for Parkinson's disease evolved after the model of this illness produced by antipsychotic drugs was fully investigated. Even our understanding of the disorders we treat whose causes are generally unknown has been enhanced by studying both the wanted and the unwanted effects of drugs.

No completely satisfactory system for reporting misadventures with drugs has yet been designed. The most common error is simply not defining what constitutes a side effect or complication of consequence. Other errors include lack of denominators (so that frequency is unknown) and lack of critical review to ensure that the report is valid. For example, a review of 7.5 years of reporting to the British Committee on Safety of Drugs revealed 102 deaths attributed to chlorpromazine. One might think that the majority of these were instances of agranulocytosis or sudden cardiac death, but such was not the case. Fifty-four patients were reported to have died from jaundice, a complication which when observed prospectively has virtually a zero death rate unless incidental to more serious illnesses. In all probability these deaths were associated with the use of chlorpromazine in patients with advanced liver failure, clearly a misuse of the drug; however, one cannot be certain that this explanation holds (Girdwood, 1974). The moral is that the reporting and discovery of side effects and complications of drugs is still rather primitive.

ANTIPSYCHOTIC DRUGS

The number of antipsychotic drugs available continues to grow, at least 160 chemicals having been given generic names and proposed for marketing.

Although the chemical structures may vary, the spectrum of pharmacological actions remains fairly constant. Some variations occur in regard to side effects and are due primarily to differences in potency.

Agranulocytosis

Agranulocytosis, a potentially fatal complication, seems to be less common than it once was. As it is most often associated with use of high-dose drugs (e.g., chlorpromazine and thioridazine), one is tempted to attribute its decreasing incidence to a declining use of these drugs. Such reasoning may be fallacious since at the moment these are the two most widely used drugs of this class in the United States. Agranulocytosis from the more potent antipsychotics (e.g., haloperidol, fluphenazine, thiothixene) is virtually unknown.

The mechanism underlying this reaction is one of direct but transient toxicity to granulopoiesis in the bone marrow, which probably affects everyone exposed to chlorpromazine but becomes of clinical importance only in rare cases (Pisciotta, 1969). Older white women in poor general health are most at risk for developing this complication. A typical case of agranulocytosis occurred in a 54-yr-old man treated with only 150 mg thioridazine for a functional anxiety syndrome. It was accompanied by hepatitis, which produced mild hepatic encephalopathy, although the case for hepatitis being secondary to drug was less certain; fortunately the patient recovered (Weiden and Buckner, 1973). What is worth emphasizing is that these powerful drugs (i.e., the antipsychotics) should not be used for trivial indications.

As there is little evidence to suggest that frequent monitoring of leukocyte counts during the first several weeks of treatment, when the complication is most likely to occur, leads to early detection, most clinicians have abandoned any such routine. A low leukocyte count prior to treatment may be an indication of reduced marrow reserve and cause greater concern. Occasional leukocyte counts should be obtained under normal circumstances and immediately after the discovery of any physical illness with fever.

Cholestatic Jaundice

Cholestatic jaundice has also declined in frequency, even as early as the late 1950s (Hollister, 1959). It now appears that the reaction may be due to precipitation of the protein and glycoprotein components of bile. Such reactions have been demonstrated *in vitro* for most tricyclic compounds with a positively charged amine side chain, including tricyclic antidepressants as well (Clarke, Maritz, and Denborough, 1972). It is possible that the reaction occurs far more frequently than is recognized clinically. Even using biopsy material, the prevalence of subclinical cholestasis was relatively infrequent, being detected in only five of 20 patients (Hollister and Hall, 1966). Further, the clinical syndrome has many earmarks of an allergic reaction: It occurs within a narrow time range after starting the drug; is accompanied by fever, eosinophilia, and rashes or other allergic manifestations; and is often promptly exacerbated by challenge doses of drug. Thus it may be that the intrinsic propensity of these drugs to precipitate bile components may not alone suffice to produce the clinical manifestations.

Not too surprisingly, patients with advanced liver disease show electro-encephalographic (EEG) evidence of aggravation of hepatic encephalopathy when exposed to chlorpromazine (Read, Laidlaw, and McCarthy, 1969). This action is shared by other sedatives, which should be used sparingly if at all in such patients. Patients with lesser degrees of liver damage tolerate antipsychotic drugs well, and uncomplicated liver disease alone should never be considered a contraindication to their use.

Neurological Disorders

The *Parkinson syndrome,* manifested most commonly by akathisia but also including classic symptoms and signs of Parkinson's disease as well as acute dystonias, is now well recognized as an unavoidable side effect of most antipsychotic drugs. It is attributed to postsynaptic blockade of dopamine receptors in the striatonigral portion of the dopaminergic system, the anti-psychotic effects being due to the same action in the mesolimbic system. Thus the mystery of why these two unique and novel actions of antipsychotic drugs should be joined is now clear.

The syndrome is readily manageable by drugs of the anticholinergic type used to treat Parkinson's disease; but as there is no depletion of dopamine involved, it is unresponsive to treatment with L-DOPA. The ease with which the syndrome is managed by antiparkinsonian drugs has led to their over-employment. Many clinicians use them prophylactically and routinely, a practice that robs the clinician of at least one pharmacological clue to proper dose levels. The syndrome is to some extent self-limiting. Several studies have indicated that antiparkinsonian drugs may be safely discontinued after several weeks (even in patients who clearly needed them at one time) without any recurrence of the Parkinson syndrome (Klett and Caffey, 1972).

Although it is often assumed that the drug-induced Parkinson syndrome occurs only in schizophrenic patients treated with high doses of antipsychotic drugs, such is not the case. Instances of a prolonged syndrome following moderate doses of these drugs used for treatment of vomiting or nervousness have been documented (Klawans, Bergen, and Bruyn, 1973). Once again, it is wise not to use potent drugs for small reasons.

The French experience that extraordinarily high doses of antipsychotic drugs may be used with minimal production of Parkinson syndrome has been confirmed by experience in the United States. This apparent paradox can best be explained by postulating that at high doses the antidopaminergic (Parkinson-producing action) and anticholinergic (antiparkinsonian) effects

of these drugs approach each other. Such a model is shown in Fig. 1. In the
case of drugs with little tendency to produce extrapyramidal motor reactions
(e.g., thioridazine and clozapine) central anticholinergic effects are relatively
more potent, and a major difference in intensity between the two opposing
pharmacological actions never occurs.

Tardive dyskinesias have been of increasing concern, their frequency of
occurrence seeming to depend on how closely one looks for the complication.
In one survey they were diagnosed in 36% of chronic mental hospital patients
(Fann, Davis, and Janowsky, 1972). They need not be in old patients

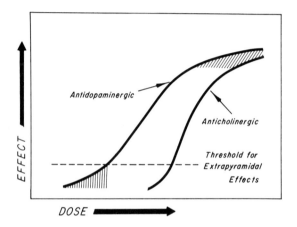

FIG. 1. A possible explanation for the paradoxical disappearance of extrapyramidal symptoms at high
doses of antipsychotic drugs is suggested by hypothetical dose-response curves for antidopaminergic
and anticholinergic actions. The balance between dopaminergic and cholinergic function is most disturbed
in the middle range of the dose-response curves. Extrapyramidal symptoms do not emerge at low doses of
antipsychotic drug. At very high doses the antidopaminergic and anticholinergic effects become close, so
extrapyramidal symptoms disappear.

(having been observed in children) nor in patients under prolonged treatment
(some develop within weeks). The fact that they may occur in nonpsychotic
patients treated with antipsychotic drugs is warning enough against using
these drugs for trivial indications (Klawans, Bergen, Bruyn, and Paulson,
1974).

Under the auspices of the American College of Neuropsychopharmacology
and the Food and Drug Administration (ACNP-FDA), a brief review of all
neurologic syndromes induced by antispychotic drugs has been presented.
The essential feature of tardive dyskinesia is repetitive involuntary movements of a choreoathetoid type involving the mouth, lips, tongue, trunk, and
extremities (ACNP-FDA Task Force, 1973). The basic mechanism proposed
to explain this syndrome is the development of dopaminergic hypersensitivity
in the striatonigral system, with a relative reduction in cholinergic function
(Klawans, 1973; Gerlach, Reisby, and Randrup, 1974). Such a formulation

explains several clinical phenomena: (1) Most if not all cases of tardive dyskinesia are preceded by the Parkinson syndrome, and occasionally there are mixed syndromes. (2) Anticholinergic drugs are not only ineffective but often unmask a latent dyskinesia. (3) Augmenting doses of antipsychotic drugs, either by using more of the same or adding another, often ameliorate the picture, at least temporarily. (4) Sudden withdrawal of an antipsychotic drug may exacerbate a latent syndrome. (5) L-DOPA makes the syndrome worse, and physostigmine may briefly ameliorate it.

Some of the proposals for managing tardive dyskinesia are more frightening

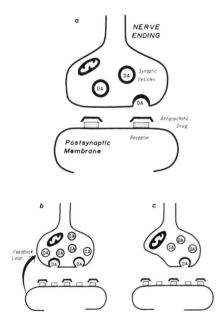

FIG. 2. Model of a dopaminergic synapse. When an antipsychotic drug is initially given (a), it blocks postsynaptic receptors and thus produces extrapyramidal effects. When an antipsychotic drug has been administered over a period of time (b), there may be activation of a feedback loop. This could lead to increased synthesis and release of dopamine, or to an increased number of dopamine receptors. This in turn could lead to loss of extrapyramidal symptoms or emergence of early dyskinesias. When an antipsychotic drug has been administered for a lengthy period of time (c), there might be damage to the presynaptic membrane. This could produce a denervation supersensitivity of receptors and cause tardive dyskinesia. (DA, dopamine)

than the complication itself (Kazamatsuri, Chien, and Cole, 1972). Figure 2 demonstrates how one may proceed from too little dopaminergic transmission in the motor system (Parkinson syndrome) to too much (tardive dyskinesia). It is obvious that the decrease in dopamine blockade might be alleviated by adding other antipsychotic drugs (or more of the same one for that matter), as shown in Fig. 3, but this approach is intrinsically hazardous. No completely satisfactory treatment is available. Reducing the dose of drug seems the most natural thing to do, but if this is done precipitously the motor disturbances may temporarily get worse. Lithium carbonate might be beneficial from two actions: (1) by increasing the intraneuronal turnover of dopamine; and (2) by decreasing receptor sensitivity. Diazepam is sometimes useful, quite possibly by inhibiting phosphodiesterase and reducing the intensity of the compensatory feedback loop. Recent reports of the use of deanol, a choline precursor, for treating L-DOPA-induced dyskinesias,

Huntington's chorea, and tardive dyskinesia have not yet been confirmed (Miller, 1974).

Neuroleptic malignant syndrome—a sometimes fatal syndrome of extrapyramidal and hypothalamic dysfunction characterized by hyperthermia, muscular rigidity, and coma—is rare. Some aspects of the syndrome resemble acute fatal catatonia (which has been rarely if ever seen since effective drugs became available) or malignant hyperpyrexia. Although the patients show markedly increased creatine phosphokinase (CPK) activity in the latter

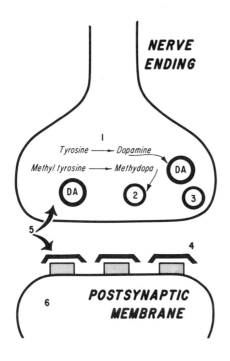

FIG. 3. Various types of pharmacological approaches to the treatment of tardive dyskinesia. These approaches involve: (1) administration of α-methyl-p-tyrosine to block synthesis of dopamine; (2) use of false transmitters to impair transmission; (3) administration of reserpine to deplete dopamine; (4) increasing the dosage of antipsychotic drug; (5) use of lithium, which might hasten dopamine degradation or diminish receptor sensitivity; (6) administration of diazepam, which might decrease feedback stimulation or diminish postsynaptic activity. Unfortunately, none of these approaches is therapeutically satisfactory. (DA, dopamine)

syndrome as well as in that due to antipsychotic drugs, the isoenzyme is different, being primarily CPK derived from muscle in the neuroleptic malignant syndrome. Such a reaction followed an initial dose of 25 mg fluphenazine enanthate in an acutely schizophrenic girl who was subsequently treated without difficulty (Meltzer, 1973). The whole question of the pertinence of increased CPK levels in schizophrenic patients, and if a disorder of skeletal muscle is related to schizophrenia, remains puzzling and intriguing.

Cardiac Complications

Much of the discussion of cardiac complications is covered in the section on antidepressants. Prolonged ventricular repolarization can be observed almost routinely in patients on substantial doses of thioridazine, and to a lesser extent in patients on other antipsychotic drugs. Both overnight fasting and oral supplements of 10 g of combined potassium salts reverse these changes, whereas giving a 100-g glucose load exacerbates them. It is believed that phenothiazines affect the electrocardiogram (ECG) by shifting potassium to the intracellular compartment (Alvarez-Mena and Frank, 1973). Other maneuvers used to reverse these drug-induced ECG abnormalities include administration of isosorbide dinitrate, ergotamine tartrate, or propranolol.

The significance of such a reversible disorder remains controversial. Regardless of its cause, any prolongation of ventricular repolarization time enhances the likelihood of re-entry rhythms. My own estimate, based on reports coming to me informally, is that during any given year 20 to 30 patients in the United States die of such arrhythmias, but these are seldom reported since the nature of the death is uncertain and the event so rare that few single centers develop an extensive experience with this complication. On the other hand, a potentially fatal complication such as agranulocytosis can scarcely be missed and accordingly is usually fully reported.

Endocrine Effects

Endocrine effects have been rather prominent since chlorpromazine first came into use. Galactorrhea is commonly observed in women chronically treated with antipsychotics (gynecomastia is sometimes seen in men); it appears to be due to an increase in circulating levels of prolactin, which is probably secondary to suppressed release of prolactin-inhibiting factor from the hypothalamus. Patients with amenorrhea tend to show variable concentrations of luteinizing hormone (LH) with absent midcycle peaks. Thus failure to menstruate may be due to a loss of the cyclic tide of LH, estradiol, and progesterone (Beumont, Gelder, Friesen, Harris, MacKinnon, Mandelbrote, and Wiles, 1974).

Sexual disturbance with loss of libido in men has been reported frequently. Chronic treatment with antipsychotics may decrease testosterone levels in men, with a rise occurring after cessation of treatment. It is questionable if such minor decreases are important in determining the level of sexual function (Beumont, Corker, Friesen, Kolakowska, Mandelbrote, Marshall, Murray, and Wiles, 1974).

Although it has been reported that chlorpromazine decreases growth hormone secretion, attempts to exploit this action as a treatment for acromegaly have been unsuccessful. Not only was the clinical condition little changed in eight patients treated with chlorpromazine (100 to 200 mg/day), but basal growth hormone levels were reduced in only one patient (Dimond, Brammer, Atkinson, Howard, and Earll, 1973). Since phenothiazines and other antipsychotic drugs are commonly used in children during early adolescence, one might have expected reports of retarded growth by now, as we saw after growing children were chronically treated with corticosteroids. However, no such observations have been reported as yet.

Cytogenetic Effects

Peripheral leukocyte cultures from patients treated with various phenothiazines, diazepam, and chlordiazepoxide show no increase in chromosomal abnormalities as compared with a matched group of untreated individuals (Cohen, Hirschhorn, and Frosch, 1969). A negative finding should be no more reassuring than a positive finding should be alarming. The present state of the art of human cytogenetics leaves much to be desired, and its clinical pertinence is far from established.

ANTIDEPRESSANT DRUGS

Adverse reactions to these agents have been well documented during the many years of their clinical employment. The literature has been extensively reviewed elsewhere (Loo and Bousser, 1972; Lambert, 1973). The prevalence of side effects from tricyclic antidepressants measured by a surveillance program involving 260 patients admitted to several hospitals while on these drugs was 15.4%. Most reactions were minor, although major reactions (e.g., toxic psychosis with hallucinations, disorientation, and agitation) occurred in 4.6% of patients (Boston Collaborative Drug Surveillance Program, 1972). In outpatients these drugs may elicit considerable drowsiness and fatigue, especially during the early stages of initiation of treatment. Variations in dosage schedules, slow increments in dose, and sometimes use of concurrent drugs have been suggested as ways to deal with these common and sometimes debilitating adverse effects.

Those drugs of several chemical classes given the epithet "tricyclics" are most often used and are of greatest interest. The monoamine oxidase (MAO) inhibitors are less frequently used, largely out of fear concerning their interactions and their unpredictable efficacy. Lithium salts have found some place in the treatment of depressions and are discussed under *Antimanic Drugs*.

Tricyclics

Cardiac Toxicity

Therapeutic doses of tricyclics were found early in the course of their investigation to produce palpitations, tachycardia, and orthostatic hypotension. Abnormalities in the ECG and arrhythmias were described somewhat later. Recent interest has focused on myocardial damage, precipitation of congestive heart failure, and sudden death.

Postural hypotension seems to be a special risk for the very young, the very old, or anyone who is debilitated. Dihydroergotamine in doses of 10 mg/day was said to be highly effective against orthostatic hypotension induced by amitriptyline without interfering with its antidepressive action (Bojanovsky and Tolle, 1974).

Ventricular tachyarrhythmias associated with phenothiazines are assumed to be due to the falling of a premature ventricular contraction during the vulnerable period of cardiac repolarization ("R on T phenomenon"). The risk is enhanced by the prolongation of repolarization produced by some drugs, notably thioridazine. Similar prolongation of repolarization (lengthened Q-T interval, prominent U-waves in the ECG) may be seen following tricyclic drugs, although generally less attention has been paid to the latter group.

The R on T phenomenon has been recognized as being associated with a high risk of *sudden death*. This phenomenon might be expected to occur with increased frequency among patients with known cardiac disease. During a 40-month period 119 of 864 hospitalized patients taking amitriptyline also had a diagnosis of cardiac disease. This group of 119 patients experienced 13 sudden deaths compared with only three such instances among a carefully matched group (Moir, Cornwell, Dingwall-Fordyce, Crooks, O'Malley, Turnbull, and Weir, 1972). Of most interest was that three died of cardiac arrest and two others were found dead without explanation; there were no deaths in the comparison group. Such deaths are especially likely to be physiological, due to the mechanism described above. A similar study in 88 patients without heart disease who received amitriptyline revealed one such instance of sudden death. None were encountered in a carefully matched comparison group (Moir, 1973). Subsequent studies by the same investigator suggested that the risk of this type of demise was greater in patients over 70 yr of age (Moir, Dingwall-Fordyce, and Weir, 1973). It has also been emphasized that the profound autonomic effects of amitriptyline should preclude its use during an acute myocardial infarction. Arrhythmias and sudden death in this situation are likely to be induced by autonomic factors (Brackenridge, 1972).

Cardiomyopathy, or heart failure, was reported in eight of 28 adverse cardiovascular reactions to tricyclics (Editorial, 1971). Cardiomyopathy was diagnosed by X-ray and ECG evidence of left ventricular hypertrophy in a 35-year-old man who had been treated for 5 years with imipramine, never in a dose larger than 100 mg/day. The cardiac enlargement regressed when the drug was withdrawn.

Three instances of *congestive heart failure* in patients without overt heart disease were believed aggravated by treatment with tricyclics. One patient received amitriptyline (300 mg/day) and another protriptyline (15 mg/day); the third received protriptyline (30 mg/day) following a much longer course that included imipramine and nortriptyline in doses of 100 mg/day (Luke, 1971). The mechanism of aggravation of congestive heart failure from tricyclics is most likely due to a decreased inotropic effect following depletion of catecholamines from the myocardium, but other mechanisms may be involved (Raisfeld, 1972).

Dysmorphogenesis

Little attention has been paid to possible dysmorphogenesis from tricyclics until a report of three possible cases from Australia (McBride, 1972). Later it turned out that the intake of drugs was not well documented. Thirty instances of mothers who took tricyclics during pregnancy in Australia and 300 others from other areas of the world were not accompanied by birth defects. These findings led to establishment of a special birth defects commission to question the relationship (Morrow, 1972).

Answers are never simple in this particular matter. Among 800 pregnancies, 19 mothers were exposed to imipramine and 28 to amitriptyline during the early weeks of pregnancy, but no definite malformations were observed (Crombie, Pinsent, and Fleming, 1972). Among a group of 15,000 pregnancies, 17 fetuses had been exposed to imipramine early on. Fourteen were normal, one had aborted, and two were abnormal (one with defective abdominal musculature and one with diaphragmatic hernia). Of 31 fetuses exposed to amitriptyline, 28 were normal, one had aborted, one was stillborn, and one showed hypospadias (Kuenssberg and Knox, 1972). The birth defects registry in Finland examined 2,784 pregnancies with matched controls (the pregnancy immediately preceding the birth of the deformed child). The mothers of only five infants with abnormalities were on tricyclics, three on imipramine, and two on amitriptyline; and in no instance was the tricyclic the sole drug. Abnormalities included cleft lip, cleft palate, meningocoele, hydrocephalus, and micrognathia. One parent on amitriptyline, with no deformities in the child, was found in the control group (Idanpaan-Heikkila and Saxen, 1973). Unless there is some compelling need to use the drugs in a pregnant woman, especially during the early stages, it should be avoided. In many of the cases reported, the drugs were used either in doses too small to be therapeutic or for indications that seemed less than adequate.

Even the use of these drugs in the perinatal period might be avoided. Three instances of distress in the newborn were reported following treatment of the mothers with tricyclics during the period prior to delivery. One infant showed signs of congestive heart failure without cardiac abnormality; another showed tachycardia and myoclonus; and the third had respiratory distress and neuromuscular spasms. These clinical manifestations were thought to result both from the adrenergic and anticholinergic effects of the drug, which readily passes the placenta (Eggermont, Raveschot, Deneve, and Casteels-Van Daele, 1972).

Psychiatric or Neurological Effects

Confusional reactions were observed in 13% of 150 patients being treated with tricyclics. The prevalence increased to 35% among patients over 40 years of age. All responded quickly to stopping the drug (Davies, Tucker, Harrow, and Detre, 1971). Older persons are particularly sensitive to the provocation of delirium by centrally acting anticholinergics. The situation may be made even worse if the patient is also receiving antipsychotics (most of which have a weakly anticholinergic effect), antiparkinsonian drugs (most of which are strongly anticholinergic), or all three types together.

The occurrence of withdrawal reactions to tricyclics has been infrequent and somewhat controversial. Three cases of apparent withdrawal followed discontinuation of large (300 to 450 mg/day) doses of tricyclics. Acute anxiety, motor restlessness, and akathisia were the predominant features (Sathananthan and Gershon, 1973).

Early reports on the use of tricyclics indicated that seizures could be a complication. The rarity of this complication is probably due to the generally conservative doses of tricyclics used. Three children who received rather large doses of tricyclics (150 mg/day in one case, 225 mg/day in the other two) experienced seizures while being treated for hyperactive-aggressive behavior. Two of the children had organic brain damage, which may have predisposed them to seizures (Brown, Winsberg, Bialer, and Press, 1973).

Visual Effects

Two instances of precipitation of narrow-angle glaucoma were encountered during treatment with tricyclics. An additional patient with known glaucoma was successfully treated with pilocarpine drops (Nouri and Cuendet, 1971). Loss of accommodation is common but of minor importance and can be remedied by prescribing glasses with magnifying lenses.

Gastrointestinal Effects

The autonomic effects of tricyclics on the gastrointestinal tract have been reviewed along with some original observations. Achalasia of the esophagus, diminished intestinal motility, and decreased gastric free acid secretion were among the effects noted (Fischbach, 1973). Adynamic ileus is another consequence of the decreased intestinal motility and may represent a potentially life-threatening situation (Clarke, 1971).

Genitourinary Effects

An experimental study revealed that 10 of 16 patients had increased bladder sphincter tonus while under treatment with tricyclics. Twelve of 31 required more fluid to evoke detrusor contraction following the onset of treatment (Appel, Eckel, and Harrer, 1971). Thus some degree of urinary retention is common in patients treated with these drugs, even though no clinical problems ensue.

The anticholinergic effects of the tricyclics produced delayed orgasm with slow ejaculation in five of seven men with sexual complaints. One of three women also reported delay in orgasm (Couper-Smartt and Rodham, 1973). It is difficult to determine how frequently sexual disturbances may follow these drugs, as patients are often reticent to discuss these problems and physicians may not recognize them as drug-related. The idea of using this side effect to treat premature ejaculation was anticipated following similar complaints during use of thioridazine.

Metabolic-Endocrine Effects

Weight gain has long been known as a concomitant of antidepressant and antipsychotic therapy. It may be part of the improved mental state, but aside from that it appears to have a physiological component. A marked craving for sweets was noted in 51 women being treated for depression with amitriptyline. When the drug was discontinued, patients lost weight. Those maintained on the drug continued to gain weight, although when the drug was discontinued they too lost weight. No abnormality was found in the fasting glucose and insulin levels or in sensitivity to insulin as measured by the intravenous insulin tolerance test (Paykel, Mueller, and De La Vergne, 1973).

Inappropriate secretion of antidiuretic hormone (ADH) was suspected in a 51-year-old woman who developed low serum osmolality and hyponatremia during two episodes of treatment with amitriptyline (Luzecky, Burman, and Schultz, 1974). Probably more often encountered is psychogenic polydipsia in patients troubled by the dry mouth that both tricyclics and phenothiazines often produce.

Hematological Effects

Two cases of nonthrombopenic purpura were observed in patients treated with tricyclics. Both responded to discontinuation of treatment (Kozakova, 1971). Agranulocytosis is a threat with tricyclics, just as it is with phenothiazines, but its prevalence is now very low.

Monoamine Oxidase Inhibitors

MAO inhibitors are not nearly so widely used as the tricyclics, and the literature on their side effects is sparse. A controlled evaluation of side effects of phenelzine was afforded by a collaborative study that evaluated this drug as an antidepressant against placebo and diazepam. During the major portion of the study patients received 45 mg/day, a moderate dose. The drug was discontinued because of side effects in only three of 110 patients; and in only one instance was the side effect serious (a patient said to have an exfoliative dermatitis which subsided despite treatment). The frequency of symptoms such as insomnia, excitement, loss of appetite, dry mouth, constipation, and headache was similar both in the placebo and in the phenelzine-treated patients at the end of 3 weeks of treatment; curiously, depression was more often mentioned as a side effect in the phenelzine patients. The major conclusion was that side effects caused few problems (Raskin, 1972).

A carefully controlled study showed that patients with impaired liver function are especially sensitive to tranylcypromine, sometimes developing obtunded consciousness and slow electroencephalograms (EEGs) similar to those found in hepatic encephalopathy. Amitriptyline was much better tolerated (Morgan and Read, 1972).

Relative impotence in three men and difficulty in achieving orgasm in two of five women were reported in a study of the use of phenelzine to treat narcolepsy (Wyatt, Fram, Buchbinder, and Snyder, 1971). Delayed ejaculation is a more common sexual disturbance.

ANTIMANIC DRUGS (Lithium salts)

The introduction of lithium as a pharmacological treatment in psychiatry revived ion therapy. For many years bromide ion was one of the most widely used and useful treatments for a variety of psychiatric disorders, including mania. Lithium has unequivocal efficacy for treating acute episodes of manic-depressive disorder and probably for preventing or diminishing the severity of recrudescences of this disorder.

The successful application of lithium treatment requires careful monitoring of plasma levels. Toxic symptoms, usually gastrointestinal or neuromuscular, required that 25% of patients with serum levels in excess of 1.4 mEq/liter be withdrawn from treatment, with little evidence for an augmented therapeutic response in patients with blood levels of this magnitude (Prien, Caffey, and Klett, 1972). Although serum lithium concentrations are largely dose-dependent, they may fluctuate in individual patients on the same dose, depending on the intake of sodium. Increased sodium intake reduced both serum lithium concentrations and side effects while increasing manic symptoms when this maneuver was done experimentally (Demers and Heninger, 1971a). Increasing sodium intake from 69 mEq to 121 to 173 mEq/day increased lithium excretion and urinary volume while reducing serum lithium levels in three patients studied experimentally (Demers and Harris, 1972). A low sodium intake or reduced urinary volume might be expected to lead to elevated levels and could be a cause of toxicity.

Neurological and Psychiatric Effects

Tremor is one of the most frequent side effects of lithium treatment, occurring at usual therapeutic dose levels. As propranolol has been reported to be effective in essential tremor, it was natural to try it for lithium-induced tremor (Kirk, Baastrup, and Schou, 1973). Its beneficial effect may be produced via the same mechanism as postulated for essential tremor—by blocking receptors sensitized to catecholamines. A variety of neurological and psychiatric abnormalities have been observed in patients treated with what are thought to be usual therapeutic levels of serum lithium. Neurological abnormalities included choreoathetosis, motor hyperactivity, ataxia, dysarthria, and aphasia. Psychiatric disturbances were generally marked mental confusion and withdrawal or bizarre motor movements (Shopsin, Johnson, and Gershon, 1970). Although lithium is said to increase seizures in epileptic patients, this was found in only one of 17 epileptic patients studied in a long-term experimental study using lithium in doses adequate to produce therapeutic levels (Erwin, Gerber, Morrison, and James, 1973).

Three patients who developed toxic-confusional states with lithium treatment received high doses of lithium but had slower than usual increases in serum lithium concentrations. The symptoms were clearly related to the blood levels, falling levels of lithium being associated with mental clearing (Agulnik, DiMascio, and Moore, 1972).

Thyroid Effects

Lithium probably decreases thyroid function in most patients exposed to the drug, but the situation is reversible or does not progress. Relatively few patients develop frank thyroid enlargement, and fewer still show symptoms of hypothyroidism. The latter is estimated to occur in no more than 15% of patients (Ayd, 1974). Sometimes hypothyroidism can progress to myxedema without goiter, as in five cases which rapidly reversed with discontinuation of treatment (Vestergaard and Poulsen, 1972). On the other hand, myxedema may occur quickly, even after as little as 7 weeks of treatment (Candy, 1972). As might be expected, iodine and lithium act synergistically (Shopsin, Shenkman, Blum, and Hollander, 1973).

Nephrogenic Diabetes Insipidus

Polydipsia and polyuria are frequent concomitants of lithium treatment, occurring at therapeutic plasma concentrations. Thus these symptoms represent true side effects rather than toxic manifestations. The principal physiological lesion involved is loss of the ability of the distal tubule to conserve water under the influence of ADH (vasopressin). Water deprivation tests in three patients during therapy with lithium showed a reduction in the ability to concentrate urine, to a striking degree in one patient (Ramsey, Mendels, Stokes, and Fitzgerald, 1972). Thus it is excessive free water clearance which causes the increased fluid intake. As the lesion is in the kidney tubule, it seems likely that ADH secretion would be normal, and such is the case. Rather, the kidney tubule in the presence of lithium shows a markedly diminished response to ADH. Although it has been thought that ADH unresponsiveness might be due to an action of lithium on ADH-sensitive adenyl cyclase in the distal tubule, experimental work suggests that ADH is specifically blocked by lithium present at the urinary surface, and the effect is not related to altered levels of cyclic adenosine monophosphate (Singer, Rotenberg, and Puschett, 1972).

Resistance to ADH has led to other attempts at therapy. Chlorithiazide has been said to be successful (Levy, Forrest, and Heninger, 1973). Such treatment is not without risk, for sodium depletion might augment lithium toxicity. In the case reported, serum lithium increased to toxic levels soon after chlorothiazine was started, necessitating a reduction in dosage. A rather unique instance of marked hyperglycemia and serum hyperosmolality accompanied diabetes insipidus in a 50-yr-old man treated for 5 yr with lithium. Large doses of insulin were required to reduce the markedly elevated plasma glucose concentrations (Martinez-Maldonado and Terrell, 1973).

Edema is a frequent side effect of lithium treatment and may be related to some effect of lithium on sodium retention. In the presence of normal or high sodium intake, both edema and increased plasma renin activity (PRA) were noted. The PRA was especially elevated in four of the six manic patients who were very agitated, suggesting that agitation alone may play a role (Demers, Hendler, Allen, and Boyd, 1972). At times edema has uncovered latent congestive heart failure (Stancer and Kivi, 1971). Although weight gain may be expected in patients who become edematous, water retention alone probably does not account for all of it. Increased thirst may lead to greater intake of calorie-containing beverages with a resultant solid weight gain due to overnutrition (Kerry, 1974).

Cardiac Effects

T-wave lowering is a frequent finding during lithium treatment (when one looks carefully). Sometimes the depression is not outside the range of normal and is only evident if one examines control tracings simultaneously. At other times the T-waves become flattened and are followed by marked U-waves, a finding sometimes seen with hypokalemia as well as during treatment with thioridazine or some of the tricyclic antidepressants (Kochar, Wang, and D'Cunha, 1971). It has been postulated that lithium may reduce the intracellular levels of potassium, but it does not have any clear effect on the serum concentrations. No evidence of myocardial damage could be found when enzyme tests were done during periods of T-wave abnormality, and the situation seems to be readily reversible (Demers and Heninger, 1971b).

Pregnancy

Concern that lithium might cause dysmorphogenesis has led to the establishment of international registries of lithium babies. After reports were received on 118 babies born to mothers who were taking lithium, it seemed clear that the prevalence of malformations noted (nine) was not appreciably higher than might be expected from such a retrospective study (Schou, Goldfield, Weinstein, and Villeneuve, 1973b). Two newborns had jaundice, two had hypotonia ("floppy"), one had a goiter, and one suffered perinatal asphyxia. Thus the issue of dysmorphogenesis is not definitely settled one way or the other. Renal clearance of lithium increases during pregnancy and reverts to lower levels immediately after delivery. A patient whose serum lithium concentration is in a good therapeutic range during pregnancy may develop toxic levels following delivery. Special care in monitoring lithium levels is needed at these times (Schou, Amdisen, and Steenstrup, 1973a).

Lithium is transferred to nursing children through breast milk, where it has a concentration about one-third to one-half that of serum (Schou and Amdisen, 1973). The phenomenon of lithium toxicity in newborns is manifested by lethargy, cyanosis, poor suck and Moro reflexes, and possibly hepatomegaly (Woody, London, and Wilbands, 1971). Rules for treating pregnant women with lithium include closely monitoring their blood lithium levels to keep them at the low end of the therapeutic range, avoiding salt restriction or diuretics, giving regular small doses, and prohibiting breast feeding (Goldfield and Weinstein, 1973).

Skin

Transient acneiform eruptions have been noted early in lithium treatment. Some of these eruptions subside with temporary discontinuation of treatment and do not recur with its resumption (Kusumi, 1971), although other times they recur promptly after treatment is restarted (Ruiz-Maldonado, Perez de Francisco, and Tamayo, 1973). Folliculitis is less dramatic and probably occurs more frequently. Twelve patients were encountered with this lesion, which resembles keratosis pilaris and is asymptomatic. It too is reversible but may recur with resumption of treatment (Rifkin, Kurtin, Quitkin, and Klein, 1973).

Miscellaneous Effects

Severe diarrhea that remitted when lithium was discontinued complicated treatment in a patient also suffering from regional ileitis (Varsamis and Wand, 1972). Curiously, lithium has been said to benefit the intestinal symptoms of patients with chronic ulcerative colitis. When variable and concurrent intestinal disorders are present, it is difficult to assess the effects of lithium on the gastrointestinal tract.

Disturbed sexual function was found in five of 33 patients treated with lithium. That erective impotency was related to lithium was clearly demonstrated in two patients treated with lithium or placebo under double-blind conditions. Substitution of placebo relieved the symptom, but impairment returned with lithium treatment (Vinarova, Uhlif, Stika, and Vinar, 1972).

ANTIANXIETY DRUGS

For practical purposes, when talking about the use of antianxiety drugs in the United States, we are concerned only with diazepam and chlordiazepoxide. These drugs are the first and third most widely prescribed therapeutic agents, far exceeding in popularity any of the others in this class. This wide acceptance must certainly be construed as evidence of their safety, as well as their efficacy. We are mainly concerned here with a few major problems.

Tolerance and Dependence

Tolerance to and dependence on drugs are closely linked. Without tolerance to a drug, physical dependence is most unlikely.

Several possible mechanisms of tolerance to a drug may be distinguished. First, "behavioral" tolerance may develop. This type is best exemplified by chronic alcoholics, who even with high plasma levels of ethanol may appear to be functioning normally. Second, "metabolic" tolerance may ensue. With continued exposure to the drug, enzymes may be induced which enhance its biotransformation to inactive metabolites. Meprobamate is an example of such a drug; its rate of hydroxylation is doubled after a week of use. When such drugs are used clinically over long periods of time, patients either experience a loss of the initial sedative effects or need to increase the dose to maintain them. If the difference between the therapeutic dose of a drug and that which may result in physical dependence is small (with meprobamate this may be as low as a factor of two to three), this type of tolerance may rapidly place the patient in danger of becoming physically dependent. Third, "immune" tolerance may develop from the formation of antibodies to the drug. Most drugs are low-molecular-weight substances not ordinarily antigenic, but when bound to protein they may act as haptens. Antibodies to many have now been demonstrated, although their role in development of tolerance is not entirely clear. Finally, tolerance may be "pharmacodynamic;" i.e., it may be based on a lessened degree of drug effect due to homeostatic or compensatory mechanisms elicited by its initial effects. As this type of tolerance is conceptually linked with physical dependence, it is discussed further below.

Two types of dependence are recognized—psychological and physiological —although the boundaries between the two are sometimes difficult to define. Psychological dependence is manifested by a strong craving for the drug but not necessarily with the appearance of physical signs of withdrawal when it is stopped abruptly. Physical dependence is defined as the appearance of psychological and physical symptoms of withdrawal, as exemplified by the

well-known withdrawal reactions that occur in heavy users of alcohol, barbiturates, or opiates. Psychological dependence is seen in all who develop
physical dependence, although the converse is not true.

One must assume that tolerance will develop during chronic exposure to
any antianxiety drug. Clear examples are observed in patients started on
modest doses of diazepam who increase the dose until they use excessive
amounts. Although such patients are often cited as examples of "abusers" of
the drug, they are more properly called "misusers." With high doses of
these drugs, the possibility of producing a withdrawal reaction on abrupt
discontinuation of dosage is real. The withdrawal reaction is attenuated in
time and tends to be milder than with shorter-acting drugs (Hollister, Motzenbecker, and Degan, 1961). Minor abstinence symptoms have been reported
after 20 weeks of uninterrupted treatment with therapeutic doses of chlordiazepoxide but not after 10 weeks of such treatment (Covi, Lipman, Pattison, Derogatis, and Uhlenhuth, 1973). For this reason, as well as for many
others, therapy with drugs of this type should follow brief, interrupted
schedules rather than sustained treatment.

Despite their extensive use, reports of serious withdrawal reactions or
abuse of the benzodiazepines are extremely rare. An interesting experiment
in which patients had access to diazepam as they saw fit, rather than as the
physician might order, showed that under such conditions patients are likely
to use less drug than might have been the case had it been prescribed on a
regular basis (Winstead, Anderson, Eilers, Blackwell, and Zaremba, 1974).
Surely these drugs must be as little likely to produce dependence as any that
can be found.

Overdoses

Overdoses may be unwitting or deliberate. The former are more common
than realized. To treat all patients with a single dose of drug is to overtreat
many, especially if the doses are repeated several times during a working
day. Further, patients take other drugs, including social drugs, that have
sedative effects. Oversedation is most hazardous when one is attempting
to perform skilled but potentially dangerous motor maneuvers, such as
driving an automobile (Hollister, 1974). The most dangerous combination
of drugs leading to oversedation is one in which an antianxiety agent (e.g.,
diazepam or meprobamate) is combined with alcohol. Doses of either drug,
which alone produced no motor impairment, clearly impaired functions when
combined (Linnoila and Mattila, 1973).

Deliberate overdoses of the benzodiazepines (which include oxazepam,
chlorazepate, and others) have been fairly easy to treat by supportive measures alone. The rare fatalities attributed to such overdoses virtually always
have been situations in which treatment was delayed or bungled, or in
which other drugs of greater toxic potential were also taken (Greenblatt and

Shader, 1974). The particular safety of these agents in overdoses is another of their great advantages over conventional sedative-hypnotic drugs.

Cytogentic Studies

In vitro studies of the effects of chlordiazepoxide on human leukocytes exposed to a variety of doses (some huge) of chlordiazepoxide revealed no evidence of chromosomal damage (Stenchever, Frankel, Jarvis, and Veress, 1970). Despite the limitations of applying such studies to the clinical situation, this experience is certainly consonant with that observed over long and extensive clinical use of this drug and others of its type.

CONCLUSIONS

Once side effects of drugs are known and their mechanisms become clear, we live with them more comfortably. To be forewarned in this case is to be truly forearmed. We can dismiss those effects of little consequence, take acceptable risks with the ones that are rare, and be alert to those which may be potentially dangerous.

Uncertainty creates malaise. With a side effect such as tardive dyskinesia, we still are not clear about its mechanisms or the implications of the persistent disorder. The same is true about the cardiac complications from antidepressants and antipsychotics, the most serious of which—sudden death—is not only rare but probably a simple increase in a normally minute natural risk. For these reasons the study of side effects of psychotherapeutic drugs will continue to be of importance in delineating their proper areas of use.

REFERENCES

ACNP-FDA Task Force (1973): Medical intelligence—drug therapy. *N. Engl. J. Med.,* 289:20–24.

Agulnik, P. L., DiMascio, A., and Moore, P. (1972): Acute brain syndrome associated with lithium therapy. *Am. J. Psychiatry,* 129:621–623.

Alvarez-Mena, S. C., and Frank, M. J. (1973): Phenothiazine-induced T-wave abnormalities. *J.A.M.A.,* 224:1730–1733.

Appel, P., Eckel, K., and Harrer, G. (1971): Veranderungen des Blasen- und Blasensphinktertonus durch Thymoleptika: Zystomanometrische Untersuchungen beim Menschen. *Int. Pharmacopsychiatry,* 6:15.

Ayd, F. J., Jr. (1974): Effects of lithium on thyroid function in man. *Int. Drug Ther. Newslett.,* 9:13–16.

Beumont, P. J. V., Corker, C. S., Friesen, H. G., Kolakowska, T., Mandelbrote, B. M., Marshall, J., Murray, M. A. F., and Wiles, D. H. (1974): The effects of phenothiazines on endocrine function. II. Effect in men and post-menopausal women. *Br. J. Psychiatry,* 124:420–430.

Beumont, P. J. V., Gelder, M. G., Friesen, H. G., Harris, G. W., MacKinnon, P. C. B., Mandelbrote, B. M., and Wiles, D. H. (1974): The effects of phenothiazines on endocrine function. I. Patients with inappropriate lactation and amenorrhoea. *Br. J. Psychiatry,* 124:413–419.

Bojanovsky, J., and Tolle, R. (1974): Dihydroergotamin gegen die Kreislaufwirkungen der Thymoleptika. *Dtsch. Med. Wochenschr.*, 99:1064–1069.

Boston Collaborative Drug Surveillance Program (1972): Adverse reactions to the tricyclic-antidepressant drugs. *Lancet*, 1:529–531.

Brackenridge, R. G. (1972): Cardiotoxicity of amitriptyline. *Lancet*, 2:929–930.

Brown, D., Winsberg, B. G., Bialer, I., and Press, M. (1973): Imipramine therapy and seizures: Three children treated for hyperactive behavior disorders. *Am. J. Psychiatry*, 130:210–212.

Candy, J. (1972): Severe hypothyroidism—an early complication of lithium therapy. *Br. Med. J.*, 3:277.

Clarke, A. E., Maritz, V. M., and Denborough, M. A. (1972): Phenothiazines and jaundice. *Aust. NZ. J. Med.*, 2:376–382.

Clarke, I. M. C. (1971): Adynamic ileus and amitriptyline. *Br. Med. J.*, 2:531.

Cohen, M. M., Hirschhorn, K., and Frosch, W. A. (1969): Cytogenetic effects of tranquilizing drugs in vivo and in vitro. *J.A.M.A.*, 207:2425–2426.

Couper-Smartt, J. D., and Rodham, R. (1973): A technique for surveying side-effects of tricyclic drugs with reference to reported sexual effects. *J. Int. Med. Res.*, 1:473–476.

Covi, L., Lipman, R. S., Pattison, J. H., Derogatis, L. R., and Uhlenhuth, E. H. (1973): Length of treatment with anxiolytic sedatives and response to their sudden withdrawal. *Acta Psychiatr. Scand.*, 49:51–64.

Crombie, D. L., Pinsent, R. J., and Fleming, D. (1972): Imipramine in pregnancy. *Br. Med. J.*, 1:745.

Davies, R. K., Tucker, G. J., Harrow, M., and Detre, T. P. (1971): Confusional episodes and antidepressant medication. *Am. J. Psychiatry*, 128:95–99.

Demers, R. G., and Harris, R. L. (1972): The effect of dietary sodium on renal lithium excretion in the manic-depressive. *Dis. Nerv. Syst.*, 33:372–375.

Demers, R. G., Hendler, R., Allen, R. P., and Boyd, J. (1972): Edema and increased plasma renin activity in lithium treated patients. *Behav. Neuropsychiatry*, 3:20–24.

Demers, R. G., and Heninger, G. R. (1971a): Sodium intake and lithium treatment in mania. *Am. J. Psychiatry*, 128:100–104.

Demers, R. G., and Heninger, G. R. (1971b): Electrocardiographic T-wave changes during lithium carbonate treatment. *J.A.M.A.*, 218:381–386.

Dimond, R. C., Brammer, S. R., Atkinson, R. L., Jr., Howard, W. J., and Earll, J. M. (1973): Chlorpromazine treatment and growth hormone secretory responses in acromegaly. *J. Clin. Endocrinol. Metab.*, 36:1189–1195.

Editorial (1971): Cardiovascular complications of tricyclic antidepressants. *N.Z. Med. J.*, 74:390.

Eggermont, E., Raveschot, J., Deneve, V., and Casteels-Van Daele, M. (1972): The adverse influence of imipramine on the adaptation of the newborn infant to extrauterine life. *Acta Paediatr. Belg.*, 26:197–204.

Erwin, C. W., Gerber, C. J., Morrison, S. D., and James, J. F. (1973): Lithium carbonate and convulsive disorders. *Arch. Gen. Psychiatry*, 28:646–648.

Fann, W. E., Davis, J. M., and Janowsky, D. S. (1972): The prevalence of tardive dyskinesias in mental hospital patients. *Dis. Nerv. Syst.*, 33:182–186.

Fischbach, R. (1973): Die vegetativen Effekte der Antidepressiva im Bereich des Gastro-Intestinaltraktes. *Wien. Med. Wochenschr.* (*123 Suppl.*), 5:3–26.

Gerlach, J., Reisby, N., and Randrup, A. (1974): Dopaminergic hypersensitivity and cholinergic hypofunction in the pathophysiology of tardive dyskinesia. *Psychopharmacologia*, 34:21–35.

Girwood, R. H. (1974): Therapeutic drug deaths in Britain. *Br. Med. J.*, 1:501–504.

Goldfield, M. D., and Weinstein, M. R. (1973): Lithium carbonate in obstetrics: Guidelines for clinical use. *Am. J. Obstet. Gynecol.*, 116:15–22.

Greenblatt, D. J., and Shader, R. I. (1974): *Benzodiazepines in Clinical Practice*, pp. 250–252. Raven Press, New York.

Hollister, L. E. (1959): Chlorpromazine jaundice. *J.A.M.A.*, 169:1235–1236.

Hollister, L. E. (1974): Psychotherapeutic drugs and driving. *Ann. Intern. Med.*, 80:413.

Hollister, L. E., and Hall, R. A. (1966): Phenothiazine derivatives and morphologic changes in the liver. *Am. J. Psychiatry*, 123:211–212.

Hollister, L. E., Motzenbecker, F. P., and Degan, R. O. (1961): Withdrawal reactions from chlordiazepoxide ("Librium"). *Psychopharmacologia*, 2:63–68.

Idanpaan-Heikkila, J., and Saxen, L. (1973): Possible teratogenicity of imipramine chloropyramine. *Lancet*, 2:282–284.

Kazamatsuri, H., Chien, C-P., and Cole, J. O. (1972): Therapeutic approaches to tardive dyskinesia. *Arch. Gen. Psychiatry*, 27:491–499.

Kerry, R. J. (1974): Lithium and weight gain. *Br. Med. J.*, 2:441.

Kirk, L., Baastrup, P. C., and Schou, M. (1973): Propranolol treatment of lithium-induced tremor. *Lancet*, 2:1086–1087.

Klawans, H. L., Jr. (1973): The pharmacology of tardive dyskinesias. *Am. J. Psychiatry*, 130:82–86.

Klawans, H. L., Jr., Bergen, D., and Bruyn, G. W. (1973): Prolonged drug-induced parkinsonism. *Confin. Neurol.*, 35:368–377.

Klawans, H. L., Bergen, D., Bruyn, G. W., and Paulson, G. W. (1974): Neuroleptic-induced tardive dyskinesias in nonpsychotic patients. *Arch. Neurol.*, 30:338–339.

Klett, C. J., and Caffey, E., Jr. (1972): Evaluating the long-term need for antiparkinson drugs by chronic schizophrenics. *Arch. Gen. Psychiatry*, 26:374–379.

Kochar, M. S., Wang, R. I. H., and D'Cunha, G. F. (1971): Electrocardiographic changes simulating hypokalemia during treatment with lithium carbonate. J. Electrocardiol, 4:371–373.

Kozakova, M. (1971): Liekova purpura po antidepresivach. *Cesk. Dermatol.*, 46:158–160.

Kuenssberg, E. V., and Knox, J. D. E. (1972): Imipramine in pregnancy. *Br. Med. J.*, 2:292.

Kusumi, Y. (1971): A cutaneous side effect of lithium: Report on two cases. *Dis. Nerv. Syst.*, 32:853–854.

Lambert, P. A. (1973): Les effets indesirables des antidepresseurs tricycliques. *Therapie*, 28:269–305.

Levy, S. T., Forrest, J. N., Jr., and Heninger, G. R. (1973): Lithium-induced diabetes insipidus: Manic symptoms, brain and electrolyte correlates, and chlorothiazide treatment. *Am. J. Psychiatry*, 130:1014–1018.

Linnoila, M., and Mattila, M. J. (1973): Drug interaction on psychomotor skills related to driving: Diazepam and alcohol. *Eur. J. Clin. Pharmacol.*, 5:186–194.

Loo, H., and Bousser, M. G. (1972): Incidents et accidents des chimiotherapies par les antidepresseurs. *Cah. Med.*, 13:777–794.

Luke, C. M. (1971): Tricyclic antidepressants and heart disease. *N.Z. Med. J.*, 74:345.

Luzecky, M. H., Burman, K. D., and Schultz, E. R. (1974): The syndrome of inappropriate secretion of antidiuretic hormone associated with amitriptyline administration. *South. Med. J.*, 67:495–497.

Martinez-Maldonado, M., and Terrell, J. (1973): Lithium carbonate-induced nephrogenic diabetes insipidus and glucose intolerance. *Arch. Intern. Med.*, 132:881–884.

McBride, N. G. (1972): Limb deformities associated with iminodibenzyl hydrochloride. *Med. J. Aust.*, 1:492.

Meltzer, H. Y. (1973): Rigidity, hyperpyrexia and coma following fluphenazine enanthate. *Psychopharmacologia*, 29:337–346.

Miller, E. M. (1974): Deanol: A solution for tardive dyskinesia? *N. Engl. J. Med.*, 291:796–797.

Moir, D. C. (1973): Tricyclic antidepressants and cardiac disease. *Am. Heart. J.*, 86:841–842.

Moir, D. C., Cornwell, W. B., Dingwall-Fordyce, I., Crooks, J., O Malley, K., Turnbull, M. J., and Weir, R. D. (1972): Cardiotoxicity of amitriptyline. *Lancet*, 2:561–564.

Moir, D. C., Dingwall-Fordyce, I., and Weir, R. D. (1973): Medicines evaluation and monitoring group: A followup study of cardiac patients receiving amitriptyline. *Eur. J. Clin. Pharmacol.*, 6:98–101.

Morgan, M. H., and Read, A. E. (1972): Antidepressants and liver disease. *Gut*, 13:697–701.

Morrow, A. W. (1972): Limb deformities associated with iminodibenzyl hydrochloride. *Med. J. Aust.*, 1:831.

Nouri, A., and Cuendet, J. F. (1971): Atteintes oculaires au cours des traitements aux thymoleptiques. *Schweiz. Med. Wochenschr.,* 101:1178–1180.

Paykel, E. S., Mueller, P. S., and De La Vergne, P. M. (1973): Amitriptyline, weight gain and carbohydrate craving: A side effect. *Br. J. Psychiatry,* 123:501–507.

Pisciotta, A. V. (1969): Agranulocytosis induced by certain phenothiazine derivatives. *J.A.M.A.,* 208:1862–1868.

Prien, R. F., Caffey, E. M., Jr., and Klett, C. J. (1972): Relationship between serum lithium level and clinical response in acute mania treated with lithium. *Br. J. Psychiatry,* 120:409–414.

Raisfeld, I. H. (1972): Cardiovascular complications of antidepressant therapy: Interactions at the adrenergic neuron. *Am. Heart J.,* 83:129–133.

Ramsey, T. A., Mendels, J., Stokes, J. W., and Fitzgerald, R. G. (1972): Lithium carbonate and kidney function: A failure in renal concentration ability. *J.A.M.A.,* 219:1446–1449.

Raskin, A. (1972): Adverse reactions to phenelzine: Results of a nine-hospital depression study. *J. Clin. Pharmacol.,* 12:22–25.

Read, A. E., Laidlaw, J., and McCarthy, C. F. (1969): Effects of chlorpromazine in patients with hepatic disease. *Br. Med. J.,* 3:497–499.

Rifkin, A., Kurtin, S. B., Quitkin, F., and Klein, D. F. (1973): Lithium-induced folliculitis. *Am. J. Psychiatry,* 130:1018–1019.

Ruiz-Maldonado, R., Perez de Francisco, C., and Tamayo, L. (1973): Lithium dermatitis. *J.A.M.A.,* 224:1534.

Sathananthan, G. L., and Gershon, S. (1973): Imipramine withdrawal: An akathisia-like syndrome. *Am. J. Psychiatry,* 130:1286–1287.

Schou, M., and Amdisen, A. (1973): Lithium and pregnancy. III. Lithium ingestion by children breast-fed by women on lithium treatment. *Br. Med. J.,* 2:138.

Schou, M., Amdisen, A., and Steenstrup, O. R. (1973a): Lithium and pregnancy. II. Hazards to women given lithium during pregnancy and delivery. *Br. Med. J.,* 2:137–138.

Schou, M., Goldfield, M. D., Weinstein, M. R., and Villeneuve, A. (1973b): Lithium and pregnancy. I. Report from the register of lithium babies. *Br. Med. J.,* 2:135–136.

Shopsin, B., Johnson, G., and Gershon, S. (1970): Neurotoxicity with lithium: Differential drug responsiveness. *Int. Pharmacopsychiatry,* 5:170.

Shopsin, B., Shenkman, L., Blum, M., and Hollander, C. S. (1973): Iodine and lithium-induced hypothyroidism: Documentation of synergism. *Am. J. Med.,* 55:695–699.

Singer, I., Rotenberg, D., and Puschett, J. B. (1972): Lithium-induced nephrogenic diabetes insipidus: In vivo and in vitro studies. *J. Clin. Invest.,* 51:1081–1091.

Stancer, H. C., and Kivi, R. (1971): Lithium carbonate and oedema. *Lancet,* 2:988.

Stenchever, M. A., Frankel, R. S., Jarvis, J. A., and Veress, K. (1970): Effect of chlordiazepoxide hydrochloride on human chromosomes. *Am. J. Obstet. Gynecol.,* 106:920–923.

Varsamis, J., and Wand, R. R. (1972): Severe diarrhea associated with lithium-carbonate therapy in regional ileitis. *Lancet,* 2:1322.

Vestergaard, P. A., and Poulsen, J. C. (1972): Myxoedema—possible side-effects of lithium? *Lancet,* 2:427–428.

Vinarova, E., Uhlif, O., Stika, L., and Vinar, O. (1972): Side effects of lithium administration. *Act. Nerv. Super.* (Praha), 14:105–107.

Weiden, P. L., and Buckner, C. D. (1973): Thioridazine toxicity: Agranulocytosis and hepatitis with encephalopathy. *J.A.M.A.,* 224:518–520.

Winstead, D. K., Anderson, A., Eilers, M. K., Blackwell, B., and Zaremba, A. L. (1974): Diazepam on demand: Drug-seeking behavior in psychiatric inpatients. *Arch. Gen. Psychiatry,* 30:349–351.

Woody, J. N., London, W. L., and Wilbands, G. D., Jr. (1971): Lithium toxicity in a newborn. *Pediatrics,* 47:94–96.

Wyatt, R. J., Fram, D. H., Buchbinder, R., and Snyder, F. (1971): Treatment of intractable narcolepsy with a monoamine oxidase inhibitor. *N. Engl. J. Med.,* 285:987–991.

Chapter 17

Drug Interactions Involving Psychotherapeutic Agents

John S. Kaufmann

The rapid increase in the number of potent new pharmacological agents during the past half-century has made available to the practicing physician an arsenal of drugs with which many of man's maladies can be cured or rendered tolerable. These advances have been accompanied by an unfortunate number of drug-induced diseases and adverse reactions. *Adverse reactions* to psychotherapeutic agents were discussed in the preceding chapter. It is equally important for the practicing physician to recognize that many *adverse drug interactions* may occur in patients receiving several drugs concomitantly.

The scope of "adverse drug interactions" depends on the manner in which the term is defined. It is recognized that when two or more drugs are used simultaneously to treat a patient, each may act independently or, to varying degrees, in concert. When two or more drugs interact in such a way that the expected response to one or more of the drugs is diminished or enhanced, or a new or unanticipated response is elicited, a significant *drug interaction* may be said to have occurred. If such an altered response exerts a deleterious effect on a patient, then the drug interaction is one of adverse nature. It would be correct, in the broadest sense, to include drug incompatibilities (physicochemical) and drug-induced changes in diagnostic laboratory procedures as types of adverse drug interations. Clearly these might result in ineffective therapy or diagnostic errors leading to poor results in patient care. These two important aspects of drug therapy have been reviewed extensively elsewhere and are not dealt with here (Lubran, 1969; Martin, 1971). It is the wise physician, however, who recognizes obvious incompatibilities and acquaints himself with the vagaries of laboratory data influenced by the drugs he elects to use!

Estimates of the frequency of adverse drug reactions vary considerably, but several surveillance studies suggest that up to 30% of hospitalized patients and approximately 3% of outpatient populations experience significant adverse drug effects (Jick, 1974; Caranasos, Stewart, and Cluff, 1974). The frequency of most adverse interactions, however, is simply unknown. It has been observed that the incidence of adverse drug reactions in hospitalized patients increases geometrically with the number of medications taken. From this, it has been inferred that drug interactions account for a large fraction

289

of such a noticeable rise. Although logic dictates that this is at least partly true, there are no prospective studies to validate the assumption.

Although some adverse drug interactions have been predicted on the basis of known pharmacological properties of new therapeutic agents, most have been observed initially only after such drugs had been used for some time by practicing physicians. Reports of apparent interactions are usually anecdotal and all too often go unrecognized for long periods of time. In addition, many practitioners are understandably reluctant to report such occurrences for reasons such as lack of "scientific" evidence, the possibility of litigation procedures evolving from such disclosure, too little time, or the erroneous assumption that the observation has already been recorded.

Psychotherapeutic agents are prescribed quite frequently by most physicians (Blackwell, 1973). Psychiatrists and other physicians involved in the treatment of patients with severe mental disease undoubtedly use antipsychotic agents with a higher frequency than do other practitioners, and pediatricians likely have a low utilization rate. Most physicians, however, prescribe sedatives, antianxiety agents, and antidepressants quite commonly. Such agents are used as therapeutic adjuncts in the overall care of patients with a variety of organic diseases, both acute and chronic. It is this setting—that of acute or chronic organic disease with its attendant emotional overlay —in which the simultaneous use of one or more psychoactive drugs and any number of other therapeutic agents most commonly occurs. It is imperative therefore that all physicians know the many pharmacological properties of each of the psychotherapeutic agents they employ. Such knowledge is essential if other drugs used in various diseases are to be rationally selected and effectively utilized.

Although certain drugs become universally accepted by physicians and maintain this status for many years, the utilization rates of most drugs rise and fall as newer and more effective agents are introduced into the therapeutic arena. This flux creates obvious difficulties for the busy practitioner, for he usually has progressively less time to acquaint himself with the pharmacological properties of new agents, yet senses a compelling need to use these "more effective" drugs for the benefit of his patients. It is reasonable to speculate that this situation would be conducive to a higher incidence of adverse interactions. Clearly a computer-backed surveillance mechanism would be of great assistance in forewarning physicians of known and suspected interactions. Of equal clarity is the realization that no such system can be assembled and used effectively until meaningful information regarding the true incidence and clinical significance of drug interactions is amassed and evaluated critically. From what source will this information necessarily arise?

Recently extensive surveillance studies have been initiated in order to determine the incidence of significant drug reactions and interactions (Jick, 1974; Miller, 1974). It is already apparent that these programs are able to identify adverse drug reactions and interactions previously unsuspected and unknown. These investigative studies, however, are currently limited in number and are expensive. Many of the larger hospitals and other medical organizations throughout the country also have instituted computerized systems capable of monitoring drug usage, and through this mechanism are able to warn physicians regarding possible adverse drug effects. Still, it is the practicing physician who must ultimately be the one who identifies and reports possible adverse drug interactions and, to a great extent, assesses the significance of them. Thus charged with this responsibility, each physician not only must know and use his chosen therapeutic agents well, but also must understand the basic mechanisms by which these drugs interact and cause adverse effects in his patients.

MECHANISMS OF DRUG INTERACTIONS IN MAN

There are two major factors that determine the response to a pharmacologically active agent. The first depends on the concentration and intrinsic activity of the drug present in the "biophase" or site of action. The second reflects the affinity for the drug by the end-organ "receptors" and the ability of the stimulated end organ to respond.

Interactions Related to Altered Pharmacokinetics

A major cause of adverse drug effects is an unexpected alteration in the concentration of a drug at its site of action. Generally it is possible to demonstrate in animals a direct relationship between the concentration of active drug in the blood and its concentration at its site of action. Although some agents exert lasting effects long after blood levels virtually have disappeared, most drugs induce responses proportional to the amount of active, free drug present in the bloodstream. Commonly when a second drug influences the response to a previously administered agent, it does so by directly or indirectly changing the concentration of free drug in the plasma. This altered drug concentration is most often a result of changes in absorption, distribution, metabolism, or excretion. The relationships of the major mechanisms which determine the concentration of active free drug in plasma are depicted in Fig. 1.

A drug may alter the absorption of another agent by reacting with it to form insoluble or nonabsorbable complexes. Drug-induced alterations in gastrointestinal motility, enzyme activity, intraluminal pH, or other determinants of drug bioavailability can lead to significant changes in therapeutic responses to subsequently administered drugs (Morrelli and Melmon, 1968, 1972; Nies, 1974).

The distribution of drugs depends on many factors. Principal among these are the binding of drugs to plasma and tissue proteins, variation in body fluid compartments, regional blood flow, and physicochemical properties of drugs which determine the mechanisms and rates of their transport into body tissues. Since the free or unbound drug present in plasma is the only form in equilibrium with active drug at the receptor site, the degree of binding and the avidity of plasma protein for a given drug are significant determinants of pharmacological responsiveness to a drug. Drugs which bind tightly to plasma proteins frequently displace other drugs that are more loosely bound (Brodie, 1965; Azarnoff and Hurwitz, 1970; Nies, 1974). In this situation

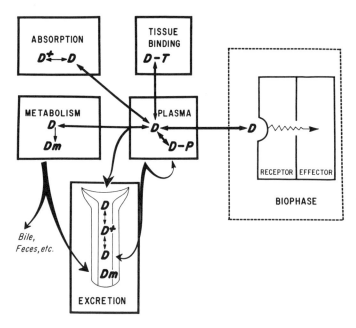

FIG. 1. Major determinants of free drug concentration. D, free drug, un-ionized. D$^+$, free drug, ionized. D-P, drug bound to plasma protein. D-T, drug bound or sequestered in various body tissues. Dm, drug metabolite(s).

the concentration of free drug of the more loosely bound species might increase significantly. This in turn could lead to enhanced pharmacological effects, increased drug metabolism and excretion, or toxicity.

The body generally regards most drugs as foreign or noxious substances to be discarded. The principal manner in which such elimination occurs is through renal excretion. For renal excretion to be effective, a drug must be soluble in aqueous media. Drugs which have a high degree of lipid solubility are characteristically able to penetrate cell membranes rapidly. Anesthetics as well as most of the psychotherapeutic agents tend to share this property and consequently readily penetrate the central nervous system (CNS). Generally lipid-soluble compounds are less effectively cleared by the kidney. Even if cleared by glomerular filtration, they tend to be reabsorbed into the bloodstream by passive diffusion from the tubular lumen. One can surmise correctly on a teleological basis that such compounds generally must be metabolized to more water-soluble compounds and/or inactive conjugates, which can then be cleared from the body by renal excretion.

Although many drugs are metabolized in various body tissues, the liver is the principal organ of drug metabolism. There are many different hepatic enzyme systems capable of metabolizing various drugs; however, one of the principal systems for enzymatic biotransformation is the mixed-function oxidases, the core of which is the P-450 cytochrome oxidase system. This enzyme system appears to be located in the "microsomal" fraction or smooth endoplasmic reticulum and is capable of oxidizing many different types of compounds.

Although the activity of certain other hepatic enzyme systems can be stimulated by a variety of compounds, it is primarily this enzyme system whose functional capacity may be stimulated or induced by several different drugs (Conney, 1967; Kuntzman, 1969). Classic examples of drugs capable of enzyme induction include many sedative-hypnotic agents such as the barbiturates. Once induction has occurred and is maintained, the enzyme system frequently displays augmented metabolism of other drugs which have little ability to induce their own metabolism. Thus "inducers" may diminish the blood levels of other drugs, thereby making it necessary for the physician to use larger doses in order to maintain a desired therapeutic effect. Moreover, if therapy with the inducing agent is stopped, the incremented dosage of the second agent, if maintained, often becomes excessive, and toxic manifestations occur (Breckenridge and Orme, 1970). It is apparent that if this latter sequence of events involved a drug such as warfarin sodium, serious hemorrhage might occur. Conversely, some drugs such as glutethimide and meprobamate stimulate their own metabolism (Conney, 1967). Indeed, it may be that tolerance to these drugs could be explained, at least in part, on the basis of induced metabolism. Thus plasma concentrations of these drugs might decrease with time, despite maintenance of the initial dosage.

In contrast to enzyme induction, there are certain drugs that may inhibit enzyme systems capable of metabolizing other drugs (Morrelli and Melmon, 1972; Nies, 1974). In this situation the plasma concentration of a drug might be increased to toxic levels by introducing a second drug that inhibits the metabolism of the first drug. For example, the CNS stimulant methylphenidate can inhibit the metabolism of various drugs, including diphenylhydantoin, phenothiazines, tricyclic antidepressants, and warfarin sodium, thereby increasing their therapeutic effect or leading to serious toxicity (Morrelli and Melmon, 1972; Nies, 1974). Hence the administration of one drug prior to or during the course of therapy with another drug may lead to significant changes in half-life and pharmacological activity, both of which would be a consequence of altered metabolic degradation.

Although a few drugs have significant elimination pathways through the lungs, skin, bowel, and biliary tract, most drugs and their metabolites are cleared through the kidney. Renal excretion of an active drug may occur by means of glomerular filtration, tubular secretion, or a combination of both. Renal blood flow and glomerular integrity are of obvious importance in the formation of the plasma ultrafiltrate. In the absence of cardiovascular abnormality or glomerular disease, drug elimination by glomerular filtration depends primarily on plasma protein binding. Thus drugs that are highly bound to proteins are not easily cleared by glomerular filtration. These drugs along with other organic acids and bases are secreted into the tubular lumen by active transport processes. The unmetabolized fractions of psychotherapeutic agents (e.g., weak bases, amphetamine, and tricyclic antidepressants) are cleared by this mechanism. Drug metabolites such as glucuronides and ethereal sulfates are also eliminated by this mechanism. Since renal plasma flow is normally four to five times greater than the glomerular filtration rate, such secretory mechanisms can be quite efficient.

Factors that alter drug excretion at this level include competition for transport mechanisms and metabolic poisons. It is apparent, then, that competitive drug interactions at the level of a kidney tubule might influence anticipated drug responses or lead to problems of toxicity. Once a drug is in the tubular lumen, factors such as pH, lipid solubility, and flow rate become important determinants of drug elimination (Morrelli and Melmon, 1972). Increased flow rate caused by osmotic diuretics exemplifies enhanced drug elimination by diminishing tubular transit time. However, the effects of changes in the pH of tubular urine is somewhat more comlex. Lipid-soluble or nonpolar compounds readily re-enter the bloodstream by passive diffusion. Drugs which are un-ionized also have enhanced lipid solubility. Therefore the clearance of weak acids and bases depends to a great degree on the pH of the tubular urine. At lower pH levels, weak acids tend to be more un-ionized, are more readily reabsorbed, and therefore have diminished clearance. The reverse is true at higher pH. Clearance of the acidic barbiturates is increased by alkalinizing the urine, for these compounds are more ionized in an alkaline environment and are less able to re-enter the bloodstream by passive diffusion through the tubular cell. For the same reasons, the weak bases, amphetamine, and tricyclic antidepressants are more ionized in acidic urine and therefore in this physicochemical state are not readily reabsorbed. Thus drugs which directly or indirectly create changes in the pH or flow of tubular urine may alter clearance rates of other drugs capable of ionization within the physiological range.

Interactions at Receptor Sites

The second major factor determining drug action (i.e., drug receptor affinity and end-organ responsiveness) is composed of a multifaceted and complex series of events. Drugs may compete directly with other drugs for receptor sites, alter pharmacophysiological phenomena which occur before and after receptor stimulation, or act directly on the end organ in such a way that the response to other drugs is altered (Morrelli and Melmon, 1972).

Alterations in receptor stimulation or end-organ response form the basis for many interactions exploited for therapeutic benefit as well as interactions leading to toxicity. For example, atropine interacts with acetylcholine by competing with this neurotransmitter for the cholinergic receptor site. Since atropine does not possess receptor-stimulating activity, an effective blockade ensues. Likewise, phentolamine competes with norepinephrine at the postganglionic α-adrenergic receptor site. Other drugs interact with enzymes at end organs or neuroeffector junctions to alter physiological responses. Such interaction is often characterized by a drug interfering with enzymes involved in either the synthesis or degradation of neurotransmitter substances.

Alteration in these functions frequently leads to a modified response to a second drug. For example, certain agents inhibit monoamine oxidase (MAO), an enzyme that degrades unbound amines within the adrenergic neuron. Thus intraneuronal accumulation of such amines may lead to exaggerated responses to both normal stimuli and drugs which might cause their release. Clearly drug interactions at receptor sites and their closely related neurotransmitter and effector components constitute a large and varied group of medically important phenomena.

INTERACTIONS INVOLVING THE PSYCHOTHERAPEUTIC AGENTS

Major Tranquilizers and/or Antipsychotic Agents

The major tranquilizers can be categorized conveniently into four major groups: (1) phenothiazines, e.g., chlorpromazine; (2) thioxanthenes, e.g., thiothixene; (3) butyrophenones, e.g., haloperidol; and (4) rauwolfia alkaloids, e.g., reserpine. Inasmuch as the rauwolfia alkaloids are seldom used for antipsychotic therapy in the United States, interactions involving rauwolfia relate primarily to its use as an antihypertensive agent.

Interactions of the major tranquilizers with other drugs are discussed in relation to CNS depressants, CNS stimulants, antihypertensive and other vasoactive compounds, and miscellaneous interactions.

Interactions With CNS Depressants

Phenothiazines potentiate the CNS depression produced by other antipsychotic agents, narcotic analgesics, minor tranquilizers, barbiturates and other sedatives, and the universally available CNS depressant alcohol (Hollister, 1972). In general, this type of interaction may be viewed as additive or potentiating in nature. Extreme care should be exercised in the concomitant use of any of these agents with the phenothiazine-type drugs and other major tranquilizers. Mechanisms of action of all of these agents were discussed in previous chapters.

Interactions With CNS Stimulants

Phenothiazine derivatives and other major tranquilizers may interact with MAO inhibitors, leading to significant hypotension (Goldberg, 1964). The ability of MAO inhibitors to lower blood pressure is postulated to result from accumulation of "false neurotransmitters," compounds that possess lower intrinsic activity than norepinephrine (Cohen, Kopin, Creveling, Musacchio, Fischer, Crout, and Gill, 1966). This feature, combined with postsynaptic adrenergic blockade by the phenothiazines, may lead to significant episodes of orthostatic hypotension and hypotensive episodes during surgery. Paradoxically the concurrent administration of MAO inhibitors and phenothiazines has also been associated with a syndrome characterized by severe extrapyramidal symptoms and hypertension (Barsa and Sanders, 1964).

The phenothiazines and amphetamines generally antagonize the effects of one another, both peripherally and centrally. There is reason to believe that amphetamines exert CNS effects both by noradrenergic and dopaminergic neuronal stimulation, resulting in release of the corresponding neurotransmitter amines (Axelrod, 1970; Carlsson, 1970). In addition, there is substantial evidence which suggests that the phenothiazines exert postsynaptic blockade on noradrenergic as well as dopaminergic receptors (Hollister, 1972). The latter mechanism is suggested particularly by the extrapyramidal manifestations resembling Parkinson's disease often seen in patients receiving phenothiazines. As noted, the amphetamines can act indirectly to release both norepinephrine and dopamine. The observed enhancement of mental alertness, increased motor activity, and dyskinesia as well as overt psychotic reactions lends credence to this concept. The ability of amphetamine to inhibit dopamine uptake by neurons in addition to norepinephrine uptake might explain its antidepressant effects. Amphetamines also act peripherally by displacement of norepinephrine from adrenergic neuronal terminals and may produce hypertension. Chlorpromazine, a phenothiazine prototype, by virtue of its sympathetic blocking capabilities, can antagonize these amphetamine-induced pressor effects.

In addition, phenothiazines (e.g., chlorpromazine) are able to inhibit the metabolism of amphetamine (Sulser and Dingell, 1968). Thus at low concentrations phenothiazines exert little α-adrenergic blockade but do significantly inhibit the metabolism of amphetamine and thereby lead to potentiation of amphetamine's pharmacological effects. At higher doses the predominant effect of the phenothiazines is that of α-adrenergic blockade and a consequent decrease in amphetamine response. It is apparent that the interaction potential of the phenothiazines and amphetamines is bimodal and dose-dependent. Clearly the concurrent use of these two drugs creates a therapeutic challenge to the practitioner and in the absence of close super-vision constitutes an overt hazard to the patient. It should be noted that the butyrophenone compound haloperidol, in contrast to most phenothiazine-like drugs, inhibits amphetamine metabolism at doses sufficient to block most of the amphetamine stimulant effects (Lemberger, Witt, Davis, and Kopin, 1970).

The older CNS stimulants such as pentylenetetrazol and picrotoxin may induce convulsive episodes in patients receiving a phenothiazine because of the latter's ability to lower seizure threshold (Jarvik, 1970). The tricyclic antidepressants also may interact adversely with the phenothiazines by one of two general mechanisms. First, the concomitant use of these agents may result in convulsive episodes precipitated by a lowered seizure threshold; second, the simultaneous use of these agents may lead to hypotensive episodes caused by the additive effects of adrenergic blockade (the phenothiazines) and ganglionic blockade (the tricyclic antidepressants).

Interactions with Other Centrally Active Agents

The major tranquilizers may interact significantly with other agents, lead-ing to adverse effects manifested by abnormal function of the nervous system. The ability of the phenothiazines and thioxanthenes to lower seizure threshold may alter patient responses to anticonvulsants. Use of the antipsychotic agents may of course enhance the CNS depressant effects of anesthetic agents and through their peripheral adrenergic blocking properties significantly aug-ment the hypotension accompanying surgical anesthesia (Martin, 1971).

Interactions with Antihypertensive Agents and Vasodilator Compounds

Numerous potentially adverse interactions with antihypertensive agents and vasoactive amines can occur during therapy with the phenothiazines. A clear understanding of the pharmacological properties of the various agents in these categories enables the physician to avoid most therapeutic pitfalls in this area. It is likely that the thiazide diuretics and the direct vasodilators (diazox-ide, hydralazine, minoxidil, etc.) exert exaggerated hypotensive effects when used concomitantly with phenothiazines as a consequence of the latter's α-adrenergic blocking properties. In addition to this α-adrenergic blockade, the phenothiazines share with the tricyclic antidepressants (but to a lesser degree) the ability to block the neuronal amine pump (Janowsky, El-Yousef, Davis, and Fann, 1973). It is this mechanism by which the action of nor-epinephrine, released by nerve stimulation, is primarily terminated. Also, it is this nonspecific amine transport mechanism by which guanethidine and other potent guanidinium antihypertensive agents are able to enter the neuron terminal (Mitchell, Cavanaugh, Arias, and Oates, 1970). The antihypertensive effects of these potent compounds depend on their ability to enter and act within the adrenergic neuron. Thus the phenothiazines may block the amine transport system and, if given to a patient also receiving guanethidine or bethanidine, prevent or reverse the intended antihypertensive effects of these agents (Janowsky, El-Yousef, Davis, Fann, and Oates, 1972).

Conversely, the phenothiazines lower blood pressure somewhat through their postsynaptic α-blocking effects. These agents potentiate the hypotensive effects of other α-blocking agents (e.g., phentolamine and phenoxybenzamine) and therefore should be used with caution in such instances. Because of the α-adrenergic blocking effect, significant hypotension brought about or enhanced by the phenothiazines may be reversibly treated by judicious use of a predominantly α-adrenergic agonist (e.g., norepinephrine, phenylephrine, or methoxamine). A lack of response to this therapeutic approach might be followed rationally by administering an agent capable of direct vasoconstriction (e.g., angiotensin). The concomitant use of phenothiazines and epinephrine is unwise because epinephrine possesses both α- and β-agonist properties of potent degree. If epinephrine is administered to a patient receiving one of the phenothiazines, the β-effect predominates and a further reduction in blood pressure may occur (Morrelli and Melmon, 1972). For the same reasons it is apparent that the use of isoproterenol in patients receiving phenothiazines should be undertaken with extreme caution, and only in circumstances of absolute necessity.

It might be reasoned from the previous discussion that the use of β-adrenergic blocking agent propranolol with a phenothiazine might be attended by either a slight rise or little change in blood pressure. Although documentation is lacking, the opposite effect likely occurs in most instances. It should be recalled that propranolol alone effectively lowers blood pressure by decreasing cardiac output as a consequence of its chronotropic and inotropic blocking properties on the heart. Thus the somewhat paradoxical hypotensive potential of both α- and β-adrenergic blocking agents in combination with phenothiazine derivatives should be considered carefully prior to concurrent use of these agents.

Interactions with Miscellaneous Compounds

It is well documented that a large variety of sedatives and hypnotics may induce hepatic microsomal metabolism. These effects are discussed specifically under that heading (*vide infra*); however, it is appropriate to note that the phenothiazine derivatives interact with several of the **barbiturates** (amobarbital, phenobarbital, etc.) in a fashion that is consistent with mutual reduction of drug activity. Evidence has accrued which indicates that chlorpromazine can induce metabolism of barbiturates (Conney, 1967), and conversely that the barbiturates may stimulate metabolism of the phenothiazines (Curry, Davis, Janowsky, and Marshall, 1970). Inasmuch as both of these agents have additive CNS depressant effects yet are able to decrease blood levels of one another by enzyme induction, accurate prediction of the combined effect of both drugs becomes exceedingly difficult if not impossible. It is apparent, however, that concurrent use of agents representing each of these drug groups must be carefully monitored. In addition, altering the dose of one drug may cause significant changes in the pharmacological effects of the other.

Haloperidol, a butyrophenone, appears also to interact with certain drugs in a manner not commonly associated with the phenothiazines. There is evidence to suggest that haloperidol's ability to induce hepatic microsomal enzyme activity can lead to accelerated inactivation of oral anticoagulants of both the coumarin and indanedione types (Formiller and Cohon, 1969). Thus patients receiving haloperidol may require unusually high doses of anticoagulants in order to achieve therapeutic drug levels. If the psychotherapeutic agent is subsequently discontinued, thus removing the stimulus for the high rate of anticoagulant metabolism, dangerously high levels of anticoagulant may result in fatal hemorrhage.

It was noted earlier that variations in drug bioavailability of orally administered medications can occur as a consequence of binding, destruction, incomplete disintegration secondary to poor drug formulations, and other alterations within the gastrointestinal tract. The vast number of such occurrences precludes their discussion; suffice it to say that inadequate response to a drug should alert the physician to this strong possibility. As an example, a diminished response to chlorpromazine associated with a decrease in blood levels has resulted from concurrent administration of antacids (Fann, Davis, Janowsky, and Smith, 1973). The extensive use of these latter agents, often without medical advice, clearly points out the necessity of a carefully monitored drug program in patients receiving psychotherapeutic agents.

Reserpine and other rauwolfia derivatives are commonly included in discussions of antipsychotic agents. The ability of these compounds to decrease neurotransmitter amines and to exert CNS depressant effects has been recognized for years; however, their use as psychotherapeutic agents has become almost nonexistent in the United States. Even the current therapeutic *raison d'etre*—its use as an antihypertensive agent—has lost much of its earlier appeal. Despite the economic asset it affords the patient, the side effects resulting from prolonged use negate its moderate degree of effectiveness. The antihypertensive effect probably results from central and peripheral adrenergic blockade associated with neuronal norepinephrine depletion. It is likely that reserpine's mechanism of action depends largely on its ability to block incorporation of dopamine, as well as previously synthesized norepinephrine, into the neuronal storage granules (Sulser and Sanders-Bush, 1971). Such depletion would impair the stimulatory effects of indirectly acting amines such as amphetamine, tyramine, and ephedrine. This property is also the probable mechanism by which reserpine exerts additive or potenti-

ating interactions with other CNS depressants and adrenergic neuronal blocking agents (Jarvik, 1970). The administration of reserpine to patients already
receiving tricyclic antidepressants or MAO inhibitors should be avoided. The
tricyclic antidepressants and MAO inhibitors result in increased neuronal
"sensitivity" to catecholamines and increased intraneuronal stores of catecholamines, respectively (*vide infra*). Thus reserpine administration could
lead ultimately to excessive sympathetic receptor stimulation and paradoxical
manic or hypertensive episodes in patients receiving these antidepressant
agents (Scientific Review Subpanel on Antihypertensives, 1973).

The use of quinidine, digitalis, or other cardioactive agents in the treatment of heart disease must be undertaken with caution in patients receiving
reserpine. Enhanced tendencies for many drug-induced arrhythmias occur in
this situation (Soffer, 1965; Scientific Review Subpanel on Psychotherapeutic
Agents, 1973). The increased risk of hypotensive episodes in patients receiving reserpine who must undergo surgery and general anesthesia is well
known. Chronic catecholamine depletion probably accounts for this response,
but adequate forewarning and appropriate presurgical anticipation of this
possibility usually permits successful anesthetic and surgical treatment
(Ominsky and Wollman, 1969).

Antidepressants

The antidepressants are comprised primarily of the MAO inhibitors and
the tricyclic antidepressants. The amphetamines and congeners are regarded
by some authorities as antidepressant agents but are more correctly classified
as stimulants. Nonetheless, drug interactions involving these three major
groups of compounds are important to the physician.

Interactions Involving MAO Inhibitors

MAO inhibitors constitute an interesting group of biologically active
compounds. They exert significant antidepressant and hypotensive effects,
but the mechanisms by which these agents act pharmacologically remain
unclear. They inhibit MAO in many organ systems, leading to notable increases in norepinephrine, epinephrine, dopamine, and 5-hydroxytryptamine
(serotonin), as well as a decrease in the excretion of their oxidative metabolites (Jarvik, 1970). It might appear obvious that this MAO inhibitory
property is the basis for the antidepressant activity of these drugs, but this
has not been clearly established.

One of the most dramatic and widely publicized drug interactions has been
that in which serious, even fatal hypertensive crises have occurred in patients
being treated with MAO inhibitors (Horwitz, Lovenberg, Engelman, and
Sjoerdsma, 1964). These misfortunes occurred following therapeutic administration of sympathomimetic amines (e.g., amphetamine and phenylpropanolamine) or after ingestion of foods containing biologically active

amines (e.g., tyramine). In the first instance, if an agent such as ampheta-mine is given to a patient receiving MAO inhibitors, it displaces the ab-normally large accumulation of norepinephrine present in the adrenergic neuron. This in turn leads to excessive α-adrenergic stimulation and a dangerously elevated blood pressure. Accumulation of norepinephrine occurs because these drugs inhibit the mitochondrial MAO, which normally de-aminates much of the free intraneuronal catecholamine. Foods associated with hypertensive episodes in patients treated with MAO inhibitors include aged cheeses, wines, beer, pickled herring, figs, and chicken liver (Pet-tinger, Mitchell, and Oates, 1968). Inasmuch as MAO inhibitors not only inhibit the breakdown of endogenous norepinephrine but also prevent the metabolism of tyramine, significant amounts of tyramine gain access to the increased store of norepinephrine, effect its release, and thus lead to a mark-edly elevated blood pressure. The pharmacological principle evinced in this interaction sequence should be applied to all other drugs that demonstrate varying degrees of MAO inhibitory activity. The antineoplastic drug pro-carbazine (Mann and Hutchison, 1967) and the antimicrobial agent furazoli-done, through its metabolite (Pettinger, Soyangco, and Oates, 1968), are compounds with different degrees of MAO inhibitory activity; therefore the duration of therapy and dosage of these compounds determine to a significant extent their potential role in interactions with biologically active amines. Clearly the simultaneous use of such agents with the MAO inhibitor anti-depressants in patients receiving other potential psychotherapeutic inter-actants should be undertaken with extreme caution.

There is evidence to suggest that administration of MAO inhibitors to parkinsonian patients being treated with L-DOPA may result in excessive accumulation of pressor amines and ensuing episodes of hypertension and palpitations (Friend, Bell, and Kline, 1965). Thus the use of drugs such as phenelzine, nialamide, tranylcypromine, and other MAO inhibitors should be avoided in such patients (Hunter, Boakes, Laurence, and Stern, 1970).

The ability of these agents to inhibit the hepatic drug-metabolizing enzymes in addition to MAO can lead, paradoxically, to enhanced CNS depression during concurrent use of these antidepressants with compounds such as alcohol, barbiturates, meperidine, chloral hydrate, and chlordiazepoxide (Goldberg, 1964). Similar inhibition of the metabolism of certain anti-cholinergic antiparkinsonian agents as well as the tricyclic antidepressants has been reported (Hollister, 1972). In the latter instance exaggerated CNS sympathetic stimulation may ensue, leading to a syndrome characterized by hyperpyrexia, convulsions, coma, and even death.

Interactions Involving Tricyclic Antidepressants

The tricyclic antidepressants, which superficially resemble the pheno-thiazines structurally, differ from these latter compounds in that the antidepressants enhance central sympathetic nervous system transmission. In addition, the tricyclics "sensitize" the peripheral adrenergic receptors to circulating catecholamines by inhibiting the neuronal amine pump (Oates, Mitchell, Feagin, Kaufmann, and Shand, 1971). They share with the phenothiazines the ability to exert a significant anticholinergic action. Curiously the tricyclic antidepressants exert a significant sedative effect similar to that observed with the phenothiazines. The degree of sedative effect displayed by different types of tricyclic antidepressants varies with the specific compound and in individual patients (Hollister, 1972). Variation in patient response to the tricyclic antidepressants can be explained, at least in part, by the wide range of plasma levels obtained in different patients following administration of the same drug dose (Alexanderson and Sjoqvist, 1971). It is reasonable to assume that there is also a corresponding difference in the extent and magnitude of adverse drug interactions occurring in patients taking these drugs. Nonetheless, certain drug interactions involving these agents have occurred frequently enough to warrant special attention. Knowledge of the previously described pharmacological properties of the tricyclic antidepressant agents enables the physician to predict most of the adverse drug interactions observed during therapy.

The deleterious effects resulting from interaction of MAO inhibitors and the tricyclic antidepressants have been discussed. This combination of drugs is to be avoided. The ability of the tricyclic antidepressants to block the adrenergic neuronal pump has led to adverse interactions in patients receiving these compounds concurrently with certain antihypertensive agents or in situations where high levels of circulating catecholamines are present. It is well established that antihypertensive effects of the potent guanidinium hypotensive agents (e.g., guanethidine and bethanidine) depend on their entry into the neuronal terminal. This transport system is inhibited by the tricyclic antidepressants as well as other agents such as cocaine and a variety of biologically active amines (Mitchell et al., 1970).

Thus the antihypertensive effect of guanethidine or bethanidine can be reversed or prevented by concurrent therapy with antidepressant drugs. Such loss of blood pressure control can occur within a few days and may result in fatal stroke, hypertensive encephalopathy, or other serious cardiovascular sequelae.

The therapeutic effect of the antihypertensive agent clonidine also is impaired by the tricyclic antidepressants (Briant, Reid, and Dollery, 1973). Clonidine is chemically dissimilar to the guanidinium hypotensive agents, and its mechanism of action apparently depends on α-receptor stimulation of cardiovascular inhibitory centers in the brainstem (Onesti, Schwartz, Kim, Paz-Martinez, and Swartz, 1971). It shares with guanethidine the ability to inhibit norepinephrine release following adrenergic stimulation; however, the mechanism by which its hypotensive action is reversed by the tricyclic antidepressants is unknown (Starke, Wagner, and Schumann, 1972).

Likewise, use of the tricyclic antidepressants enhances the "sensitivity" of sympathetic receptors, probably by inhibiting the neuronal reuptake of norepinephrine (Oates et al., 1971). Thus administration of directly acting pressor agents (e.g., phenylephrine or phenylpropanolamine) may result in significant and dangerous elevations in blood pressure. It is likely that the inadvertent administration of tricyclic antidepressants to patients with occult pheochromocytoma has resulted in similar responses owing to the high level of endogenous catecholamines produced by these tumors (Kaufmann, 1974).

The anticholinergic properties of the tricyclic antidepressants should be considered when they are used in patients receiving drugs with similar properties. Concomitant use of these agents can lead to additive effects in patients receiving anticholinergic compounds for gastrointestinal diseases or antiparkinsonian drugs. Clearly anticholinergic side effects (e.g., constipation, urinary retention, mydriasis, and the more serious risk of tachyarrhythmias in patients with cardiac disease) would be more likely to become serious problems in such instances.

Interactions Involving Amphetamines and Congeners

The use of amphetamines and congeners as antidepressants is usually unwarranted. It is true that these agents are effective psychomotor stimulants when used for short periods, but their utility as true antidepressant agents is limited. In addition, the rapid development of psychic dependence and tolerance frequently leads to their abuse. Such abuse in turn may lead to acute psychosis or an increased risk of profound mental depression, particularly following discontinuation of the drug after prolonged, high-dose administration. Thus the manifestations and potential for serious drug interactions related to the amphetamines depend on both dosage and duration of drug administration. Some of the significant interactions of these agents with other psychotherapeutic drugs were already described (see *Interactions With CNS Stimulants,* above). It is important for the practicing physician to remain aware of these interactions, for, even as medical usage decreases, the illicit market for stimulants (e.g. amphetamines and cocaine) continues to grow. In addition, amphetamines are capable of reversing the antihypertensive effects of guanethidine and related compounds (Day and Rand, 1963). Administration of these stimulants to patients being treated with guanethidine results in displacement of the hypotensive agent from its intraneuronal site of action, hastens its renal clearance, and leads to loss of blood pressure control.

Sedatives, Hypnotics, and Antianxiety Agents

The sedative-hypnotic agents constitute a large group of drugs used primarily to reduce anxiety and to induce sleep. The effectiveness of these compounds in allaying anxiety associated with psychotic disorders is not out-standing, but short-term use in neurotic disorders and situational anxieties is well established. These drugs include such agents as chloral hydrate, bar-biturates, glutethimide, meprobamate, methaqualone, methyprylon, and the newer benzodiazepine derivatives such as diazepam. All of these agents are CNS depressants, but their mechanisms of action are not well defined. Current concepts regarding their pharmacological mechanisms were discussed in preceding chapters. It is clear, nonetheless, that all of these agents can interact in an additive manner, leading to CNS depression, coma, and death if sufficient amounts are administered concurrently. Also, the depressant effects of the major tranquilizers are frequently potentiated by the simul-taneous use of the sedative drugs. Chronic use of these agents leads to po-tential interactions that are not readily apparent.

As indicated earlier, most of the barbiturates and congeners are able to stimulate the hepatic microsomal enzymes, thereby metabolizing a large number of drugs, many of which bear little structural or pharmacological similarity. This augmentation in the rate of metabolic biotransformation of oral anticoagulants, griseofulvin, chlorpromazine, diphenylhydantoin, and possibly tricyclic antidepressants may reach a degree sufficient to diminish their therapeutic effectiveness (Cucinell, Conney, Sansur, and Burns, 1965; Levy, O'Reilly, Aggeler, and Keech, 1970; Morrelli and Melmon, 1972). At-tempts to compensate for this by increasing dosage may lead to toxicity in the event therapy with the "inducing" agent is discontinued. Therefore when the stimulus for increased drug metabolism is removed there should be a con-comitant reduction in dosage of the drug in question, thereby avoiding toxic concentrations and adverse effects.

Interactions involving chloral hydrate and oral anticoagulants have been reported with varying manifestations. Chloral hydrate is metabolized in part to trichloracetic acid, and displacement of bound warfarin sodium from plasma proteins by this metabolite has been reported to result in augmented anticoagulant effect and hemorrhage (Sellers and Koch-Weser, 1970). Chronic use of the drug was reported in earlier studies to result in enzyme induction leading to accelerated breakdown of the anticoagulant and di-minished therapeutic effect (Cucinell, Odessky, Weiss, and Dayton, 1966). It should be noted that MAO inhibitors can inhibit the metabolism of chloral hydrate, leading to increased CNS depression by the latter agent.

Certain types of drugs are able to increase their own metabolism, which can lead to tolerance. Glutethimide and meprobamate are known to possess this ability and have been alluded to previously. The role of this mechanism in the alteration of pharmacological effects of most other psychotherapeutic agents apparently is not significant in man. The antihistamines are known to exert soporific effects, and their simultaneous administration with any of the CNS depressants may lead to dangerously excessive sedation (Hollister, 1972). Conversely, these agents share with the barbiturates possible enzyme induction capabilities; consequently these agents may effectively and mutually cancel such additive effects. It is apparent that this represents yet another interaction possibility that is poorly documented but of potential importance because of the frequency with which the interactants are prescribed. The benzodiazepine derivatives (e.g., chlordiazepoxide and diazepam) have been used extensively and have proved to be remarkably free of interaction potential. Generally, except for the additive depressant properties shared with other known CNS depressants, these agents do not display characteristic abilities to alter either pharmacokinetic parameters or end-organ responses of most other drugs (Hollister, 1972).

Miscellaneous Compounds

Lithium

The more effective and predictable use of lithium carbonate in reducing exacerbations of manic-depressive disorders has been primarily the result of more frequent and accurate measurements of blood levels of this drug. Avoidance of levels above 2.0 mEq/liter results in a significant decrease in adverse effects attributable to this agent (Schou, 1968). Renal excretion of lithium is fairly predictable, but decreased clearance occurs in the presence of moderately severe and severe hyponatremia. Thus the excessive use of diuretic agents coupled with a sodium-restricted diet may lead to lithium toxicity related to iatrogenic hyponatremia (Davis and Fann, 1970).

Alcohol

Although alcohol is seldom formally used by physicians as a psychotherapeutic agent, its widespread use and ready availability make it a significant factor in adverse interactions with commonly prescribed psychotherapeutic drugs. The physician must remind himself constantly of this potential source of therapeutic mishap, as well as that present in "over-the-counter" medications. Alcohol enhances the CNS depressant effects of the major and minor tranquilizers, sedative-hypnotic agents, antihistamines, and anesthetic agents when used concurrently. Furthermore, through its vasodilating effects alcohol may lead to hypotension in patients receiving phenothiazines, thus augmenting the latter drugs' postsynaptic adrenergic blocking properties. The ability of alcohol to induce microsomal enzymes in patients who *chronically* imbibe significant amounts of ethanolic beverages has led to enhanced degradation and consequent diminution in therapeutic effects of diphenylhydantoin, tolbutamide, warfarin sodium, barbiturates, and meprobamate. Conversely, *acute* intoxication with alcohol leads to inhibition of these enzymes, thus causing potentially fatal toxicity through exaggeration of the known pharmacological effects of these agents (Rubin, Gang, Misra, and

Lieber, 1970). The ethanol-induced syndrome of abdominal cramps, vomiting, and mental aberration resulting from accumulation of acetaldehyde in patients taking disulfiram is a classic drug interaction that has been used therapeutically (Kalant, 1962). In this instance disulfiram blocks the enzymatic breakdown of acetaldehyde derived from ethanol and thus leads to such an oppressive reaction that patients are reluctant to consume additional spirits.

CONCLUSION

The magnitude of potential problems related to adverse drug interactions need not impart a sense of futility to the physician. Clearly there are numerous possibilities for such interactions in the use of psychotherapeutic agents. The preceding discussion has been based on the concept that most adverse drug interactions are predictable and therefore preventable.

In order to treat patients with maximum safety and effectiveness, the physician must know his drugs well, select them carefully, and prescribe the least amount required to attain his therapeutic goal. Despite such care, he must remain alert for evidence that suggests drug interaction. Failure to obtain an expected result, an exaggerated therapeutic response, or the occurrence of a toxic reaction should serve as a warning to the practitioner. A systematic review of the pharmacokinetic determinants of a drug's effective concentration may offer a tenable explanation and suggest an appropriate change in therapy.

Many examples of interactions involving psychotherapeutic agents and other drugs at their respective sites of action have been reviewed. It has not been the intent of this review to be replete in this regard, but rather to emphasize those interactions which have been shown to be clinically important or those which exemplify pharmacophysiological principles applicable to a specific drug class.

It is worthwhile to reiterate that it is the conscientious, observant clinician who must continue to alert other members of the medical community to possible adverse drug reactions and interactions. Surveillance systems undoubtedly will document the incidence of such mishaps and forewarn of possible interactions, both known and suspected. In the final analysis, however, it is the responsibility of the practitioner to observe, assess, and report the clinical significance of the initial adverse interaction. Evaluation of drug interactions involving psychotherapeutic agents is especially difficult, but in no other area of drug therapy is it more necessary and rewarding.

ACKNOWLEDGMENTS

This work was supported in part by the Pharmaceutical Manufacturers Association Foundation. Dr. Kaufmann is a recipient of a PMAF Faculty Development Award in Clinical Pharmacology.

REFERENCES

Alexanderson, B., and Sjoqvist, F. (1971): Individual differences in the pharmaco-kinetics of monomethylated tricyclic antidepressants: Role of genetic and environmental factors and clinical importance. *Ann. N.Y. Acad. Sci.,* 179:739–751.

Axelrod, J. (1970): *Amphetamines and Related Compounds,* edited by F. Costa and S. Garattini. Raven Press, New York.

Azarnoff, D. L., and Hurwitz, A. (1970): Drug interactions. *Pharmacol. Physicians,* 4:1–7.

Barsa, J., and Sanders, J. C. (1964): A comparative study of tranylcypromine and pargyline. *Psychopharmacologia,* 6:295–298.

Blackwell, B. (1973): Psychotropic drugs in use today. *J.A.M.A.,* 225:1637–1641.

Breckenridge, A., and Orme, M. (1970): Clinical implications of enzyme induction. *Ann. N.Y. Acad. Sci.,* 179:421–431.

Briant, R. H., Reid, J. L., and Dollery, C. T. (1973): Interaction between clonidine and desipramine in man. *Br. Med. J.,* 1:522–523.

Brodie, B. B. (1965): Clinical effects of interaction between drugs: Displacement of one drug by another from carrier or receptor sites. *Proc. R. Soc. Med.,* 58:946–955.

Caranasos, G. J., Stewart, R. B., and Cluff, L. E. (1974): Drug-induced illness leading to hospitalization. *J.A.M.A.,* 228:713–717.

Carlsson, A. (1970): *Amphetamines and Related Compounds,* edited by F. Costa and S. Garattini. Raven Press, New York.

Cohen, R. A., Kopin, I. J., Creveling, C. R., Musacchio, J. M., Fischer, J. E., Crout, J. R., and Gill, J. R., Jr. (1966): False neurochemical transmitters. *Ann. Intern. Med.,* 65:347–362.

Conney, A. H. (1967): Pharmacologic implications of microsomal enzyme induction. *Pharmacol. Rev.,* 19:317–367.

Cucinell, S. A., Conney, A. H., Sansur, M., and Burns, J. J. (1965): Drug interactions in man. I. Lowering effect of phenobarbital on plasma levels of bishydroxycoumarin (Dicumarol) and diphenylhydantoin (Dilantin). *Clin. Pharmacol. Ther.,* 6:420–429.

Cucinell, S. A., Odessky, L., Weiss, M., and Dayton, P. G. (1966): The effect of chloral hydrate on bishydroxycoumarin metabolism: A fatal outcome. *J.A.M.A.,* 197:366–368.

Curry, S. H., Davis, J. M., Janowsky, D. S., and Marshall, J. H. L. (1970): Factors affecting chlorpromazine plasma levels in psychiatric patients. *Arch. Gen. Psychiatry,* 22:209–215.

Davis, J. M., and Fann, W. E. (1970): Lithium. *Annu. Rev. Pharmacol.,* 11:285–303.

Day, M. D., and Rand, M. J. (1963): Evidence of a competitive antagonism of guanethidine by dexamphetamine. *Br. J. Pharmacol.,* 20:17–28.

Fann, W. E., Davis, J. M., Janowsky, D. S., and Schmidt, D. (1973): The effect of antacids on blood levels of chlorpromazine. *Clin. Pharmacol. Ther.,* 14:135.

Formiller, M., and Cohon, M. S. (1969): Coumarin and indanedione anticoagulants—potentiators and antagonists. *Am. J. Hosp. Pharm.,* 26:574–582.

Friend, D. G., Bell, W. R., and Kline, N. S. (1965): The action of L-dihydroxyphenylalanine in patients receiving nialamide. *Clin. Pharmacol. Ther.,* 6:362–366.

Goldberg, L. I. (1964): Monoamine-oxidase inhibitors. *J.A.M.A.,* 190:456–462.

Hollister, L. E. (1972): Psychiatric and neurologic disorders. In: *Clinical Pharmacology,* edited by K. L. Melmon and H. F. Morelli. Macmillan, New York.

Horwitz, D., Lovenberg, W., Engelman, K., and Sjoerdsma, A. (1964): Monoamine oxidase inhibitors, tyramine, and cheese. *J.A.M.A.,* 188:1108–1110.

Hunter, K. R., Boakes, A. J., Laurence, D. R., and Stern, G. M. (1970): Monoamine oxidase inhibitors and L-dopa. *Br. Med. J.,* 3:388.

Janowsky, D. S., El-Yousef, M. K., Davis, M. K., Fann, W. E., and Oates, J. A. (1972): Guanethidine antagonism by antipsychotic drugs. *J. Tenn. Med. Assoc.,* 65:620–622.

Janowsky, D. S., El-Yousef, M. K., Davis, J. M., and Fann, W. E. (1973): Antagonism of guanethidine by chlorpromazine. *Am. J. Psychiatry,* 130:808–812.

Jarvik, M. E. (1970): Drugs used in the treatment of psychiatric disorders. In: *The Pharmacological Basis of Therapeutics*, Ed. 4, edited by L. S. Goodman and A. Gilman. Macmillan, New York.

Jick, H. (1974): Drugs—remarkably nontoxic. *N. Engl. J. Med.*, 291:824–828.

Kalant, H. (1962): Some recent physiological and biochemical investigations on alcohol and alcoholism. *Q. J. Stud. Alcohol*, 23:52–93.

Kaufmann, J. S. (1974): Pheochromocytoma and tricyclic antidepressants. *J.A.M.A.*, 229:1282.

Kuntzman, R. (1969): Drugs and enzyme induction. *Annu. Rev. Pharmacol.*, 9:21–36.

Lemberger, L., Witt, E. D., Davies, J. M., and Kopin, I. (1970): The effects of haloperidol and chlorpromazine on amphetamine metabolism and amphetamine stereotype behavior in the rat. *J. Pharmacol. Exp. Ther.*, 174:428–433.

Levy, G., O'Reilly, R. A., Aggeler, P. M., and Keech, G. M. (1970): Pharmacokinetic analyses of the effect of barbiturate on the anticoagulant action of warfarin in man. *Clin. Pharmacol. Ther.*, 11:372–377.

Lubran, M. (1969): The effects of drugs on laboratory values. *Med. Clin. North Am.*, 53:211–222.

Mann, A. M., and Hutchison, J. L. (1967): Manic reaction associated with procarbazine hydrochloride therapy of Hodgkin's disease. *Can. Med. Assoc. J.*, 97:1350–1353.

Martin, E. W. (1971): *Hazards of Medication*. Lippincott, Philadelphia.

Miller, R. R. (1974): Hospital admissions due to adverse drug reactions: A report from the Boston Collaborative Drug Surveillance Program. *Arch. Intern. Med.*, 134:219–223.

Mitchell, J. R., Cavanaugh, J. H., Arias, L., and Oates, J. A. (1970): Guanethidine and related agents. III. Antagonism by drugs which inhibit the norepinephrine pump in man. *J. Clin. Invest.*, 49:1596–1604.

Morelli, H. F., and Melmon, K. L. (1968): The clinician's approach to drug interactions. *Calif. Med.*, 109:380–389.

Morelli, H. F., and Melmon, K. L. (1972): Drug interactions. In: *Clinical Pharmacology*, edited by K. L. Melmon and H. F. Morrelli. Macmillan, New York.

Nies, A. S. (1974): Drug interactions. *Med. Clin. North Am.*, 58:965–975.

Oates, J. A., Mitchell, J. R., Feagin, O. T., Kaufmann, J. S., and Shand, D. G. (1971): Distribution of guanidinium antihypertensives—mechanism of their selective action. *Ann. N.Y. Acad. Sci.*, 179:302–308.

Ominsky, A. J., and Wollman, H. (1969): Hazards of general anesthesia in the reserpinized patient. *Anesthesiology*, 30:443–446.

Onesti, G., Schwartz, A. B., Kim, K. E., Paz-Martinez, V., and Swartz, C. (1971): Antihypertensive effect of clonidine. *Circ. Res. (Suppl. 2)*, 28/29:53–69.

Pettinger, W. A., Mitchell, J. R., and Oates, J. A. (1968): Cardiovascular effects and toxicity of psychotropic agents in man. In: *Psychopharmacology. A Review of Progress, 1957–67*, edited by D. H. Efron. Public Health Service Publication No. 1836. Government Printing Office, Washington, D.C.

Pettinger, W. A., Soyangco, F. G., and Oates, J. A. (1968): Inhibition of monoamine oxidase in man by furazolidone. *Clin. Pharmacol. Ther.*, 9:442–447.

Rubin, E., Gang, H., Misra, P. S., and Lieber, C. S. (1970): Inhibition of drug metabolism by acute ethanol intoxication. *Am. J. Med.*, 49:801–806.

Schou, M. (1968): Lithium in psychiatric therapy and prophylaxis. *J. Psychiatr. Res.*, 6:67–95.

Scientific Review Subpanel on Antihypertensives (1973): *Evaluation of Drug Interactions—1973*. American Pharmaceutical Association, Washington, D.C.

Scientific Review Subpanel on Psychotherapeutic Agents (1973): *Evaluation of Drug Interactions—1973*. American Pharmaceutical Association, Washington, D.C.

Sellers, E. M., and Koch-Weser, J. (1970): Potentiation of warfarin induced hypoprothrombinemia by chloral hydrate. *N. Engl. J. Med.*, 283:827–831.

Soffer, A. (1965): Digitalis intoxication, reserpine, and double tachycardia. *J.A.M.A.*, 191:777.

Starke, K., Wagner, J., and Schumann, H. J. (1972): Adrenergic neuron blockade by clonidine: Comparison with guanethidine and local anesthetics. *Arch. Int. Pharma-codyn. Ther.*, 195:291–308.

Sulser, F., and Dingell, J. V. (1968): Potentiation and blockade of the central action of amphetamines by chlorpromazine. *Biochem. Pharmacol.*, 17:634–636.

Sulser, F., and Sanders-Bush, E. (1971): Effect of drugs on amines in the CNS. *Annu. Rev. Pharmacol.*, 11:209–230.

Subject Index

Acetophenazine (Tindal); *see also*
   Phenothiazines
   dosage, 28
   geriatric response to, 24, 240-241, 242
Acetylation, drug *see* Drug therapy,
   Genetic Factors
Acetylcholine
   affective disorder states and, 118,
     183-184
   effect of atropine, 295
   tricyclics' action on, 119
Acromegaly, antipsychotics and, 273
S-Adenosylmethionine, methyl donor in
   brain, 7
Adrenergic blocking agents
   drug interactions with, 297-298, 300
   effect on geriatrics, 259
   role in mania, 183-184
Adrenergic effect of tricyclics in
   dysmorphogenesis, 276
Affective disorders
   biologic substratum for, 117, 118
   electrolyte basis for, 185
   neurotransmitters role in, 149,
     175-191
Agoraphobia, drug therapy for, 64,
   67-68
Agranulocytosis, drug-induced, 137, 268
Akathisia, drug-induced, 22-23, 54
Alcohol
   drug interactions with, 55, 86, 99,
     295-296, 301, 305-306
   as therapy, 254, 256
Alcoholic state
   addiction, therapy for, 45-46
   depression, therapy for, 103
   withdrawal, therapy for, 52, 76, 77,
     84-85
Alzheimer's disease, senile dementia
   similar to, 256
Amantidine, haloperidol-induced side
   effects controlled by, 54
Amine hypothesis of affective disorders,
   149, 200
   in depression, 177, 181-189
   in mania, 176-181
   reserpine's role in, 116, 267
Aminobutyric acid receptors, butyrophenones action on, 55

Amitriptyline (Elavil); *see also* Tricyclics
   action of, 92, 118-120
   blood levels, 135
   chemical structure and synthesis, 131
   chemical use, 112-113, 132, 133,
     143-144
   in anxiety, 71, 139, 140
   in geriatrics, 247-249
   in pediatrics, 217
   response variables for, 114, 115
   dosage, 132-134, 145
   efficacy, compared with other therapy,
     37, 38, 130
   side effects, 136, 137, 247, 275-279
Amobarbital
   drug interactions with, 298-299
   geriatric response to, 253
   meprobamate vs., 94, 95
D-Amphetamine (dexedrine); *see also*
     Amphetamines
   clinical effects of, 167
   dosage, 171
D, L-Amphetamine (Benzedrine); *see also*
     Amphetamines
   clinical effects, 167
   dosage, 171
   pediatric use, 213
Amphetamines, 161-173
   addiction, 45-46, 48
   basic pharmacology, 161-164
   clinical pharmacology, 164-165
   dosage, 171
   drug interactions with, 170, 171,
     296-297, 299-300, 301, 303
   excretion, 294
   history, 161
   psychiatric uses, 165-168
     in geriatrics, 255-256
     in pediatrics, 222-223
   side effects, 9, 32, 33, 168-170, 171
   for study of amine metabolism in
     mania, 178
Analeptics, geriatric use of, 255-256
Analgesics
   carisoprodol effective as, 103
   drug interactions with, 295-296
Anesthetic agents, drug interactions with,
   305-306

Hydrazines, 151, 153
17-Hydroxycorticosteroid, urinary
  excretion of during depression, 110
5-Hydroxyindoleacetic acid (5-HIAA),
  114, 116, 180
Hydroxynorephedrine and sympathetic
  transmission failure, 169
5-Hydroxytryptamine (5-HT), see Serotonin
Hydroxyzine, 20, 52
Hyperactive children, drug therapy for, 209-236
Hyperkinesia, see Minimal brain dysfunction
Hypertension
  amphetamine-induced, 168-169, 170
  MAO-inhibitors and, 149-150
Hypnotic agents
  antianxiety action as secondary effect,
    77
  benzodiazepines as, 74, 76, 85-86
  drug interactions with, 303-305
  geriatric psychotherapy and, 238,
    252-255
  pediatric use, 220
  propanediols useful as, 93, 100-101
Hypochondria
  in anxious neuroses, 101
  in geriatric patients, 245, 248, 250
  meprobamate useful for, 96
Hypothyroidism drug-induced, 251-252

Imipramine (Presamine, Tofranil),
  142-143; see also Tricyclics
  action of, 92, 118-120
  chemical structure and synthesis, 131
  clinical effects, 132
  dosage for, 132-134, 145
  efficacy, 130, 154
    vs. ECT, 37
    vs. lithium, 111, 197, 199
  response variables, 114, 115
  side effects, 137, 247, 275, 276
  use, 14, 96, 112, 113, 142-143
    in geriatrics, 241, 247, 249
    in pediatrics, 211, 215, 217-219
Inapsine, see Droperidol
Indoleamine hypothesis of affective
  disorders, 116-118, 176, 180
Indoleamine-N-methyltransferase, 7-8
Indoles, pediatric use of, 225
Insomnia; see also Hypnotic agents
  amphetamine-induced, 169
  drug therapy, 74, 76, 80, 94-95,
    100-101
Interneurons, meprobamate's effect on,
  91-92
Involutional melancholia therapy, 41, 166,
  250
Ion therapy, see Lithium

Iprindole, tricyclic action vs., 119
Iproniazid (Marsilid); see also MAO-
    inhibitors
  antidepressant action, 120-121
  efficacy, 130, 150
  history, 127
  side effects, 156
Isocarboxazid (Marplan); see also MAO-
    inhibitors
  derivation, 151
  efficacy, 130
  usefulness, 154, 219
Isoniazid, metabolism and response
  variables for, 115
Isoproterenol, drug interactions with,
  298
Isosorbide dinitrate to reverse drug-
  induced ECG abnormalities, 273
Isoxsuprine, geriatric response to, 256

Jaundice, cholestatic, drug-induced,
  268-269

L-DOPA, see Levodopa
Learning theory
  anxiety and, 62, 63, 68
  benzodiazepines, effects on condi-
    tioned behavior, 75
Leukocytosis, a side effect of tricyclics, 137
Leukopenia, a side effect of tricyclics, 137
Levoamphetamine, pediatric use of, 215
Levodopa (L-DOPA)
  drug interactions with, 301
  manic-depressive symptomatology
    related to, 111-112, 117
  psychosis-evoking action, 9
  use, 211, 226-227, 243, 267, 269,
    271
Levomepromazine, 21
Librium, see Chlordiazepoxide
Limbic system, 76, 92
Lithane, see Lithium carbonate
Lithium bromide, 194
Lithium carbonate (Eskalith, Lithane,
    Lithonate)
  blood levels, 201-202
  dosage, 205
  drug interactions with, 305
  half-life, 251
  history, 193-195
  mode of action, 119, 200-201
  side effects, 202-203, 251-252
  therapeutic effects of
    for depression, 111-114, 196-197,
      204
    for dyskinesia, 271, 272, 279-283

Organic brain syndrome, (OBS) chronic,
drug therapy for, 241-257
Oxazepam (Serax); *see also* Benzodiazepines
basic pharmacology, 73-74
conflict reducing properties, 75
dosage schedule, 81, 88
hostility affected by, 82-83
Oxygenation, hyperbaric, geriatric
response to, 258

Panic attacks and phobic anxiety syndrome,
64, 65, 66, 143
Papaverine, geriatric response to, 256,
257
Parachlorophenylalanine (PCPA),
181
Paranoid-schizophrenic syndrome,
amphetamine-induced, 170
Pargyline (Eutonyl); *see also* MAO
inhibitors, 130, 149
Parkinson's disease, drug therapy for,
226, 267
Parkinson syndrome, drug-induced, 8-9,
14-15, 22, 54, 269-272
Parnate, *see* Tranylcypromine
Pediatric psychotherapeutic drugs, 209-236
administration and special considerations, 210-213
antianxiety drugs, 220-221
antiautistic drugs, 47-48
antidepressants, 210, 217-219
antipsychotics, 47-48, 210,
221-225
hallucinogens, 227
hynotics and anticonvulsants, 220
L-DOPA, 226-227
lithium, 225-226
megavitamins, 227
psychomotor stimulants, 212, 213-216
sedatives, 212, 219-220
triiodothyronine, 228
Pemoline, *see* Magnesium pemoline
Pentobarbital
absorption and distribution, 98
geriatric response to, 252
side effects, 95
sleep cycle altered by, 100-101
Pentylenetetrazol
drug interactions with, 297
geriatric response to, 255-256
Perphenazine
analogue, 31-36
side effects, 21
use, 28, 52, 139, 140
Personality disorders, phenothiazines
as therapy for, 20
Pertofrane, *see* Desipramine

Phenelzine (Nardil); *see also* MAO
inhibitors
clinical effects, 153
derivation, 151
efficacy, 37, 113, 130, 154
metabolism, 115, 153
side effects, 156-157, 278-279
use, 154-155, 219
Phenethylamine related to affective disorder states, 117-118
Pheniprazine (Catron); *see also* MAO
inhibitors, efficacy of, 37, 130
Phenobarbital
drug interactions with, 298-299
meprobamate vs., 94, 95
Phenothiazines, 13-30
action on amine transport, 8-9, 117-120
analogues, 31-43
basic pharmacology, 14-15
chromatography testing with,
7
clinical use, 15-21, 62, 69, 71, 137,
139-140, 170, 221-223, 224, 241,
243, 253, 273
cytogenetic effects, 274
drug interactions with, 293, 295-300
drugs compared with, 47, 79, 196
side effects, 20-28, 243-244, 273,
275
Phenoxybenzamine
drug interactions with, 298
use, 170
Phentolamine
drug interactions with, 295, 298
use, 170
Phenylbutazone, geriatric response to,
239
Phenylephrine
drug-induced hypotension reversed by,
298
drug interactions with, 303
Phenylpropanolamine, drug interactions
with, 303
Pheochromocytoma, amphetamines
contraindicated in presence of, 171
Phobia; *see also* Neuroses
phobic avoidance, 66
phobic-obsessive-compulsive, 102
school, 218, 220-221
Photosensitivity, side effect of
chlorpromazine, 24
Physostigmine
anticholinergic effect, 10, 116, 138
dyskinesia treated with, 271
effect of manic patients, 183-184
Picrotoxin, drug interactions with, 297
Pilocarpine drops, for drug-induced
glaucoma, 277